APPLIED MEMORY

APPLIED MEMORY

MATTHEW R. KELLEY
EDITOR

Nova Science Publishers, Inc.
New York

For permission to use material from this book please contact us:
Telephone 631-231-7269; Fax 631-231-8175
Web Site: http://www.novapublishers.com

LIBRARY OF CONGRESS CATALOGING-IN-PUBLICATION DATA

Applied memory / Matthew R. Kelley (editor).
p. cm.
ISBN 978-1-60692-143-2 (hardcover)
1. Memory. I. Kelley, Matthew, 1962-
BF371.A56 2008
153.1'2--dc22

2008032511

Published by Nova Science Publishers, Inc. ✦ New York

Dedication

I would like to dedicate this book to my wife (Susanna), my children (Alexander & Quentin), and my parents (Robin & Terry), who honor me everyday with their boundless love and support.

CONTENTS

PREFACE

The idea for *Applied Memory* originated while teaching core courses in human memory and cognition. After weeks of examining benchmark memory phenomena (e.g., effects of phonological similarity, irrelevant speech, generation) and critiquing influential theories of memory by eminent researchers (e.g., John Anderson, Alan Baddeley, Bennet Murdock, James Nairne, and Richard Shiffrin), students inevitably asked the 'application' question: How does this research affect *me* and *my* everyday life?

Many scholars find the 'application' question frustrating and take the opportunity to remind students that the goal of research is not to demonstrate real-world relevance, but instead to elucidate the processes and mechanisms that underlie cognition. Students, however, rarely are dissuaded by this argument—and why should they be? The question of personal relevance is certainly valid, even if not always of theoretical import. Indeed, many researchers focus exclusively on applied questions and a variety of journals are dedicated to disseminating high quality applied research on memory and cognition (e.g., *Applied Cognitive Psychology*; *Journal of Experimental Psychology: Applied*). Perusal of such journals reveals extensive coverage of certain applied topics, such as legal, courtroom, and forensic applications (e.g., memory for victims, eyewitness, jurors; recovered and implanted memories). Less common, however, are applied explorations of the benchmark memory phenomena described earlier.

The goal of the *Applied Memory* volume was to highlight many interesting and creative applications of basic memory phenomena that are underrepresented, or even unrepresented, in the literature. Authors were charged with the task of reviewing relevant basic and applied research and offering new empirical investigations into the applications of these benchmark phenomena. To this end, *Applied Memory* consists of 17 chapters that explore the influences of generation, irrelevant speech, verbal overshadowing, isolation, part-set cuing, reminiscence, hypermnesia, placebos, mental state, metamemory knowledge, flashbulb events, and traumatic events on memory in everyday settings, as well as applications of source memory, social memory, involuntary autobiographical memory, dream memory, and strategic memory regulation. The volume was designed as a resource for basic and applied memory researchers and as a supplementary text in graduate or upper-level undergraduate courses in cognitive psychology, human memory, or applied psychology.

Matthew R. Kelley, Ph.D.
Lake Forest College

In: Applied Memory
Editor: Matthew R. Kelley
ISBN 978-1-60692-143-2

Chapter 1

IRONIC EFFECTS OF CENSORSHIP: GENERATING CENSORED LYRICS ENHANCES MEMORY

***Matthew R. Kelley*[*1], *Brittany A. Goldman*[1], *James E. Briggs*[2], *and James W. Chambers*[3]**
[1] Lake Forest College
[2] University of Wisconsin at Milwaukee
[3] Wheaton College, IL, USA

ABSTRACT

Three experiments explored the generation effect—mnemonic advantage for self-generated information—in the applied setting of lyrical censorship. Participants listened to an original song in which a subset of nouns were either partially or completely censored and then completed a recognition memory test consisting of heard, censored, and distractor items. Overall recognition accuracy did not differ for censored and heard items, despite the fact that the censored items were never presented. More importantly, when the data were made conditional upon successful generation of the censored item during encoding, the standard generation effect was observed—ironically, recognition accuracy was significantly higher for the generated censored items compared to the heard items. Source memory did not differ from chance and participants showed a strong bias towards indicating than any 'recognized' word was 'heard.' Overall, these results suggest that by omitting certain words from songs, censors might actually make those words more memorable.

INTRODUCTION

In the human memory literature, the *generation effect* refers to the mnemonic advantage for to-be-remzembered (TBR) information that is self-generated (e.g., Mulligan and Lozito, 2004; Slamecka and Graf, 1978). Typically, generation is manipulated by presenting words in

* Corresponding author

an incomplete or deficient format (e.g., word stems, word fragments, letter transposition) so that participants are required to actively and overtly generate the TBR material; retention of these generated words is then compared to retention of words that were originally presented intact and required only that participants read the material (e.g., Gardiner, 1988; Nairne and Widner, 1987). The mnemonic benefits of self-generation have been well documented in the laboratory using a wide variety of materials, designs, and procedures, including using pictures (e.g., Kinjo and Snodgrass, 2000; Lohaus and Lachnit, 2001), explicit recall and recognition tests (e.g., Burns, 1990; Hirshman and Bjork, 1988), implicit memory tests (e.g., Mulligan, 2002; Nicolas, Ehrlich, and Facci, 1996), within-list and between-list designs (e.g., Serra and Nairne, 1993; Slamecka and Katsaiti, 1987).

Although the vast majority of generation effect research has employed traditional laboratory materials and procedures, a growing number of researchers have begun to examine the generation effect in applied settings, such as in the classroom and the marketplace (e.g., de Winstanley and Bjork, 2004; Lutz, Briggs, and Cain, 2003; Reardon and Moore, 1996; Thompson and Barnett, 1981). For instance, Foos, Mora, and Tkacz (1994) reported a reliable generation effect for students who generated their own outlines after reading a 2,300 word text, as compared to students who were given an experimenter-generated outline. In a study examining memory for advertisements, Sengupta and Gorn (2002) omitted key elements from certain advertisements and found elevated recall for the ads that required generation. Given the robust nature and broad influence of the generation phenomenon, one may wonder whether generation also is relevant within other contexts, such as with lyrical censorship.

Musicians and the music industry commonly practice self-censorship in which they proactively censor words or lyrics that may be deemed profane, obscene, or offensive (Corbett, 1994). Typically, lyrics are censored by completely or partially omitting the profane material; however, other techniques such as a backward masking (presenting the word in reverse) are increasingly common (Corbett, 1994). Regardless of the specific censorship technique employed, one could imagine that listeners would be able to generate some of the censored words on their own using the context of the song as a guide. If indeed this is the case, then one might expect a generation effect for the censored lyrics in which the words that were self-generated (censored words) would be remembered better than the other non-generated (heard) words from the song. That is, in contrast to its original intent, censorship might actually encourage substantial cognitive processing and promote retention of censored material.

To date, no existing research has attempted to examine the generation phenomenon within the context of lyrical or musical censorship. However, evidence from two disparate lines of research indicates that memory enhancement following lyrical censorship is plausible. First, McDaniel (1984) explored the generation effect using written story stimuli. Participants read stories in which some idea units were degraded because certain letters from important words were deleted, whereas other idea units remained intact. Across three experiments, he showed that participants recalled significantly more idea units when they required generation. To the extent that song lyrics are similar to stories, people should be able to use contextual information to generate missing lyrics and their retention of this information may be enhanced.

Moreover, extant evidence in the form of the phonemic restoration effect suggests that humans are able to naturally generate missing auditory information (Samuel, 1981; 1996). For instance, in a study by Warren and Warren (1980), participants heard several sentences in which a critical phoneme within a word was replaced by the sound of a cough. Despite the missing phoneme, participants' comprehension of the sentences was unaffected. Furthermore, participants rarely realized that a sound was missing; they reported having heard the entire word. Similarly, Cooper et al. (1987) examined whether comprehension of a text was affected by missing phonemic information. In their study, participants listened to several paragraphs in which certain key content words were omitted and replaced by silence. Although these key words were critical to the accurate comprehension of the text, Cooper et al. (1987) found that comprehension of the paragraphs was not impaired by the missing words. Based on the convergence of McDaniel's (1984) demonstration of a generation effect in story recall and the phonemic restoration effect (e.g., Cooper et al., 1987), a positive generation effect for censored lyrics seems reasonable, if not likely.

The current experiments were designed to determine whether people are able to generate and subsequently remember censored lyrics within the context of an aurally presented song. In each experiment, participants listened to an original song that contained a variety of censored nouns (either partially censored or completely censored). Whereas most censored lyrics represent a small pool of emotional or controversial words (e.g., profanities, drug- or violence-related terms), the current study used a variety of common everyday nouns as the target stimuli. We reasoned that the use of common nouns would provide a stronger test of the generation effect (i.e., set of censored items is not known a priori; larger pool of potential targets) and would allow easier comparisons between the current study and traditional investigations of the generation effect using similar stimuli. In addition, we were able to minimize any potential ethical conflicts associated with the presentation of profane material.

Following the song, participants completed a three-alternative, forced-choice recognition test in which participants were asked to identify whether (a) they remembered "hearing" the word in the song, (b) they remembered that the word was "censored" from the song, or (c) the word did not appear in the song. In other words, participants made a source judgment along with their recognition judgment. According to the leading explanations of the generation effect—the multifactor account (e.g., Hirshman and Bjork, 1988; Hunt and McDaniel, 1993; Mulligan, 2001; Nairne, Riegler, and Serra, 1991) and the processing account (e.g., Jacoby, 1983; Mulligan, 2004)—source memory should be impaired for censored items relative to not censored items. The multifactor account suggests that generation encourages extra item-specific processing, which enhances item retention, while disrupting the processing and subsequent retention of other types of information (e.g., order, intertarget relational, context, source). Although the processing account offers the same prediction, the explanation is markedly different as it does not appeal to a processing trade-off. Instead, generated and non-generated information are assumed to encourage different types of processing during encoding; the former promotes greater item processing while the latter promotes greater perceptual processing. This enhanced perceptual processing should benefit source recollection solely for non-generated (heard) items.

EXPERIMENT 1

Experiment 1 explored the influence of lyrical censorship on memory using intentional (expected) and incidental (unexpected) memory tests. In the incidental condition, participants were told that they would hear a song and would be asked to rate the song on a variety of characteristics, such as pleasantness of lyrics, vocals, and instrumentals. We reasoned that the incidental condition would be roughly analogous to how people normally listen to a song outside the laboratory (i.e., determining whether they like a song's music and lyrics), and hence, would have high ecological validity and realism. In the intentional condition, on the other hand, participants were informed of both the pleasantness ratings and the subsequent recognition test—a manipulation more congruous with traditional explorations of the generation effect (e.g., Slamecka and Graf, 1978). Of central interest were the recognition and source judgments for the censored and heard words, as well as the influence of test expectation.

Method

Participants. Eighty students from an introductory psychology course at Lake Forest College earned extra-credit for their participation in this task. Groups of 4 or fewer participants were tested in sessions lasting approximately 15 minutes. Stimuli were presented and controlled with an IBM-compatible computer.

Materials and Design. The authors created an original song about a budding relationship between a man and a woman. The song consisted of 306 words, of which 30 non-offensive, high-frequency nouns were drawn from the Kucera and Francis (1967) norms (average frequency 241.72; range 107-787; average word length 5.38; range 4-7). In a given version of the song, 15 of these nouns were censored (e.g., market, voice, family) and 15 were presented intact (e.g., island, hand, friend); the words were counterbalanced such that each word served as a censored and non-censored words equally often across participants. Along with the 30 nouns used in the song, 30 other matched, high frequency nouns were selected to serve as distractors in the recognition memory test (average frequency 178.72; range 101-470; average word length 5.81; range 4-7). The song was recorded using a male vocalist who was accompanied by an acoustic guitar and a keyboard.

We factorially manipulated the type of censorship (partial vs. complete) and whether the participants expected a memory test or not (intentional vs. incidental) using a between-subjects design. In the completely censored conditions, the entire word was eliminated from the song (silence), whereas in the partially censored conditions, the word's initial phoneme remained audible (e.g., the 't' sound in 'tree'). In the intentional conditions, participants were instructed that, once the song was complete, they would 1) complete a short questionnaire about how much they enjoyed the song, and 2) complete a recognition test for the words in the song. In the incidental condition, participants were instructed only about the short questionnaire, but did not expect a memory test.

Procedure. Participants began the experiment by reading a brief set of instructions (intentional or incidental). Following the instructions, participants listened to the song (approximately 6 minutes) and then recorded their opinions about certain aspects of the song. They were asked to rate, on a 5-point Likert scale, how interesting, pleasant, and realistic the song was, as well as whether the presence of censored items affected their enjoyment of the song. Next, participants completed the three-alternative, forced-choice recognition test, which consisted of viewing 60 words, one at a time, and deciding whether 1) they heard the word in the song, 2) they knew that the word was censored from the song, or 3) the word was neither heard nor censored. Of these 60 words, 30 were new distracting items, 15 were censored during the original song presentation, and 15 were heard normally. Following the test, participants were debriefed as to the exact nature of the experiment.

Results and Discussion

Overall Recognition and Discrimination. Overall recognition performance was analyzed with a 2 (intent: intentional vs. incidental) x 2 (generation type: partial vs. complete) x 3 (stimulus type: not censored, censored, neither) mixed-factor analysis of variance (ANOVA). Figure 1 displays the average performance on the recognition test in each of these experimental conditions. The ANOVA revealed a significant main effect of stimulus type, $F(2, 152) = 222.97, p < .01$. Consistent with past research showing equivalent performance for intentional and incidental learning tasks (e.g., Hyde and Jenkins, 1973; Postman, 1964), there was no significant main effect of intent. The main effect of generation type also failed to reach significance, as did all of the interactions (all $p > .05$).

A Newman-Keuls post-hoc analysis revealed a common pattern of results across every intent and generation condition—recognition accuracy was statistically equivalent for censored and non-censored words and performance in both conditions far exceeded the false alarm rate for distractor items. This pattern held true for the intentional-partial condition [(.75=.72)>.38], the intentional-complete condition, [(.73=.72)>.43], the incidental-partial condition [(.69=.69)>.40], and the incidental-complete condition [(.68=.66)>.40]. Thus, it appears that the experiment did not produce a traditional generation effect, yet participants were able to accurately recognize censored words at the same rate as words they actually heard. Importantly, overall recognition accuracy for these censored items (.70) was significantly higher than the false alarm rate for distractors (.40).

In addition to examining recognition accuracy, participants' discriminability (d') was measured using the signal detection method. The d' measure considers the relationship between recognition accuracy (hit rate) and false alarm rate, such that higher d' values reflect better discrimination performance. Figure 2 displays the d' statistics as a function of intent, generation type, and stimulus type (not censored vs. censored). An ANOVA revealed no significant main effects or interactions, which suggests that participants were able to discriminate distractor items from censored and not censored items equally well in each condition. This finding is not surprising given the nearly identical recognition accuracy for censored and not censored words.

Source Discrimination. A separate 2 (intent) x 2 (generation type) x 3 (stimulus type) x 2 (source judgment: censored vs. not censored) ANOVA examined the pattern of source judgments across the various conditions (see Figure 1). The ANOVA revealed a reliable main effect for stimulus type, once again showing that performance was higher for not censored and censored words than for false alarms, $F(2, 152) = 222.971, p < .01$. The main effect of source judgment was also statistically significant, $F(1, 76) = 360.432, p < .01$, which shows that participants were much more likely to report that the words they 'recognized' were words that were 'not censored' in the song. The analysis also yielded a reliable interaction between stimulus type and source judgment, $F(2, 152) = 37.393, p < .01$. A Newman-Keuls analysis revealed that participants made a greater proportion of 'not censored' judgments to not censored stimuli (.58) than to censored stimuli (.52) and distractor stimuli (.29).

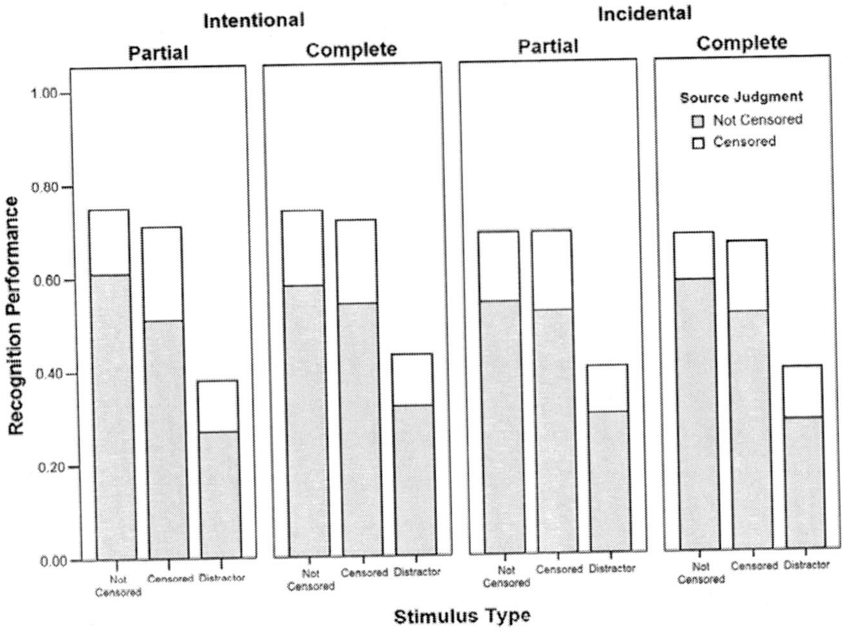

Figure 1. Recognition performance and source judgments as a function of intent condition, censorship type, and stimulus type in Experiment 1.

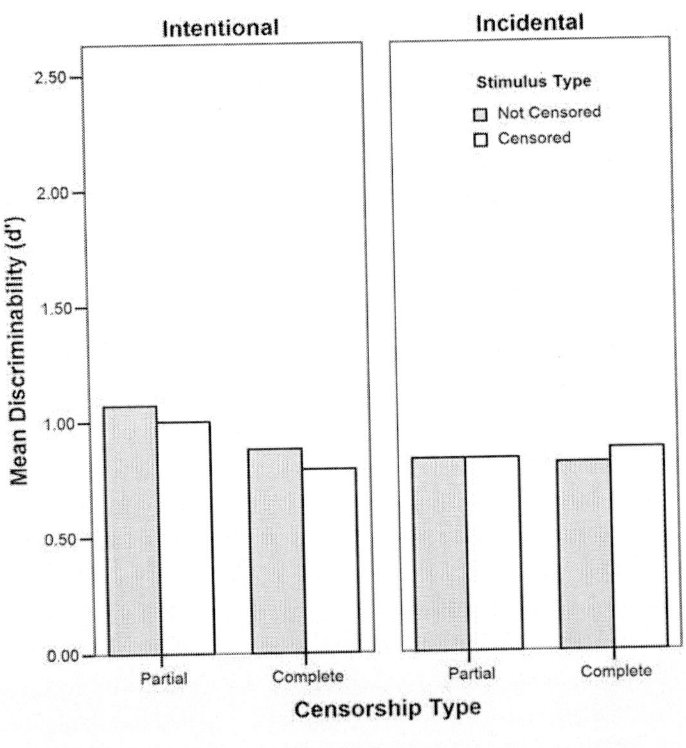

Figure 2. Discriminability (d') as a function of intent condition, censorship type, and stimulus type in Experiment 1.

Alternatively, the proportion of 'censored' judgments did not differ for censored and not censored stimuli (.17=.14), but both were significantly higher than the proportion of 'censored' judgments made for distractor stimuli (.11). All remaining main effects and interactions failed to reach significance (all $p>.05$).

Consistent with the predictions of the multifactor and processing accounts, participants appeared to ascribe source information more accurately for the not censored (heard) stimuli. However, with participants exhibiting such a strong source bias toward 'not censored' responses, the issue is not so clear cut. Indeed, in cases with such robust bias, one encounters the problems of determining whether overall source memory exceeded chance levels and then disentangling source memory from source bias. The former issue can be addressed by computing the ACSIM measure (Murnane and Bayen, 1996) which is determined by calculating the sum of the censored items called 'censored' and the not censored items called 'not censored' and dividing this score by all censored and not censored items that were 'recgonized.' The ACSIM measures were .51, .54, .56, and .52 for the intentional-partial, intentional-complete, incidental-partial, and incidental-complete conditions, respectively. Given that a series of one-sample t-tests, using Bonferroni correction for a family of tests, revealed that none of these measures was differed significantly from chance, it appears that participants were unable to effectively use source information in this task. Moreover, the aforementioned differences in the proportions of source responses are easily explained by assuming that participants (a) were unable to distinguish among the two sources, (b) assumed all recognized items were 'not censored,' and (c) occasionally made 'censored' source judgments because it was an available option.

Limitations. In traditional laboratory studies of the generation effect, experimenters ensure that each to-be-generated item, in fact, is generated by the participant (e.g., by using talk aloud protocols or providing the participants with a generation rule). In an attempt to maintain high ecological validity in the present study, participants were *not* asked to explicitly generate the missing information during the encoding/listening phase, leaving them free to spontaneously and privately self-generate the censored words. An unfortunate consequence of this design, however, is that we cannot know (a) which words, if any, were generated during encoding; (b) whether these generated words were remembered or forgotten at test; and (c) what percentage of the recognized words were simply guessed at test.

If participants successfully generated a portion of the censored words during encoding, then the mnemonic benefit of generation effect may have been underestimated in Experiment 1. For instance, a participant who remembered 11 of the 13 words that she correctly generated during encoding would enjoy a conditional accuracy of 85%, as compared to an absolute accuracy of 73% (11 out of 15 total stimuli). Thus, by making the data conditional upon generation during encoding, one might find a generation advantage.

EXPERIMENT 2

Experiment 2 was designed to address the major limitation of Experiment 1 by having participants indicate when they generated a censored word during the encoding phase. Participants began the task by listening to the same original song that contained a selection of censored nouns (partial or complete omission) used in first experiment. Then, they listened to each line of the song individually and were asked to indicate with a yes/no button press (a) whether the line contained a censored item, and (b) whether they were able to determine the censored item's identity. Thus, participants did not actually report the identity of the censored item, but instead stated whether they believed that they successfully generated the missing word. Although we cannot be certain that a given word was generated correctly, we reasoned that this processes maintained a better sense of realism in the generation process (e.g., spontaneously and privately generating censored lyrics while listening to music) than other potential methods (e.g., having participants shadow each non-censored word of the song and generate each censored word). All participants were informed of the ensuing forced-choice recognition test prior to the song's presentation. The conditionalized data were of primary importance in this study, as they allowed estimates of how often words were generated during encoding, how often generated words were remembered at test, and the extent to which guessing contributed to overall performance.

Method

Participants. Sixty-eight students from an introductory psychology course at Lake Forest College earned extra-credit for their participation in this task. Groups of 4 or fewer participants were tested in sessions lasting approximately 15 minutes. Stimuli were presented and controlled with an IBM-compatible computer.

Materials and Design. The materials and design were identical to those employed in Experiment 1, with the one exception—the incidental condition was eliminated.

Procedure. The procedure was identical to that used in Experiment 1, with the following additions. Upon hearing the entire song once, participants listened to the song again, one line at a time. After each line, participants were asked, "Did the phrase contain a censored (or omitted) word?" and pressed either a yes or no button. Following a yes response, they were asked, "Were you able to determine the identity of the censored item? That is, could you still tell what the word was supposed to be, even though it was censored?" At the conclusion of the line-by-line presentation, participants completed the opinion survey and the forced-choice recognition test, as detailed in Experiment 1.

Results and Discussion

Overall Recognition and Discrimination. Overall recognition performance was analyzed with a 2 (generation type: partial vs. complete) x 3 (stimulus type: not censored, censored, neither) mixed-factor ANOVA (see left half of Figure 3). As in the first experiment, only the main effect of stimulus type reached statistical significance, $F(2, 132) = 351.581, p < .01$. A Newman-Keuls post-hoc analysis revealed that recognition accuracy was statistically equivalent for censored and non-censored words and performance in both conditions far exceeded the false alarm rate for distractor items, which held true for the partial condition [(.65=.67)>.23] and the complete condition [(.61=.58)>.23].

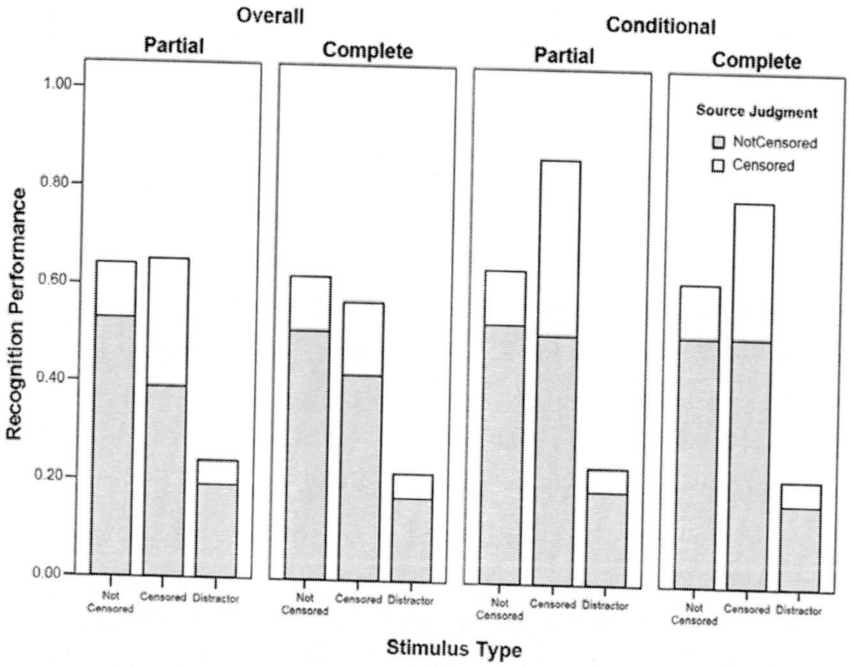

Figure 3. Overall and conditional recognition performance and source judgments as a function of censorship type and stimulus type in Experiment 2.

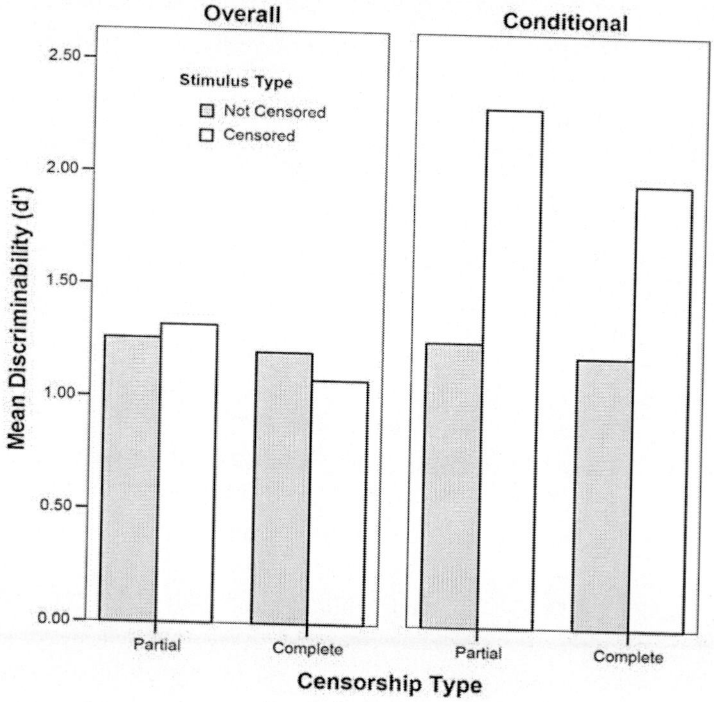

Figure 4. Overall and conditional discriminability (d') as a function of censorship type and stimulus type in Experiment 2.

Figure 4 (left half) shows the overall d' statistics as a function of generation type and stimulus type (not censored vs. censored). As in Experiment 1, the present ANOVA revealed no significant main effects or interactions, which suggests that participants were able to discriminate distractor items from censored and not censored items equally well in each condition. The current patterns of results are consistent with those reported in Experiment 1, albeit with reduced hit and false alarm rates and enhanced discrimination ability in Experiment 2. Overall, participants were able to accurately recognize censored words at the same rate as words they actually heard, but did not produce a traditional generation effect.

Overall Source Discrimination. The overall pattern of source judgments was examined using a 2 (generation type) x 3 (stimulus type) x 2 (source judgment: censored vs. not censored) ANOVA (see left half of Figure 3). The ANOVA revealed reliable main effects of stimulus type, $F(2, 132) = 351.581, p < .01$, and source judgment, $F(1, 66) =197.178, p < .01$. As in Experiment 1, participants were much more likely to designate a 'recognized' word as having a 'not censored' source. The ANOVA also indicated a reliable interaction between stimulus type and source judgment, $F(2, 132) = 48.536, p < .01$. A Newman-Keuls analysis revealed that participants made significantly more 'not censored' judgments to not censored stimuli (.52) than to censored stimuli (.41) and distractor stimuli (.18). Alternately, participants made significantly more 'censored' judgments to censored stimuli (.21) than to not censored stimuli (.11) and distractor stimuli (.05). This latter pattern differed from Experiment 1, which showed similar proportions of 'censored' judgments for censored and not censored stimuli. All remaining main effects and interactions failed to reach significance (all $p>.05$). Consistent with Experiment 1, the ACSIM measures were not statistically different than chance (.61 ànd .55 for partial and complete, respectively), which suggests that participants were unable to accurately discriminate among the two sources.

Conditional Recognition and Discrimination. In an attempt to more closely examine the direct influence generation on retention, data inclusion was made conditional upon participant reports of successful item generation during encoding. During encoding, participants in the partial condition indicated that they were able to determine the identities of 60% of the censored items, as compared to 37% in the complete condition.

To calculate the conditional recognition performance for censored words, we determined the proportion of censored words 'generated' during encoding that was subsequently remembered on the recognition test. Conditional data were not necessary for the 'not censored' and 'neither' stimulus types. Recognition performance was analyzed with a 2 (generation type: partial vs. complete) x 3 (stimulus type: not censored, censored, neither) mixed-factor ANOVA. Figure 4 (right half) displays the average performance on the recognition test in each of these experimental conditions.

The ANOVA revealed that only the main effect of stimulus type was significant, $F(2, 132) = 461.744, p < .01$. A Newman-Keuls post hoc analysis revealed a traditional generation effect—recognition accuracy for generated censored items *exceeded* that of not censored items by .21, and both exceeded the false alarm rate. Similar patterns of performance emerged for both the partial [.88>.65>.23] and complete [.80>.61>.23] censorship conditions. Moreover, a 2 (generation type: partial vs. complete) x 2 (stimulus type: not censored vs. censored) ANOVA comparing d' performance indicated a significant main effect of stimulus type, $F(1, 66) = 81.798, p < .01$, which reflects superior discrimination of censored items as compared to not censored items (see right half of Figure 4). These results demonstrate an ironic effect of censorship, namely, that omitting words from a song can make those words more memorable and more discriminable.

Conditional Source Discrimination. The pattern of source judgments for the conditional data was examined using a 2 (generation type) x 3 (stimulus type) x 2 (source judgment: censored vs. not censored) ANOVA (see right half of Figure 4). The ANOVA showed reliable main effects of stimulus type, $F(2, 132) = 461.744, p < .01$, and source judgment, $F(1, 66) = 172.992, p < .01$. As in the overall analysis, participants were much more likely to report that the words they 'recognized' were words that were 'not censored' in the song. The ANOVA also revealed a reliable interaction between stimulus type and source judgment, $F(2, 132) = 21.516, p < .01$. A Newman-Keuls post-hoc analysis revealed no difference between the proportions of 'not censored' judgments made to not censored stimuli (.52) and to censored stimuli (.51), while both exceeded the proportion made to distractor stimuli (.18). Participants made significantly more 'censored' judgments to censored stimuli (.32) than to not censored stimuli (.11) and distractor stimuli (.05). All remaining main effects and interactions failed to reach significance (all $p > .05$). The ACSIM measures of .54 and .47 for the partial and complete conditions did not differ significantly from chance performance, which again reflects a lack of source discrimination.

Limitations. As mentioned previously, in an attempt to maintain a sense of realism in the generation process, participants in Experiment 2 were not asked to report the identities of the censored items. Instead, they simply stated whether they believed that they successfully generated the censored item. By not identifying the words, we cannot be sure that participants generated the appropriate items during song presentation, which may influence estimates of both the proportion of items generated during encoding and subsequent recognition performance. While generation rate may have been overestimated in Experiment 2, conditional recognition performance for censored items may have been underestimated. That is, if a participant erroneously generated 'food' instead of 'friend' during encoding, she would indicate successful generation but would fail to recognize 'friend' on the test and conditional performance would wrongly decline. Of course, two wrongs could also make a right (i.e., erroneous generation of 'food' during encoding, false alarm to 'friend' at test; appears to be successful generation and recognition). Clearly, relying solely on participant self reports of internal generation is problematic.

EXPERIMENT 3

Experiment 3 was designed to address the major limitation of Experiment 2 by having participants shadow the song's lyrics during the presentation phase. That is, participants were asked to repeat every 'heard' word and generate every 'censored' word that they encountered. Accordingly, conditionalized data were computed for both censored and not censored items based on shadowing/generating accuracy. Although shadowing solves the problem of relying on participant self reports of successful generation, the process is more intrusive, less ecologically valid, demands more resources (which may negatively impact generation rate), and the generation is less realistic (e.g., less spontaneous, not private). Still, the shadowing manipulation should provide an unambiguous answer to the question of central interest—namely, are generated censored words remembered better than not censored words?

Method

Participants. Thirty-two students from an introductory psychology course at Lake Forest College earned extra-credit for their participation in this task. Participants were tested individually in sessions lasting approximately 15 minutes. Stimuli were presented and controlled with an IBM-compatible computer.

Materials and Design. The materials and design were identical to those employed in Experiment 2, with the two additions. First, a 30 second clip of the theme song from the television show *Cheers* was used in a shadowing practice session. Also, an experimenter was in the room with the participant and recorded shadowing/generating accuracy on a sheet of paper that displayed the song lyrics.

Procedure. The procedure was similar to that used in Experiment 1, with the following additions. Prior to hearing the experimental song, participants were given shadowing practice. Then, participants were asked to shadow the experimental song while an experimenter recorded shadowing/generating accuracy. At the conclusion of the shadowing task, participants completed the opinion survey and the forced-choice recognition test, as detailed in Experiment 1.

Results and Discussion

Overall Recognition and Discrimination. Overall recognition performance was analyzed with a 2 (generation type: partial vs. complete) x 3 (stimulus type: not censored, censored, neither) mixed-factor ANOVA (see left half of Figure 5). Consistent with first two experiments, only the main effect of stimulus type reached statistical significance, $F(2, 60) = 139.112, p < .01$. A Newman-Keuls post-hoc analysis revealed that recognition accuracy was statistically equivalent for censored and non-censored words and performance in both conditions far exceeded the false alarm rate for distractor items, which held true for the partial condition [(.66=.63)>.29] and the complete condition [(.69=.67)>.33]. Figure 6 (left half) shows the overall d' statistics as a function of generation type and stimulus type (not censored vs. censored). Similar to Experiment 1 and 2, this ANOVA revealed no significant main effects or interactions. Participants were able to discriminate distractor items from censored and not censored items equally well in each condition. Overall, participants were able to accurately recognize censored words at the same rate as words they actually heard, but did not produce a traditional generation effect.

Overall Source Discrimination. The overall pattern of source judgments was examined using a 2 (generation type) x 3 (stimulus type) x 2 (source judgment: censored vs. not censored) ANOVA (see left half of Figure 5). The ANOVA revealed reliable main effects of stimulus type, $F(2, 60) = 139.112, p < .01$, and source judgment, $F(1, 30) =133.820, p < .01$. As in the first two experiments, participants were much more likely to designate a 'recognized' word as having a 'not censored' source. The ANOVA also indicated a reliable interaction between stimulus type and source judgment, $F(2, 60) = 36.241, p < .01$. A Newman-Keuls analysis revealed that participants made significantly more 'not censored' judgments to not censored stimuli (.58) than to censored stimuli (.49) and distractor stimuli

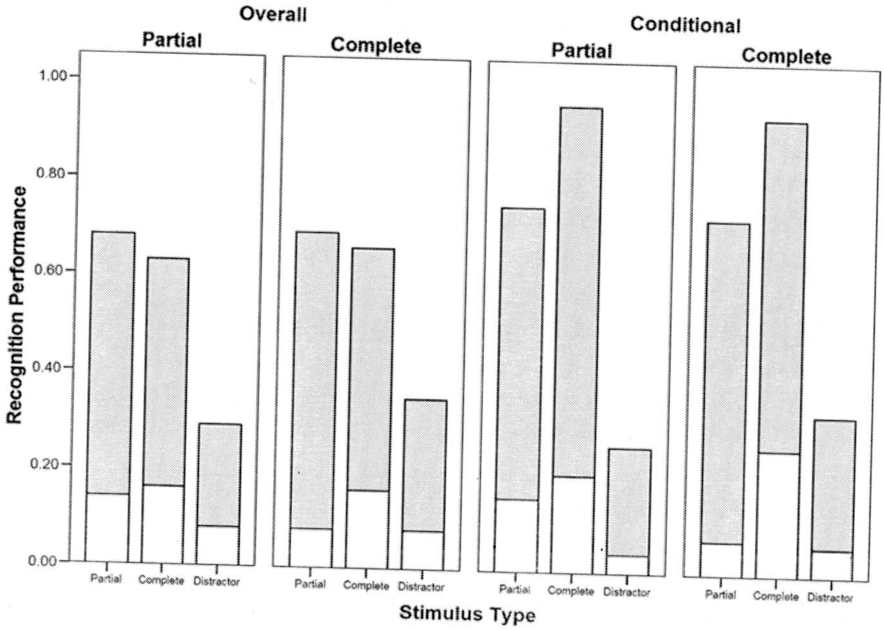

Figure 5. Overall and conditional recognition performance and source judgments as a function of censorship type and stimulus type in Experiment 3.

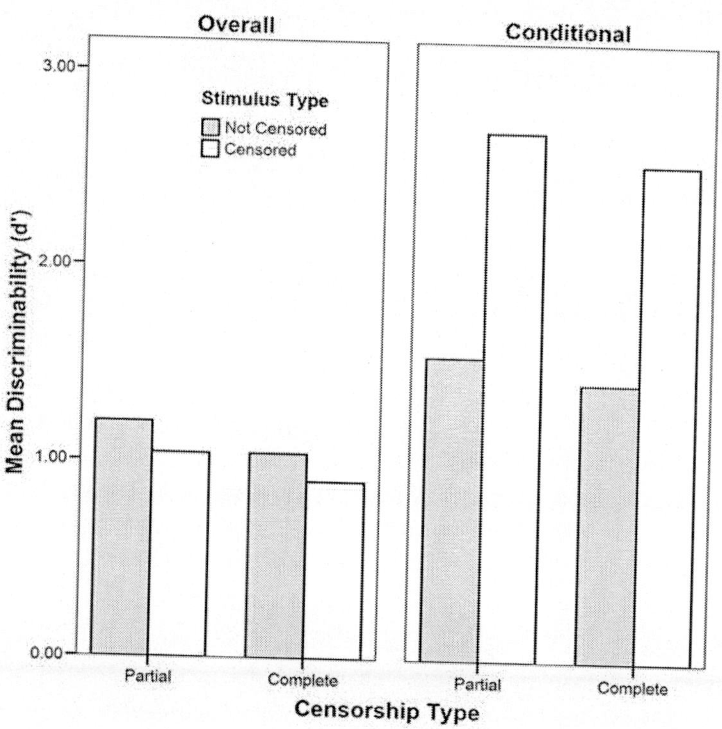

Figure 6. Overall and conditional discriminability (d') as a function of censorship type and stimulus type in Experiment 3

(.24). In contrast, participants made significantly more 'censored' judgments to censored stimuli (.16) than to not censored stimuli (.11) and distractor stimuli (.08). All remaining main effects and interactions failed to reach significance (all $p>.05$). Consistent with Experiments 1 and 2, the ACSIM measures of .53 and .56 for the partial and complete conditions did not differ significantly from chance, which suggests that participants failed to effectively utilize any available source information in this task.

Conditional Recognition and Discrimination. In the present analyses, data inclusion was made conditional upon successful shadowing of non-censored items and successful generation and shadowing of censored items. The shadowing task proved challenging for participants, as evidenced by not censored shadowing rates of 73% and 70% and generation rates of 46% and 31% for the partial and complete conditions, respectively.

To calculate the conditional recognition performance for not censored and censored words, we determined the proportion of not censored and censored words shadowed/generated during encoding that were subsequently remembered on the recognition test. Conditional data were not necessary for the 'neither' stimulus type. Recognition performance was analyzed with a 2 (generation type: partial vs. complete) x 3 (stimulus type: not censored, censored, neither) mixed-factor ANOVA. Figure 6 (right half) displays the average performance on the recognition test in each of these experimental conditions.

The ANOVA revealed that only the main effect of stimulus type was significant, $F(2, 60) = 195.770, p < .01$. A Newman-Keuls post hoc analysis revealed a traditional generation effect—recognition accuracy for generated censored items *exceeded* that of not censored items by .21, and both exceeded the false alarm rate. Similar patterns of performance were evident for both the partial [.96>.75>.29] and complete [.94>.73>.34] censorship conditions. A 2 (generation type: partial vs. complete) x 2 (stimulus type: not censored vs. censored) ANOVA comparing d' performance indicated a significant main effect of stimulus type, $F(1, 30) = 46.651, p < .01$, which reflects superior discrimination of censored items as compared to not censored items (see right half of Figure 6). These results confirm the ironic effect of censorship noted in Experiment 2—that is, censored words that were generated during encoding were both more memorable and more discriminable than comparable not censored (heard) words.

Conditional Source Discrimination. The pattern of source judgments for the conditional data was examined using a 2 (generation type) x 3 (stimulus type) x 2 (source judgment: censored vs. not censored) ANOVA (see right half of Figure 5). The ANOVA showed reliable main effects of stimulus type, $F(2, 60) = 50.817, p < .01$, and source judgment, $F(1, 30) = 166.890, p < .01$. As in the overall analysis and previous experiments, participants were much more likely to report that the words they 'recognized' were words that were 'not censored' in the song. The ANOVA also revealed a reliable interaction between stimulus type and source judgment, $F(2, 60) = 12.907, p < .01$. A Newman-Keuls post-hoc analysis revealed no difference between the proportions of 'not censored' judgments made to not censored stimuli (.72) and to censored stimuli (.64), while both exceeded the proportion made to distractor stimuli (.25). Participants made significantly more 'censored' judgments to censored stimuli (.23) than to not censored stimuli (.10) and distractor stimuli (.05). All remaining main effects and interactions failed to reach significance (all $p>.05$). As with all the previous studies, the ACSIM measures of .47 and .55 for the partial and complete conditions were not statistically different from chance.

Conclusion

College-aged students were able to successfully generate censored words from an aurally presented song, with a higher rate of generation for partially censored as compared to completely censored items. Although overall recognition accuracy did not differ for censored and heard items, when the data were made conditional upon successful generation of the censored item during encoding, an ironic effect of censorship was revealed—recognition accuracy was significantly higher for the generated censored items compared to the heard items. In other words, the present study demonstrated a standard generation effect within the applied context of lyrical censorship. These results are consistent with past research which showed that, despite deleting and obscuring single phonemes (e.g., Warren et al., 1980) or entire words (e.g., Cooper et al, 1987), people were able to effectively generate the missing information as evidenced by no reduction in performance on subsequent comprehension tests.

Although generated items enjoyed a mnemonic benefit in this study, the act of generating the censored lyrics proved to be a challenging task for participants, who produced generation rates of 60%, 46%, 37%, and 31% for the partial and complete conditions in Experiments 2 and 3, respectively. With such low rates of generation, the conditional analyses were necessary to unmask the direct influence of generation on memory for censored lyrics. Of course, this procedure opens the door to item selection artifacts—that is, one could argue that successfully generated items were intrinsically easier than unsuccessfully generated items and, therefore, the mnemonic benefit was a function of ease and not due to the generation process. To address this possibility, a series of separate item analyses were performed on the conditional data from the partial and complete conditions of Experiment 2 and 3. Three values were calculated for each of the 30 nouns: (a) the item's generation rate, (b) the proportion correct when the item was not censored, and (c) the proportion correct when the item was censored.

Intrinsic ease was operationalized by performing a quartile split on the generation rate data, where items in highest and lowest quartiles represented the intrinsically easy and difficult ends of the continuum, respectively. Sign tests were used to compare not censored and censored recognition performance across the items. Quartile membership and sign test results were remarkably similar across the partial and complete conditions of each experiment. For the sake of simplicity and to minimize repetition, we combined all of the data into one grand item analysis; the results are displayed Table 1. Of the 30 words, 24 showed a standard generation effect (censored > not censored), four showed the opposite, and there were two ties ($p<.01$). Positive generation effects were clearly the modal response in each quartile, with the four opposite performance patterns spread equally across the upper-middle and lower quartiles, and one tie each in the highest and upper-middle quartiles. Hence, there is no evidence that the present data represent item selection artifacts.

With regard to source memory, when participants recognized a word in the present experiments, they were more likely to report that they "heard" the word, regardless of whether the word was actually heard or censored. Analyses of the raw proportions of correct source judgments offered evidence that the sources of non-censored items were remembered better than censored items. However, ACSIM measures suggested that overall source memory did not differ from chance and that the non-censored advantage may have been driven by the 'heard' bias.

Table 1. Item analysis for conditional data, collapsed across partial and complete conditions from Experiments 2 and 3

Item	Generation Rate	Proportion Correct Not Censored	Proportion Correct Censored
Face	.88	.81	.94
Heart	.79	.86	.94
Couple	.73	.93	.93
Town	.73	.64	.73
Voice	.69	.52	.91
Feeling	.65	.83	.95
Hand	.63	.55	.84
Memory	.58	.55	.67
Friend	.54	.78	.82
Woman	.52	.92	1.00
Story	.50	.84	.84
Family	.48	.90	.85
Wife	.44	.85	.91
Island	.42	.60	.46
Company	.42	.37	.74
Father	.38	.46	1.00
Mother	.38	.81	.85
Years	.37	.80	1.00
Need	.33	.53	.72
Hour	.31	.71	.75
Market	.31	.58	.63
Music	.31	.35	.79
Person	.29	.64	.79
World	.29	.47	.64
Faith	.27	.53	.33
Country	.25	.66	.71
Volume	.25	.24	.47
Week	.23	.45	.49
History	.19	.57	.90
Union	.15	.50	.42

FUTURE DIRECTIONS

If the primary goal of censorship is to discourage, or prohibit, cognitive awareness or processing of profane or objectionable material, then these current findings certainly suggest that lyrical censorship does not achieve always its desired results. Of course, lyrical censorship is not designed with college-aged students in mind and it is not surprising that college students are able to generate omitted information from context alone (e.g., Cooper et al, 1987; McDaniel, 1984). Of greater interest is whether younger children are able to generate the censored information. Indeed, previous research with children has shown that generation ability (for word fragments) increases substantially from age 7 to 11 (McFarland,

Duncan, and Bruno, 1983). Given that the standard generation effect generalizes to younger populations, one might expect a similar mnemonic benefit for generated censored items, although with a reduced generation rate. Other variables also might influence the generation and retention of censored items, including: type of censored material (e.g., common words, emotional words, traditionally censored words), type of memory test (e.g., recognition, recall, relearning); type of censorship (e.g., omission, over-dub, backward); level of familiarity with the song; and the availability of context information. Clearly, further research with different populations and procedures is required before we can assess the generality of these ironic effects of censorship.

Author Note

This research was sponsored by a Psi Chi Faculty Advisor Research Grant (Psi Chi National Office; Chattanooga, TN) and the Hotchkiss Fellows Program for Junior Faculty at Lake Forest College. Special thanks to Emily Blegen, Joanna Bovee, Jerrica Cerda, Dustin Koch, Stacey Parrot, & Gretchen Yehl for their assistance with data collection.

References

Burns, D. J. (1990). The generation effect: A test between single- and multifactor theories. *Journal of Experimental Psychology: Learning, Memory, and Cognition, 16,* 1060-1067.

Corbett, J. (1994). *Extended play: Sounding off from John Cage to Dr. Funkenstein.* Durham, NC: Duke University Press.

Cooper, W. E., Tye-Murray, N., and Nelson, L. J. (1987). Missing words and the comprehension of spoken text. *Acta Psychologica, 65,* 13-24.

de Winstanley, P. A., and Bjork, E. L. (2004). Processing strategies and the generation effect: Implications for making a better reader. *Memory and Cognition, 32,* 945-955.

Foos, P. W., Mora, J. J., and Tkacz, S. (1994). Student study techniques and the generation effect. *Journal of Educational Psychology, 86,* 567-576.

Gardiner, J. M. (1988). Generation and priming effects in word-fragment completion. *Journal of Experimental Psychology: Learning, Memory, and Cognition, 14,* 495-501.

Hirshman, E., and Bjork, R. A. (1988). The generation effect: Support for a two-factor theory. *Journal of Experimental Psychology: Learning, Memory, and Cognition, 14,* 484-494.

Hunt, R. R., and McDaniel, M. A. (1993). The enigma of organization and distinctiveness. *Journal of Memory and Language, 32,* 421-445.

Hyde, T. S., and Jenkins, J. J. (1973). Recall of words as a function of semantic, graphic, and syntactic orienting tasks. *Journal of Verbal Learning and Verbal Behavior, 12,* 471-480.

Kinjo, H., and Snodgrass, J. G. (2000). Does the generation effect occur for pictures? *American Journal of Psychology, 113,* 95-121.

Jacoby, L. L. (1983). Remembering the data: Analyzing interactive processes in reading. *Journal of Verbal Learning and Verbal Behavior, 22,* 495-508.

Lohaus, D., and Lachnit, H. (2001). Generation effects with pictorial material. *Psychologische Beitrage, 43,* 787-802.

Lutz, J., Briggs, A., and Cain, K. (2003). An examination of the value of the generation effect for learning new material. *Journal of General Psychology, 130,* 171-188.

McFarland, C. E., Duncan, E., and Bruno, J. M. (1983). Developmental aspects of the generation effect. *Journal of Experimental Child Psychology, 36,* 413-428.

McDaniel, M. A. (1984). The role of elaborative and schema processes in story memory. *Memory and Cognition, 12,* 46-51.

Mulligan, N. W. (2001). Generation and hypermnesia. *Journal of Experimental Psychology: Learning, Memory, and Cognition, 27,* 436-450.

Mulligan, N. W. (2002). The effects of generation on conceptual implicit memory. *Journal of Memory and Language, 47,* 327-342.

Mulligan, N. W. (2004). Generation and memory for contextual detail. *Journal of Experimental Psychology: Learning, Memory, and Cognition, 30*, 838-855.

Mulligan, N. W., and Lozito, J. P. (2004). Self-generation and memory. In B. H. Ross (Ed.) *The psychology of learning and motivation: Advances in research and theory, Vol 45* (pp. 175-214). San Diego, CA: Elsevier Academic Press

Murnane, K., and Bayen, U. J. (1996). An evaluation of empirical measures of source identification. *Memory and Cognition, 24,* 417-428.

Nairne, J. S., and Widner, R. L. (1987). Generation effects with nonwords: The role of test appropriateness. *Journal of Experimental Psychology: Learning, Memory, and Cognition, 13*, 164-171.

Nairne, J. S., Riegler, G. L., and Serra, M. (1991). Dissociative effects of generation on item and order retention. *Journal of Experimental Psychology: Learning, Memory, and Cognition, 17,* 702-709.

Nicolas, S., Ehrlich, M., and Facci, G. (1996). Implicit memory and aging: Generation effect in a word-stem completion test. *Cahiers de Psychologie Cognitive/Current Psychology of Cognition, 15,* 513-533

Postman, L. (1964). Short-term memory and incidental learning. In A. W. Melton (Ed.), Categories of human learning. New York: Academic Press.

Reardon, R., and Moore, D. J. (1996). The greater memorability of self-generated versus externally presented product information. *Psychology and Marketing, 13,* 305-320.

Samuel, A. G. (1981). Phonemic restoration: Insights from a new methodology. *Journal of Experimental Psychology: General, 110,* 474-494.

Samuel, A. G. (1996). Phoneme restoration. *Language and Cognitive Processes, 11,* 647-653.

Sengupta, J., and Gorn, G. J. (2002). Absence makes the mind grow sharper: Effects of element omission on subsequent recall. *Journal of Marketing Research, 39,* 186-201.

Serra, M., and Nairne, J. S. (1993). Design controversies and the generation effect: Support for an item-order hypothesis. *Memory and Cognition, 21,* 34-40.

Slamecka, N. J., and Graf, P. (1978). The generation effect: Delineation of a phenomenon. *Journal of Experimental Psychology: Human Learning and Memory, 4,* 592-604.

Slamecka, N.J., and Katsaiti, L.T. (1987). The generation effect as an artifact of selective displaced rehearsal. *Journal of Memory and Language, 26,* 589-607.

Thompson, C. P., and Barnett, C. (1981). Memory for product names: The generation effect. *Bulletin of the Psychonomic Society, 18(5),* 241-243.

Warren, R. M., and Warren, R. P. (1980). Auditory illusions and confusions. *Scientific American, 223,* 30-36.

In: Applied Memory
Editor: Matthew R. Kelley

ISBN 978-1-60692-143-2

Chapter 2

STUDYING WITH MUSIC: IS THE IRRELEVANT SPEECH EFFECT RELEVANT?

Justin Kantner
Department of Psychology, University of Victoria
Victoria, BC, Canada

ABSTRACT

The detrimental impact of background speech on short-term serial recall, known as the irrelevant speech effect, has a long history as a valuable theoretical tool, but its applications have received less attention. Two experiments attempted to determine whether the effect would extend to the practice of studying for an exam in the presence of background music containing lyrics. In Experiment 1, participants listened to vocal or instrumental music while studying for a serial recall test under conditions designed to mimic a realistic study-test experience. Despite several methodological departures from the traditional irrelevant speech paradigm, the results were consistent with a classic irrelevant speech effect. In Experiment 2, highly naturalistic study materials and test questions were used to determine the generality of the irrelevant speech effect beyond short-term serial recall. Vocal music hurt test performance relative to instrumental music under these conditions, but only when the study materials consisted of a chart; when the materials were prose paragraphs, no irrelevant speech effect was found. Explanations for this pattern of results are considered in terms of processing strategies at study, and further aspects of a realistic examination of studying with background music are discussed.

INTRODUCTION

The irrelevant speech effect—the tendency for ambient human speech to impair short-term serial recall—began, and has remained, a quintessential laboratory phenomenon in the human memory literature (e.g., Colle & Welsh, 1976; Salamé & Baddeley, 1982). Generated almost exclusively within a single task domain using simple, highly controlled stimulus materials, irrelevant speech effect data are channeled largely towards theory development and assessment. Among the classic memory phenomena with long, fruitful careers under laboratory scrutiny (e.g., the phonological similarity effect, the word length effect, articulatory suppression), the irrelevant speech effect is perhaps one of those most intuitively suited to real-world application. Despite its identity as a short-term serial recall phenomenon, the effect speaks to an utterly pervasive facet of everyday life—namely, environmental sound distraction. Thus, its practical implications for cognitive performance in applied settings are presumed to be considerable (Banbury, Tremblay, Macken, & Jones, 2001; Beaman, 2005; Jones, 1999).

The present investigation asks whether background music containing vocals can impair efforts to study for an exam by causing an irrelevant speech effect. The scenario of listening to music while studying for an exam has seldom been touched upon in past research, despite the fact that it bears a strong resemblance to a typical irrelevant speech experiment in many respects. Background music is analogous to the irrelevant speech played in traditional experiments, and both natural and experimental study tasks involve committing information to memory in the presence of a task-irrelevant auditory stream. Moreover, the population most often studied in irrelevant speech experiments is the one to which the current application is most directly relevant: college students. Exam preparation is a nearly perpetual matter for undergraduates, and listening to background music while studying is a popular habit. Given that the primary (if not exclusive) goal of studying is to encode information into memory ahead of an anticipated test, the potential of lyrics in vocal background music to constitute irrelevant speech, and thus to disrupt memorization, is a significant applied question.

The Irrelevant Speech Effect in the Laboratory

The vast majority of work on the irrelevant speech effect has concerned the effect of irrelevant speech on immediate (or short-term) serial recall. In a typical experiment, short lists of simple stimuli such as digits, letters, or words are presented one-at-a-time. Following the offset of the final list item (or a short delay thereafter), participants attempt to recall the list items in their presentation order. When human speech is played during list presentation, or during a subsequent pre-test rehearsal period (Miles, Jones, & Madden, 1991), serial recall performance suffers. This decrement—the irrelevant speech effect—has been reported with magnitudes ranging from 5% to 50% in the literature (Neath, 2000). In this short-term serial recall paradigm, the irrelevant speech effect is an extremely robust phenomenon, replicated numerous times with a wide variety of materials, designs, and procedures (e.g., Colle, 1980; Colle & Welsh, 1976; Ellermeier & Zimmer, 1997; Hanley & Broadbent, 1987; Jones, 1994; Jones, Madden, & Miles, 1992; Neath, Surprenant, & LeCompte, 1998; Salamé & Baddeley, 1982, 1986, 1989; Surprenant, LeCompte, & Neath, 2000).

One of the intriguing aspects of the irrelevant speech effect is that the speech can be deleterious to memory without being related in any way to the to-be-remembered material (hence the term "irrelevant"). Indeed, the first published report of the effect by Colle and Welsh (1976) demonstrated that it can be produced even when the speech is in a foreign language. In general, the content of the speech does not have much bearing on the magnitude of the effect (e.g., Buchner, Irmen, & Erdfelder, 1996), though some exceptions have been reported (Buchner & Erdfelder, 2005; Buchner, Rothermund, Wentura, & Mehl, 2004; Neely & LeCompte, 1999). The effect is largely indifferent to the phonological overlap of the irrelevant speech and the to-be-remembered material (Jones & Macken, 1993, 1995; though see Salamé & Baddeley, 1982) and the volume at which the speech is played (Colle, 1980; Salamé & Baddeley, 1987). In sum, the evidence to date characterizes the irrelevant speech effect as a highly consistent phenomenon, robust with respect to numerous physical and psychological manipulations, and resistant, even, to habituation (Hellbrück, Kowano, & Namba, 1996; Tremblay & Jones, 1998).

The impenetrability of the effect has fostered great interest in its cognitive substrates. Examinations of the effect and its interactions with other classic short-term memory phenomena, such as the phonological similarity effect, the word length effect, and articulatory suppression have led to important insights as to the factors that affect short-term memory (e.g., Jones, Macken, & Nicholls, 2004; Neath, Farley, & Surprenant, 2003). The irrelevant speech effect has played an important role in model development; these models, in turn, have driven an ongoing debate as to how the effect is best explained (see Baddeley, 2000, Jones & Tremblay, 2000, and Neath, 2000, for one exchange, and Baddeley & Larsen, 2003, and Macken & Jones, 2003, for another).

An early and highly influential account of the effect was provided by Baddeley's Working Memory framework (Baddeley, 1986; Baddeley & Hitch, 1974; Salamé & Baddeley, 1982), which holds that irrelevant speech gains automatic access to a Phonological Store, where it interferes with to-be-remembered information also in the store. By contrast, the Object-Oriented Episodic Record (O-OER) model (Jones, 1993; Jones & Macken, 1993; Jones, Macken, & Murray, 1993) posits that interference from irrelevant speech occurs via automatically generated "pointers" that represent the serial order of any dynamic stimulus stream. The pointers from irrelevant speech interfere with those from the to-be-remembered information, which causes the loss of serial order information. Alternatively, the Feature Model, originally proposed by Nairne (1988, 1990) and augmented to account for the irrelevant speech effect by Neath (2000), characterizes the disruption in terms of feature adoption (i.e., the features of the irrelevant speech become part of the representation of to-be-remembered information) and divided attention (i.e., between the to-be-remembered information and the to-be-ignored speech). These varying conceptions of the phenomenon—and of short-term memory, more generally—give rise to competing predictions regarding its interaction with a host of stimulus manipulations.

A close examination of these theories and their predictions is beyond the scope of this work (see Neath & Surprenant, 2003, for a review). This purpose of the present chapter is to establish the generality of the irrelevant speech effect to a more realistic study-test scenario than is usually in place in irrelevant speech experiments—specifically, studying for an exam with music playing in the background. If background speech impairs serial recall performance, then background music containing speech (i.e., lyrics) could reasonably be expected to have a similar effect in this applied setting.

Music as Irrelevant Speech

While a number of studies have explored the effects of music on cognitive performance (e.g., Fogelson, 1973; Freeburne & Fleischer, 1952; Furnham & Bradley, 1997; Hallam, Price, & Katarsou, 2002; Ransdell & Gilroy, 2001), few have tested the potential for music to produce an irrelevant speech effect. Demonstration of a musical irrelevant speech effect requires at least one vocal and one non-vocal (i.e., instrumental) background condition, so that memory performance in each may be compared. Past studies employing this design have provided strong evidence that vocals in music do produce a memory deficit closely resembling an irrelevant speech effect. Boyle and Coltheart (1996) presented participants with 50 10-item lists, half of which contained rhyming words and half of which contained non-rhyming words. Serial recall was initiated after each list. Study and recall of each list were accompanied by one of five auditory conditions: silence, instrumentals from Gilbert and Sullivan songs, singing plus instrumentals from the same songs, singing from those songs alone, and the lyrics from those songs read as normal speech. Boyle and Coltheart (1996) found that each condition containing speech (singing, singing plus instrumentals, and speech) significantly impaired serial recall performance, and to roughly the same degree. Instrumental music produced a directional but non-significant deficit in performance. Similarly, Salamé and Baddeley (1989) tested serial recall of random digit strings while participants listened to instrumental or vocal versions of opera pieces. Vocal music significantly lowered performance relative to both instrumental music and silence.

Salamé and Baddeley (1989) discussed the implications of their findings for settings such as school and the workplace, and suggested that further research should test the generalizability of their findings in such environments. The most direct extension of the Salamé and Baddeley (1989) paradigm beyond serial recall, however, was arguably that of Martin, Wogalter, and Forlano (1988), published one year earlier. In their Experiment 2, Martin et al. (1988) tested vocal versus instrumental music conditions while having participants read short passages on various topics (e.g., the propagation of sound, the creative process) from a GRE practice guide. Reading comprehension of each passage was tested after a 30-sec delay interval. The music consisted of the song "You Light Up My Life" by Joe Brooks; in the instrumental condition, the music from the song was played without lyrical accompaniment, while in the lyrics conditions, the words to the song were either sung or read by a vocalist from the university's music department, with and without backing instrumentation. Reading comprehension test scores were 6-7% lower for passages read in the lyrics conditions than for those read in the instrumental or silence conditions, a significant difference (Martin et al., 1988). Although these results do not indicate a large effect size, and are limited to a single experiment utilizing a single musical piece, they dovetail with those of Boyle and Coltheart (1996) and Salamé and Baddeley (1989) in suggesting that vocal music can cause an irrelevant speech effect. Further, they suggest that the effect might be felt under conditions more closely approximating a realistic study and test procedure than those generally used in irrelevant speech experiments.

EXPERIMENT 1

The goal of Experiment 1 was to begin to bridge the gap between the traditional irrelevant speech paradigm and a naturalistic examination of the effects of vocal music on studying for an exam. Therefore, Experiment 1 was built upon the list-learning, serial recall design of the Boyle and Coltheart (1996) and Salamé and Baddeley (1989) studies, but added several features meant to reflect a more realistic learning scenario. First, the nature of the stimuli was changed. Lists in typical irrelevant speech experiments are composed of simple materials such as digits, letters, and words. Not only are such stimuli decidedly more elemental than those that would be learned in any university course, their inter-relationships differ from those of regular learning materials in ways likely to modulate the impact of irrelevant speech. That is, digit, letter, and word stimuli usually have no meaningful semantic relationship to one another. Lists of unrelated items are particularly vulnerable to irrelevant speech effects, because participants are likely to rely on phonological processing strategies such as subvocal rehearsal to facilitate learning (Jones & Tremblay, 2000). By contrast, related items may be processed in terms of meaning, leading to a diminished irrelevant speech effect. Hanley and Bakopoulou (2003) directly manipulated the learning strategy used by participants, instructing some to adopt a phonological rehearsal strategy and others to process items semantically. While the phonological group demonstrated a classic irrelevant speech effect (with an additive effect of phonological similarity), the semantic group exhibited a small, non-significant irrelevant speech effect, and no additional decrement from phonological similarity.

These results hold clear implications for the question of whether irrelevant speech in music will be detrimental to learning exam material. While the stimulus lists used in most irrelevant speech research consist of unrelated items, learning material in academic coursework is predominantly composed of highly inter-related information. The latter, then, might elicit semantic processing and be less prone to interference through irrelevant speech. In Experiment 1, study lists were composed of actual names, periods, or scientific terms organized according to a particular sequential order. For example, one list, labeled "20th Century U.S. Presidents (in the order they held office)" contained the items ROOSEVELT, TRUMAN, EISENHOWER, KENNEDY, JOHNSON, NIXON, and FORD. Thus, the items of each list adhered to a meaningful consecution, made apparent by the preceding list label.

Second, the music played was intended to approximate what current undergraduates might listen to independently. That is, modern themes and instrumentation were emphasized, and an array of songs was chosen, in order to simulate the experience of listening to a CD, iPod, or radio station while studying. The selection of songs was at the discretion of the researcher, and no claim is made that the songs used in the experiment are, themselves, commonly listened to by the participants. Indeed, the objective was to choose songs performed by current recording artists that were generally not "household names" amongst 18-22 year-olds, so as to minimize individual differences in familiarity with the music.

For the non-lyrical comparison condition, instrumental tracks were chosen from predominantly vocal albums of roughly the same genre as those used in the lyrics condition. This selection strategy was intended to help gather a set of instrumental songs with similar instrumentation, tempo, and length to those of the vocal songs. The highly complex nature of the range of songs used made precise matching of the vocal and instrumental tracks along these dimensions infeasible, but this was considered a reasonable exchange for the ecological validity of the materials.

Third, whereas most irrelevant speech experiments involve repeated study-test cycles wherein lists are recalled either immediately or shortly after presentation, academic exam preparation generally entails repeated review of all to-be-remembered material, followed by a single test. To simulate these factors in Experiment 1, participants studied each of eight lists on three separate occasions, and received only one test, on all of the lists, following the study phase.

Finally, music was played only at study; tests were taken in silence. This aspect of the format again mimicked that of academic testing, and ensured that participants would not derive a musical benefit of state-dependent memory at test (Balch, Bowman, & Mohler, 1992). In a third (control) condition, both study and test were undertaken in silence.

Method

Participants. Participants were 82 undergraduates at the University of Victoria who took part in the experiment in exchange for bonus credit in an introductory psychology course. Twenty-eight participated in the lyrics condition, 27 participated in the instrumental condition, and 28 participated in the silence condition. All were fluent in English.

Materials. Eight lists of seven items each were created by the author. Lists were composed of real-life examples of names and terms occurring in a natural sequence. The eight lists were 20th Century U.S. Presidents (in the order they held office), Metallic Elements (in order of appearance in the Periodic Table), Layers of the Atmosphere (from highest to lowest altitude), the Caesars (in the order they ruled), Canadian Provinces (in the order of their incorporation into Canada), Geological Eras (from most recent to least recent), and Shakespearean Plays (in order of date of first performance). The full lists appear in Appendix A.

Vocal music selections were assembled by the author and consisted of various tracks from recent albums loosely definable as rock or pop. Songs were selected that contained contemporary instrumentation (e.g., drums and guitars) and themes but were not likely to be known to most first- or second-year University of Victoria undergraduates. These songs contained innocuous lyrics and instrumentals that were not likely to be perceived as overly heavy or grating. Ten vocal music tracks were used in the experiment, half containing male vocals and half containing female vocals. Ten non-vocal music selections were chosen on the basis of their similarity to the vocal tracks in instrumentation, tempo, and genre. In most cases, these tracks were drawn from instrumental pieces on albums predominantly composed of vocal rock or pop songs. A list of the songs used in the experiment appears in Appendix B. The music was played at a moderate volume level through stereo headphones.

Instructions and lists were presented via E-Prime software. Paper test forms were created and were completed with pen or pencil.

Procedure. Participants were tested one-at-a-time, with an experimenter present throughout the session. Instructions informed participants that they would study eight lists of seven items each and that they should try to learn each in its proper order. Participants were encouraged to approach the task as though they were studying for an exam on which the order of the lists would be tested. Each list was preceded by a label in a blue font indicating the topic of the list to follow and the organizational structure of the list (e.g., "20th Century U.S. Presidents (in the order they held office)"). Participants pressed the space bar after reading the list topic to initiate the presentation of the list. Each list item appeared in black lettering in the center of the computer screen for 2 sec. Following the presentation of the final item of a given list, the screen went blank for 3 sec, followed by the topic of the next list. While the list items appeared in their fixed order, the lists themselves appeared in a random order.

After the presentation of all eight lists, a screen appeared indicating that the lists would be presented again and that the task was to continue to memorize them in order. The procedure of this second study block was identical to that of the first study block, except that the lists were presented in a new random order.

Following the second study block, a screen appeared indicating that each list would be presented for a final time, and that participants should make their best effort to memorize the order of each before the subsequent test. They were also encouraged to try and anticipate items in the third study block before they appeared on the screen as a check on their knowledge. The third study block was identical to the first two, except that the lists were presented a new random order, and the parenthetical component of the list topic was dropped, such that only the topic itself appeared on the screen (e.g., "20th Century U.S. Presidents").

All participants wore headphones throughout the study phase. Participants in the lyrics condition heard a randomly ordered assortment of as many of the ten vocal music songs as fit within the duration of the study session. Participants in the instrumental condition heard an assortment of the instrumental tracks, while participants in the silence condition heard nothing.

Following the third study block, participants removed the headphones and received test instructions. These instructions created a delay of roughly 30 sec between the end of the study phase and the administration of the test. Participants were then given a test sheet containing eight rows with seven blanks each. The first list to be recalled was indicated via the appearance of that list's topical label in the center of the screen. After participants had written down the items from the list to their satisfaction, they pressed the space bar to bring up the next list to be recalled. The eight lists were probed in a random order and subjects were given as much time as needed to recall each one.

Upon conclusion of the test, all participants were asked how many of the lists they felt they could have ordered with 100% accuracy before taking part in the experiment. None reported more than one such list out of the eight studied. Of the nine participants reporting extra-experimental knowledge of one list, four were in the lyrics condition, four were in the instrumental condition, and one was in the silence condition.

Results and Discussion

Prior to analysis, the data of three participants were removed due to exceedingly low test scores and/or a failure to understand task instructions. Thus, the analyses that follow are based on the data from 27, 26, and 27 participants in the lyrics, instrumental, and silence conditions, respectively.

Mean accuracy as a function of serial position is plotted for each of the three conditions in Figure 1. As is evident from inspection of the figure, performance in all three conditions was superior for the items at the beginning and end of the lists, yielding the classic bow-shaped serial position curve well known to characterize memory for order (Murdock, 1960). A repeated measures ANOVA with serial position (1-7) as a within-subjects factor and listening condition (lyrics, instrumental, or silence) as a between-subjects factor revealed a highly significant main effect of serial position, $F(6, 456) = 45.4$, $p < .001$. The serial position effect did not interact with listening condition ($F < 1$).

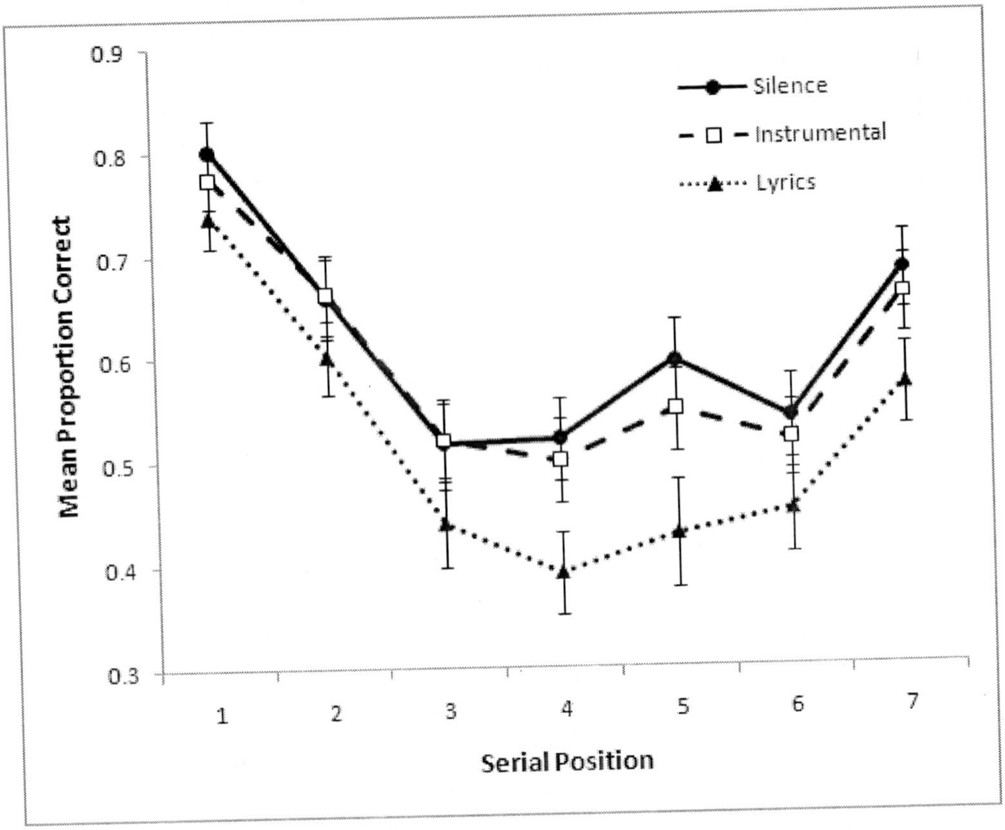

Figure 1. Serial recall performance as a function of item list position (1-7) and listening condition during study in Experiment 1. Error bars represent one standard error of the mean.

Participants in the lyrics condition performed less accurately than those in the other two conditions at every list position. Collapsed across serial positions, the mean percentage of correct responses was 61.6 for the silence group, 59.8 for the instrumental group, and 51.7 for the lyrics group. The main effect of listening condition was significant, $F(2, 76) = 3.372$, $p < .05$. Planned comparisons confirmed that the silence, $t(50) = 2.02$, $p < .05$, and instrumental, $t(51) = 1.86$, $p < .05$, groups were significantly more accurate than the lyrics group, but did not differ significantly from one another, $t(51) = 0.83$, $p = .53$.

In short, these results mirror those of more traditional irrelevant speech experiments in two important respects. First, all three conditions displayed bow-shaped serial position curves, a well-established pattern of accuracy in the irrelevant speech paradigm. Second, performance in the lyrics condition was impaired relative to the instrumental and silence conditions at a magnitude quite consistent with more typical irrelevant speech studies. That this correspondence between past results (e.g., Boyle & Coltheart, 1996; Salamé & Baddeley, 1989) and those of the current study was observed despite substantial design modifications in the present experiment suggests that the irrelevant speech effect may indeed generalize to the practice of studying with background music.

EXPERIMENT 2

The results of Experiment 1 suggest that lyrics in music can function as irrelevant speech and can impair serial recall performance. While the current experiment represents an extension of past work on the irrelevant speech effect, there are still many respects in which it does not reflect the circumstances of realistic exam preparation, nor a realistic academic test. Perhaps the most obvious is that students are not usually tested solely on rote serial recall. Instead, they are given questions that call for multiple types of mnemonic judgments, such as free recall (as in the fill-in-the-blank or short answer questions) and recognition (as in true/false or multiple choice questions).

Whether irrelevant speech would impact performance on these types of tasks, given naturalistic study materials, is an open question. The O-OER model (Jones, 1993) predicts that only tasks with a serial component (i.e., serial rehearsal of study items) will be subject to an irrelevant speech effect. Neither the Phonological Store hypothesis (Salamé & Baddeley, 1982) nor the Feature Model (Neath, 2000) makes this explicit prediction (Farley, Neath, Allbritton, & Surprenant, 2007). Generally, however, the evidence has favored the hypothesis that seriation is necessary for an irrelevant speech effect (Farley et al., 2007).

LeCompte (1994) demonstrated irrelevant speech effects in free recall, cued recall, and recognition using letter and word stimuli, which suggests that that the effect extends well beyond serial recall to tasks eliciting no serial processing. Beaman and Jones (1997), however, have argued that such tasks may elicit a serial rehearsal strategy, even though the goal is not serial recall per se (see also Jones and Tremblay, 2000). That is, although participants are not asked to memorize the order of to-be-remembered items, they may find rehearsal according to presentation order the best mnemonic strategy at their disposal.

By this view, the effects of irrelevant speech in music may be felt when studying for tests other than serial recall. To the extent that seriation is a prominent component of study strategies, one might expect irrelevant speech to have a negative impact on free recall, recognition, and other types of tests often represented on academic exams. Whether or not students engage in serial processing, however, may depend largely on the nature of the study materials. The serial rehearsal strategy encouraged by a list learning task, for example, may not be adopted in more natural learning situations, such as when one is studying from a textbook. Moreover, the processing strategy chosen is likely to follow from one's expectations as to the nature of the test questions. In a typical irrelevant speech experiment (and in the current Experiment 1), participants study with fore knowledge of the exact nature of the test, and, in effect, the questions to be asked. Such is not generally the case for undergraduates outside the laboratory.

In Experiment 2, participants studied three topics: Caesars, Canadian Prime Ministers, and geological eras. Information about the Caesars and Prime Ministers was presented via multiple pages of text interspersed with pictures, a format meant to approximate the appearance of pages from a textbook. Information about the geological eras was presented in chart format, with the names of the eras and their associated flora and fauna laid out in a list-like fashion. In each case, the material to be learned was distinctly serial in nature: the Caesars and Prime Ministers were discussed, and the geological eras were listed, in temporal order. In the former two cases, however, the information was embedded in prose. If prose presentation obviates or otherwise discourages the use of a serial processing strategy necessary for the emergence of an irrelevant speech effect, music containing lyrics should pose no disadvantage to the study of the Caesars and Prime Ministers, but might still be expected to diminish recall of the geological eras. Memory for the different topics was assessed with serial reconstruction, fill-in-the-blank, multiple choice, and recognition questions. Participants were given no foreknowledge of the general format of the test, nor the individual questions; they were simply told to try their best to learn as much of the material as possible in the time allotted.

Another shortcoming with respect to the ecological validity of Experiment 1 was addressed in Experiment 2: the delay between study and test. Although this interval (approximately 30 sec) was considerably longer in Experiment 1 than is usually the case in irrelevant speech experiments, it was unrealistic in that students are not usually given exams so soon after study. While some review often occurs immediately before the test, students often prepare in the days leading up to the exam (particularly the day before). Thus, a stronger test of the practical implications of the irrelevant speech effect would hold study and test sessions on separate days. In Experiment 2, participants were tested twice: immediately after study, and on the following day. The first test served as an immediate measure of memory and as a means of preparation for the second test. The longer-term effects of irrelevant speech under conditions such as those of Experiment 2 remain to be established, though Knez and Hygge (2002) reported a detrimental effect of background conversation on recall from a text passage after a two-hr delay. Whether the effects of irrelevant speech would maintain after an approximately 24-hr delay is an open question.

Finally, the method of sound delivery was changed in Experiment 2. Participants in Experiment 1 listened to music through headphones, perhaps rendering the music particularly difficult to ignore. To the extent that students would normally play music through a more ambient, less invasive medium (e.g., external speakers) while studying, Experiment 1 may have exaggerated its impact. In Experiment 2, music was played through speakers and was audible throughout the testing room.

Method

Participants. Participants were 42 undergraduates at the University of Victoria who took part in the experiment in exchange for bonus credit in an introductory psychology course. All were fluent in English. Twenty-two participated in the lyrics condition and 20 participated in the instrumental condition. A silence condition was not included in Experiment 2.

Study Materials. Three topics for study were chosen by the author: the early Caesars, 20th Century Canadian Prime Ministers, and geological eras. Caesar materials were adapted from a Wikipedia article summarizing the writings of the historian Suetonius (http://en.wikipedia.org/wiki/Lives_of_the_Twelve_Caesars). Text and pictures from the article pertaining to the first six Caesars were fashioned into a document consisting of six sections, one for each of the Caesars discussed. Each section began with a picture of a bust of the Caesar along with his name, followed by four to six paragraphs (approximately 400-700 words) of history and anecdotes related to the Caesar. The Caesars were presented in the order of their rule from earliest to latest; this ordering was evident from the consecutive nature of events described in the text. Pictures of associated figures referred to in the text (e.g., Mark Antony) were interspersed throughout the document. The Caesar material contained 10 pages in all, printed back-to-back and stapled together into a packet.

Prime Minister materials were drawn from the website "The Prime Ministers of Canada" (www.primeministers.ca) and were arranged similarly to the Caesar information. Six pages were constructed, each containing the name, years in office, and picture of a 20th Century Canadian Prime Minister, followed by a brief sketch (150-200 words) of the Prime Minister's term. As with the Caesar material, the Prime Ministers were presented in chronological order.

The geology materials consisted of a single-page chart from the website "Enchanted Learning" (www.enchantedlearning.com). A portion of the chart containing information about the 12 most recent periods of geological history was used in the experiment. The periods were listed in order from latest (at the top of the chart) to earliest (at the bottom). The chart indicated the flora and fauna associated with each period, the years of history encompassed by the period, and the geological Era and Eon to which each period belonged. All information was conveyed in single words and short phrases; no prose was included.

Test Materials: Day 1. A separate paper-and-pencil test for each of the three study topics was constructed. Each test began with a question requiring serial reconstruction of the names or periods studied. In the Caesars test, for example, the six Caesars were listed vertically in a random order with blanks next to each; participants were to enter a number 1-6 into each blank to indicate the order in which the Caesars held power. The question was analogous in the Prime Minister and geology tests; on the geology test, six of the 12 studied periods were included, so that each of the three tests called for the serial reconstruction of six items.

Following the reconstruction question on each test were seven fill-in-the-blank (FIB) and six multiple choice (MC) questions written by the author. Each FIB question could be answered with a single Caesar, Prime Minister, or period name. MC questions contained four alternatives, each the name of a Caesar, Prime Minister, or period.

The Caesar and Prime Minister tests contained an additional section testing recognition of the pictures presented in the study materials. In this section, the six Caesar busts (or Prime Minister portraits) from the study materials were randomly intermixed with six new items from each category. New Caesar busts were gathered from various locations on the internet; new Prime Minister portraits were taken from the website mentioned above. Participants were to indicate whether or not they had seen each item during study by writing "yes" or "no" beneath the picture. As there were no pictures in the geology materials, no recognition section was included on the geology test.

Both the questions within each section and the response options within each question (where applicable) appeared on the test in a random order. The test was identical across participants.

Test Materials: Day 2. The three Day 1 tests were combined into a single test to be given on Day 2. The questions and correct answers were identical to those included on the Day 1 test, but with new random orderings of the serial reconstruction items, multiple choice options, and faces on the recognition test. The reconstruction questions appeared on the front page of the test, followed by the FIB, MC, and recognition sections. Within the FIB and MC sections, questions from each of the three topics were randomly intermixed.

Music Materials: The music was identical to that used in Experiment 1 (see Appendix A). The songs were played in a random order using Windows Media Player, and were heard through standard external computer speakers.

Procedure: Day 1. Participation took place in groups of one to three, with an experimenter present at all times. Participants were seated in positions roughly equidistant from the computer speakers, and such that they were not easily able to view each other's test answers. Instructions characterized the task as one with which the participants were quite familiar: studying for an exam. Materials for each of the three topics were introduced, and participants were told that they would be given 15 min to study all three before receiving a test on their contents. It was emphasized that 15 min would not be sufficient to learn all of the material thoroughly, and that the interest of the experiment was simply in how much they could learn in the time allotted. No particular direction was given as to how the materials were to be studied, but participants were asked to devote some time to each of the three topics. The music (either vocal or instrumental) was playing when participants entered the room and continued throughout the study phase, but was never mentioned by the experimenter.

After 15 min had elapsed, the music was stopped and the study materials were collected. The three tests were then passed out to each participant, with instructions that only 10 min would be given to work on all three. Participants were asked to answer as many questions as possible while striving for accuracy, and were advised against dwelling on any given question.

At the end of the 10-min test period, the study materials were handed back, the music was re-initiated, and a review phase began. Participants were instructed to use the study materials to check their test answers, and to mark any corrections to the right or left of the corresponding answer blank (but not to change their original answers). Seven min were given for the review. The entire session lasted approximately 40 min.

Procedure: Day 2. Participants returned roughly 24 hr after the first session and were again tested in groups of one to three. The second session consisted solely of the administration of the Day 2 test. The test was distributed following a brief description of its general composition. Participants were given up to 15 min to complete the test, and were encouraged to take any extra time after finishing to check their answers as thoroughly as possible. Background music was not played at any point in the session.

Results and Discussion

The data of one participant who did not follow test instructions and another who achieved an extremely low Day 1 test score were removed prior to analysis, leaving 22 and 18 participants in the lyrics and instrumental conditions, respectively. Caesar, Prime Minister, and geology test scores were computed by averaging the proportion of correct responses on the serial reconstruction, FIB, and MC portions of the tests. Overall test scores were then calculated as the mean of the Caesar, Prime Minister, and geology test scores. Results from the recognition section did not figure into the final test scores due to the incidental nature of that test (i.e., participants were most likely not trying to commit the pictures to memory while studying), as well as the fact that the geology test did not contain a recognition section. However, the recognition results are reported below.

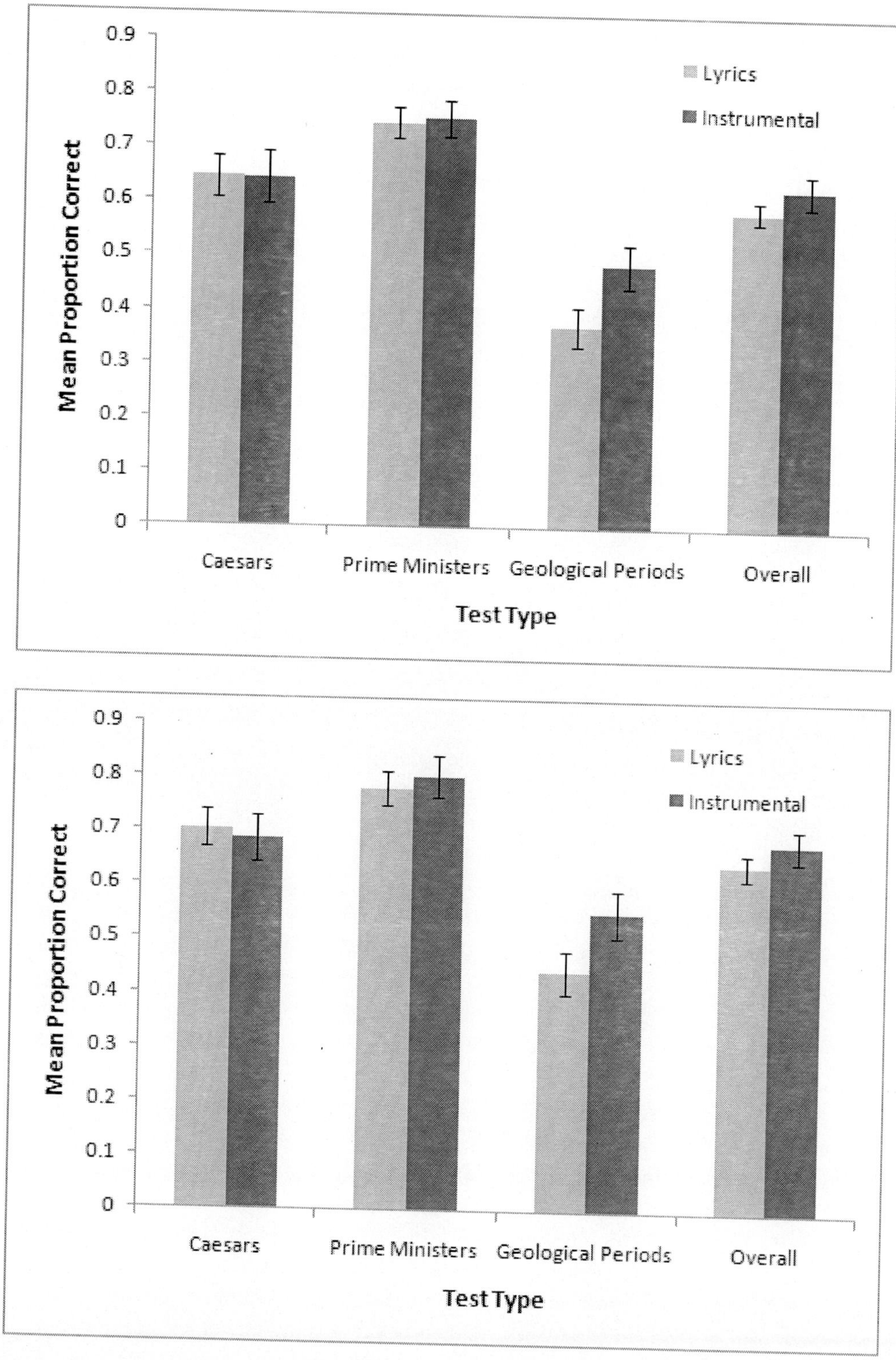

Figure 2. Test performance in Experiment 2 on Day 1 (top panel) and Day 2 (bottom panel). Error bars represent one standard error of the mean.

An additional repeated measures ANOVA was conducted to assess the performance of the instrumental and lyrics groups on the different types of test questions (serial reconstruction, FIB, and MC). This analysis revealed no interaction between listening condition and question type, $p = .75$. Planned comparisons yielded no significant differences between the listening conditions on any type of test question (all $ps > .25$), although there was a directional tendency towards better serial reconstruction performance in the instrumental condition. The only individual comparison yielding a significant difference between listening conditions concerned performance on MC geology questions, which was higher in the instrumental condition, $t(38) = 2.847$, $p < .01$. Although the instrumental group held moderate advantages in serial reconstruction of Prime Ministers (6.7%) and geological periods (10.5%), these differences did not reach significance, due in part to considerable variability in the data.

Finally, recognition test performance, measured as the hit rate minus the false alarm rate collapsed across the Caesar and Prime Minister tests, did not vary between the instrumental and lyrics groups, $p = .49$.

Day 2. The pattern of results on the second test closely followed that of the first test. Once again, the instrumental group held a slight overall performance advantage (68.3% to 64.3%), but this advantage failed to reach significance, $F(1,38) = 1.102$, $p = .30$. Listening condition did not interact with test type, $p = .14$, nor did it interact with question type, $p = .24$. Instrumental and lyrics participants performed equally on Caesar and Prime Minister tests (both $ps > .60$), but, as in the Day 1 test, the lyrics group performed more poorly on the geology test, $t(38) = 1.842$, $p < .08$. No other comparisons between the two groups approached significance, with the exception of superior performance for the instrumental group on FIB questions, $t(38) = 1.892$, $p < .07$.

These data were marked by a high degree of variability. The predominant source of this variability may have been strong individual differences in the ability to extract to-be-tested information from study materials in the brief time given. However, the naturalistic aims of the study required a lack of strict experimental control in several facets of the design, any of which could conceivably have contributed individual difference-based variability to the data. For example, participants likely varied in their study strategies (see General Discussion), pre-experimental familiarity with the topics studied, and personal reaction to the musical selections.

Despite this variability, the central result of Experiment 2 seems clear-cut: music with lyrics was detrimental to performance only on the geology test. Geology test scores were higher in the instrumental condition for all three question types on both administrations of the test, a consistency not seen in any other relevant aspect of the data. The magnitude of the vocal music detriment was virtually identical on Days 1 and 2 (11.3% and 11.0%, respectively), although the Day 2 result was only near-significant. Given that Caesar and Prime Minister test scores never differed by more than 2.5% across listening conditions, the effects observed on the geology test are compelling. Generally, they indicate that vocal music can cause an irrelevant speech effect while studying under relatively naturalistic circumstances. Moreover, they implicate the nature of the study materials as a critical determinant of the effects of the irrelevant speech: the geology materials were the only ones composed of a chart, and not paragraphs of prose. Explanations of these results are considered below.

General Discussion

The object of the present experiments was to test a practical implication of the irrelevant speech effect; namely, that studying while listening to background music containing lyrics could impair memory for the studied material, thus lowering exam performance. To that end, both experiments were designed to more closely mimic an authentic study-test experience than traditional irrelevant speech experiments. In Experiment 1, lists were composed of names and terms following a meaningful, naturally occurring sequence. Furthermore, modern music was used and multiple reviews of the study lists were followed by a single test session, during which no music was played. Despite these departures from the established irrelevant speech paradigm, the overall pattern of results in Experiment 1 bore all the markings of an irrelevant speech effect: the presence of lyrics in music was associated with an approximately 8% decrease in accurate serial recall relative to instrumental music, and an approximately 10% decrease relative to silence. These trends parallel those of two other studies using music as irrelevant speech (Boyle & Coltheart, 1996; Salamé & Baddeley, 1989), even though both of those studies tested immediate serial recall after a single presentation of each list, and used lists of items with no systematic semantic relationship to one another.

One might have expected that repeated exposure to each list in Experiment 1 would have allowed participants in the lyrics condition to overcome the handicap posed by the vocal content of the music, yielding a weakened irrelevant speech effect. By contrast, the data suggest that the lyrics continued to interfere with serial encoding during each study presentation, resulting in a classic irrelevant speech effect. One might also have expected that the meaningful connections between the list items in Experiment 1 would have inspired a more semantic (and less phonological) processing orientation at study, rendering the lists less vulnerable to interference by irrelevant speech (e.g., Jones & Tremblay, 2000). The results suggest, however, that the strategy or combination of strategies chosen by participants did not diminish the detrimental impact of the lyrics. Considering that the naturalistic aspects of the Experiment 1 design failed to prevent the occurrence of an irrelevant speech effect, the present results may be taken as evidence that the effect can be produced by vocal background music, and can impact the efficacy of study efforts.

Experiment 2 was designed to test these implications under highly realistic conditions. While all study materials remained serially structured, they appeared in a prose format accompanied with illustrations, mimicking the style of a textbook, or as a chart. Tests were given immediately and approximately 24 hr after study, and were designed to emulate the format of a university exam. The results indicated that vocal music only reduced performance on the portion of the test for which the study material was a chart (geological periods); test scores on the topics studied with prose materials (Caesars and Prime Ministers) were virtually identical in the lyrics and instrumental conditions. Interestingly, this pattern of results held for multiple choice and fill-in-the-blank questions as well as questions calling for the reconstruction of order. The general pattern of results also held both immediately following study and after a 24-hr delay. In terms of the interfering effects of lyrics, then, the critical factor appeared to be the format of the study materials: information studied in prose format was resistant to the effects of irrelevant speech, while information studied in a chart format was not.

Why would irrelevant speech interfere with memory for information gleaned from a chart, but not from prose? An intuitive explanation is that the rich, elaborative nature of prose encourages semantic processing, while the list-like features of a chart elicit the phonological processing strategy known to be more vulnerable to effects of irrelevant speech (e.g., Hanley & Bakopoulou, 2003; Jones & Tremblay, 2000; Salamé & Baddeley, 1986). A second possibility is that the discrete, hierarchical structure of information presented in the chart encouraged serial processing, while the continuous nature of the prose rendered such processing less likely. This explanation may be particularly well-suited to account for the present data, as serial processing is a benchmark concomitant (if not prerequisite) of the irrelevant speech effect (e.g., Jones, 1993). Performance on the serial reconstruction portions of the Caesar and Prime Minister tests clearly indicates that order information was learned from prose, but such learning may not have arisen from explicitly serial study processing (e.g., serial rehearsal).

Whether either or both of the above explanations bear on the current results remains speculative until more is understood about the strategies engaged by participants at study. Indeed, the importance of strategy as a mediator of the irrelevant speech effect has received attention in the short-term serial recall irrelevant speech literature (e.g., Baddeley, 2000; Baddeley & Larsen, 2003; Hanley & Bakopoulou, 2003; Salamé & Baddeley, 1986), and might be of greater consequence under the more complex demands of exam studying. Participants appear to utilize a range of strategies even when faced with a simple serial recall task. Hanley and Bakopoulou (2003) explicitly manipulated study strategies by having participants engage in phonological or semantic processing of letter stimuli (discussed above), but included a third condition in which participants were free to choose their own strategies. These participants reported using five different strategies, classified as phonological (27% of participants), semantic (18%), a mixture of phonological and semantic (14%), representing each letter with a word and rehearsing the words subvocally (14%), and merging letters into short words or nonsense syllables and repeating these subvocally (27%). Each of these strategies likely entails a unique balance of phonological and semantic processing, and thus, potentially, a unique level of susceptibility to irrelevant speech effects. The results of the current experiments undoubtedly reflect a distribution of approaches as well. Assessing the strategic approach of participants under circumstances such as those of Experiment 2 is therefore an important direction for future research. To the extent that the nature of the study materials modulates processing strategy, it modulates susceptibility to the irrelevant speech effect.

Several other factors that might influence the extent of musical irrelevant speech effects on exam studying are not addressed by the present research. For example, a number of participants in Experiment 2 asked whether they would be allowed to take notes as they studied. While this option was not extended in the current experiments, it is a pervasive learning strategy, and should be incorporated into future experiments. Studying from notes, which often bear more resemblance to outlines and charts than to prose materials, might be more susceptible to irrelevant speech effects than other methods. The role of past experience studying with music is another factor left unexamined by the current experiments. Many participants in Experiment 1 claimed that they commonly listened to music while studying, and that they were proficient at "tuning it out" such that it did not affect their study efforts (though several others admitted to studying with music in spite of their sense that it was a hindrance to learning). Evidence that the irrelevant speech effect is resistant to habituation

(Hellbrück et al., 1996; Tremblay & Jones, 1998) would seem to argue against the claim that one can develop immunity to the effect, but this possibility has not been tested in the current context. A related question concerns the role of past experience with the music itself. While participants in the current experiments listened to songs that were largely unfamiliar to them, students often choose highly familiar (and highly enjoyed) songs as background music while studying. If such music is more easily ignored than novel music, the lower demand on attentional resources might reduce susceptibility to irrelevant speech effects (e.g., Neath, 2000).

The practice of studying with background music takes place in a complex real-world context. The role of the experiments reported in this chapter has been to suggest that the often laboratory-bound irrelevant speech effect can extend beyond its normal empirical range and hold influence in such a context. Future research will help determine when this influence is benign, and when it may cost a letter grade.

APPENDIX A

20th Century U.S. Presidents (in the order they held office)
Roosevelt
Truman
Eisenhower
Kennedy
Johnson
Nixon
Ford

Canadian Provinces (in the order they became part of Canada)
Nova Scotia
Manitoba
British Columbia
Prince Edward Island
Yukon
Alberta
Newfoundland

Metallic Elements (in order of appearance in the Periodic Table)
Chromium
Manganese
Iron
Cobalt
Nickel
Copper
Zinc

Shakespearean Plays (in order of date of first performance)
Henry VI
Richard III
Two Gentlemen of Verona
King John
As You Like It
The Merry Wives of Windsor
The Winter's Tale

The Caesars (the first seven)
Augustus
Tiberius
Caligula
Claudius
Nero
Vespasian
Titus

Layers of the Atmosphere (lowest to highest altitude)
Troposphere
Stratosphere
Mesosphere
Thermosphere
Ionosphere
Magnetosphere
Exosphere

Geological Eras (most recent to least recent)
Quarternary
Neogene
Paleogene
Cretaceous
Jurassic
Triassic
Permian

APPENDIX B

Songs used in the Lyrics condition
Alison Krauss – Baby, Now That I've Found You
Cowboy Junkies – Crescent Moon
Eels – I Like Birds
Eels – Packing Blankets
Last Forever – Hide and Seek

Sean Lennon – Bathtub
Sean Lennon – Breeze
Sean Lennon – Spaceship
Shawn Colvin – The Facts about Jimmy
The Sundays – Here's Where the Story Ends

Songs used in the Instrumental condition
311 – Colors
Alice In Chains – Whale & Wasp
Eels – Dusk: A Peach in the Orchard
Eels – Going to Your Funeral Part II
Orbital – New Style
Sting – Saint Agnes and the Burning Train
Stone Temple Pilots – No Memory
The Appleseed Cast – Doors Lead to Questions
The Appleseed Cast – View of a Burning City
U2 – Bass Trap

References

Baddeley, A. (1986). *Working memory.* New York, NY: Clarendon Press/Oxford University Press.

Baddeley, A. D. (2000). The phonological loop and irrelevant speech effect: Some comments on Neath (2000). *Psychonomic Bulletin & Review, 7*(3), 544-549.

Baddeley, A.D., & Hitch, G. (1974). Working memory. In G.H. Bower (Ed.), *The psychology of learning and motivation: Advances in research and theory* (Vol. 8, pp. 47-89). New York: Academic Press.

Baddeley, A., & Larsen, J. D. (2003). The disruption of STM: A response to our commentators. *The Quarterly Journal of Experimental Psychology A: Human Experimental Psychology, 56*(8), 1301-1306.

Balch, W. R., Bowman, K., & Mohler, L. A. (1992). Music-dependent memory in immediate and delayed word recall. *Memory & Cognition, 20*(1), 21-28.

Banbury, S. P., Tremblay, S., Macken, W. J., & Jones, D. M. (2001). Auditory distraction and short-term memory: Phenomena and practical implications. *Human Factors, 43*(1), 12-29.

Beaman, C. P. (2005). Auditory distraction from low-intensity noise: A review of the consequences for learning and workplace environments. *Applied Cognitive Psychology, 19*(8), 1041-1064.

Beaman, C. P., & Jones, D. M. (1997). Role of serial order in the irrelevant speech effect: Tests of the changing-state hypothesis. *Journal of Experimental Psychology: Learning, Memory, and Cognition, 23*(2), 459-471.

Boyle, R., & Coltheart, V. (1996). Effects of irrelevant sounds on phonological coding in reading comprehension and short-term memory. *The Quarterly Journal of Experimental Psychology A: Human Experimental Psychology, 49*(2), 398-416.

Buchner, A., & Erdfelder, E. (2005). Word frequency of irrelevant speech distractors affects serial recall. *Memory & Cognition, 33*(1), 86-97.

Buchner, A., Irmen, L., & Erdfelder, E. (1996). On the irrelevance of semantic information for the 'irrelevant speech' effect. *The Quarterly Journal of Experimental Psychology A: Human Experimental Psychology, 49*(3), 765-779.

Buchner, A., Rothermund, K., Wentura, D., & Mehl, B. (2004). Valence of distractor words increases the effects of irrelevant speech on serial recall. *Memory & Cognition, 32*(5), 722-731.

Colle, H. A. (1980). Auditory encoding in visual short-term recall: Effects of noise intensity and spatial location. *Journal of Verbal Learning & Verbal Behavior, 19*(6), 722-735.

Colle, H. A., & Welsh, A. (1976). Acoustic masking in primary memory. *Journal of Verbal Learning & Verbal Behavior, 15*(1), 17-31.

Ellermeier, W., & Zimmer, K. (1997). Individual differences in susceptibility to the 'irrelevant speech effect.'. *Journal of the Acoustical Society of America, 102*(4), 2191-2199.

Farley, L. A., Neath, I., Allbritton, D. W., & Surprenant, A. M. (2007). Irrelevant speech effects and sequence learning. *Memory & Cognition, 35*(1), 156-165.

Fogelson, S. (1973). Music as a distractor on reading-test performance of eighth grade students. *Perceptual and Motor Skills, 36*(3), 1265-1266.

Freeburne, C. M., & Fleischer, M. S. (1952). The effect of music distraction upon reading rate and comprehension. *Journal of Educational Psychology, 43*(2), 101-109.

Furnham, A., & Bradley, A. (1997). Music while you work: The differential distraction of background music on the cognitive test performance of introverts and extroverts. *Applied Cognitive Psychology, 11*(5), 445-455.

Hallam, S., Price, J., & Katsarou, G. (2002). The effects of background music on primary school pupils' task performance. *Educational Studies, 28*(2), 111-122.

Hanley, J. R., & Bakopoulou, E. (2003). Irrelevant speech, articulatory suppression, and phonological similarity: A test of the phonological loop model and the feature model. *Psychonomic Bulletin & Review, 10*(2), 435-444.

Hanley, J. R., & Broadbent, C. (1987). The effect of unattended speech on serial recall following auditory presentation. *British Journal of Psychology, 78*(3), 287-297.

Hellbrück, J., Kuwano, S., & Namba, S. (1996). Irrelevant speech and human performance: Is there long-term habituation? *Journal of the Acoustical Society of Japan, 17,* 239-247.

Jones, D. M. (1993). Objects, streams, and threads of auditory attention. In A. D. Baddeley, & L. Weiskrantz (Eds.), *Attention: Selection, awareness, and control: A tribute to Donald Broadbent.* (pp. 87-104). New York, NY, US: Clarendon Press/Oxford University Press.

Jones, D. M. (1999). The cognitive psychology of auditory distraction: The 1997 BPS Broadbent lecture. *British Journal of Psychology, 90*(2), 167-187.

Jones, D. M. (1994). Disruption of memory for lip-read lists by irrelevant speech: Further support for the changing state hypothesis. *The Quarterly Journal of Experimental Psychology A: Human Experimental Psychology, 47*(1), 143-160.

Jones, D. M., & Macken, W. J. (1993). Irrelevant tones produce an irrelevant speech effect: Implications for phonological coding in working memory. *Journal of Experimental Psychology: Learning, Memory, and Cognition, 19*(2), 369-381.

Jones, D. M., & Macken, W. J. (1995). Phonological similarity in the irrelevant speech effect: Within- or between-stream similarity? *Journal of Experimental Psychology: Learning, Memory, and Cognition, 21*(1), 103-133.

Jones, D. M., Macken, W. J., & Murray, A. C. (1993). Disruption of visual short-term memory by changing-state auditory stimuli: The role of segmentation. *Memory & Cognition, 21*(3), 318-328.

Jones, D. M., Macken, W. J., & Nicholls, A. P. (2004). The phonological store of working memory: Is it phonological and is it a store? *Journal of Experimental Psychology: Learning, Memory, and Cognition, 30*(3), 656-674.

Jones, D. M., Madden, C., & Miles, C. (1992). Privileged access by irrelevant speech to short-term memory: The role of changing state. *The Quarterly Journal of Experimental Psychology A: Human Experimental Psychology, 44*(4), 645-669.

Jones, D. M., & Tremblay, S. (2000). Interference in memory by process or content? A reply to Neath (2000). *Psychonomic Bulletin & Review, 7*(3), 550-558.

Knez, I., & Hygge, S. (2002). Irrelevant speech and indoor lighting: Effects of cognitive performance and self-reported affect. *Applied Cognitive Psychology, 16*(6), 709-718.

LeCompte, D. C. (1994). Extending the irrelevant speech effect beyond serial recall. *Journal of Experimental Psychology: Learning, Memory, and Cognition, 20*(6), 1396-1408.

Macken, W. J., & Jones, D. M. (2003). Reification of phonological storage. *The Quarterly Journal of Experimental Psychology A: Human Experimental Psychology, 56*(8), 1279-1288.

Martin, R. C., Wogalter, M. S., & Forlano, J. G. (1988). Reading comprehension in the presence of unattended speech and music. *Journal of Memory and Language, 27*(4), 382-398.

Miles, C., Jones, D. M., & Madden, C. A. (1991). Locus of the irrelevant speech effect in short-term memory. *Journal of Experimental Psychology: Learning, Memory, and Cognition, 17*(3), 578-584.

Murdock, B. B. (1960). The distinctiveness of stimuli. *Psychological Review, 67*(1), 16-31.

Nairne, J. S. (1988). A framework for interpreting recency effects in immediate serial recall. *Memory & Cognition, 16*(4), 343-352.

Nairne, J. S. (1990). A feature model of immediate memory. *Memory & Cognition, 18*(3), 251-269.

Neath, I. (2000). Modeling the effects of irrelevant speech on memory. *Psychonomic Bulletin & Review, 7*(3), 403-423.

Neath, I., Farley, L. A., & Surprenant, A. M. (2003). Directly assessing the relationship between irrelevant speech and articulatory suppression. *The Quarterly Journal of Experimental Psychology A: Human Experimental Psychology, 56A*(8), 1269-1278.

Neath, I., & Surprenant, A. M. (2003). *Human memory: Second Edition*. Belmont, CA: Wadsworth/Thomson Learning.

Neath, I., Surprenant, A. M., & LeCompte, D. C. (1998). Irrelevant speech eliminates the word length effect. *Memory & Cognition, 26*(2), 343-354.

Neely, C. B., & LeCompte, D. C. (1999). The importance of semantic similarity to the irrelevant speech effect. *Memory & Cognition, 27*(1), 37-44.

Ransdell, S. E., & Gilroy, L. (2001). The effects of background music on word processed writing. *Computers in Human Behavior, 17*(2), 141-148.

Salamé, P., & Baddeley, A. D. (1982). Disruption of short-term memory by unattended speech: Implications for the structure of working memory. *Journal of Verbal Learning & Verbal Behavior, 21*(2), 150-164.

Salamé, P., & Baddeley, A. D. (1986). Phonological factors in STM: Similarity and the unattended speech effect. *Bulletin of the Psychonomic Society, 24*(4), 263-265.

Salamé, P., & Baddeley, A. D. (1987). Noise, unattended speech and short-term memory. *Ergonomics, 30*(8), 1185-1194.

Salamé, P., & Baddeley, A. D. (1989). Effects of background music on phonological short-term memory. *The Quarterly Journal of Experimental Psychology A: Human Experimental Psychology, 41*(1), 107-122.

Surprenant, A. M., LeCompte, D. C., & Neath, I. (2000). Manipulations of irrelevant information: Suffix effects with articulatory suppression and irrelevant speech. *The Quarterly Journal of Experimental Psychology A: Human Experimental Psychology, 53*(2), 325-348.

Tremblay, S., & Jones, D. M. (1998). Role of habituation in the irrelevant sound effect: Evidence from the effects of token set size and rate of transition. *Journal of Experimental Psychology: Learning, Memory, and Cognition, 24*(3), 659-671.

In: Applied Memory
Editor: Matthew R. Kelley

ISBN 978-1-60692-143-2

Chapter 3

VERBALIZING MUSICAL MEMORIES

***Charity Brown*[*1], *Toby J. Lloyd-Jones,*[2] *and Katherine Moor*[1]**
[1]Department of Psychology
University of Leeds, Leeds, UK
[2] Department of Psychology, Swansea University,
Wales, UK

ABSTRACT

Verbal overshadowing is the phenomenon whereby describing a perceptual memory, such as one's memory for a face, can impair recognition. Verbal interference is not limited to the particular face that is described, but can extend to other non-described faces presented within a similar context (Brown and Lloyd-Jones, 2003). Moreover, verbal overshadowing is found to occur in a variety of domains concerned with perceptual expertise and effects of verbal overshadowing may arise when perceptual/non-verbal expertise outweighs verbal expertise. In this chapter, we focus upon establishing the effects of verbal overshadowing within a specific domain of auditory memory, namely music recognition. We examine whether verbal interference will generalise across multiple non-described musical segments, following a single musical segment description. We also test whether vulnerability to verbal overshadowing is associated with level of musical expertise. Participants listened to 12 to-be-remembered musical segments and then described (or not, in the control condition) another musical segment. Subsequently they discriminated the 12 original musical segments from 12 distracters in a 'yes/no' recognition decision. Verbal overshadowing was evident for music recognition; description participants were significantly less accurate in the recognition test than no description participants. Effects of verbal overshadowing were evident across both musicians and non-musicians. We argue that these findings are consistent with verbalisation producing a general shift in participants 'processing style' from a predominantly perceptual/global to verbal/local processing style which is less effective for discriminating between highly similar perceptual stimuli (Schooler, 2002). Further, the vulnerability of both musicians and non-musicians to verbal overshadowing is consistent with accounts of music perception which propose that global processing is a necessary and perhaps automatic aspect of music perception.

* Corresponding author.

INTRODUCTION

Language is the primary tool for communicating and sharing our experiences with others. However, language does not always adequately capture our meaning, thoughts or experiences. Indeed, there are many aspects of our environment which we are unable to communicate accurately to others in words. For instance, we may find ourselves at a loss as to how to describe our memory for a beautiful scene, an exotic taste or a sublime melody. This apparent ineptness of language has led researchers to consider how describing perceptual experiences may influence our subsequent behaviour.

A perceptual task which has received much interest in this respect is recognising faces. Here, a disparity between visual and verbal ability is evident in that whilst our capacity for face recognition is typically good, descriptions of faces are often vague and imprecise (Ellis, Shepard and Davies, 1980). Numerous studies have now shown that verbally describing a face can prove detrimental for subsequent attempts to recognise that face, a phenomenon termed 'verbal overshadowing' (for a review, see Schooler, 2002). For instance, in a seminal study of eyewitness memory, Schooler and Engstler-Schooler (1990) asked participants to describe (or not, in the control condition) the facial features of a bank robber they had viewed in a video event. Participants who had provided a description of the face were subsequently less likely to identify the robber's face from a line-up of similar looking faces. More recently, a meta-analysis of verbal overshadowing studies has revealed a small but reliable negative effect of verbalization on face recognition ($Zr = .12$; Meissner and Brigham, 2001).

Much research concerning verbal overshadowing has occurred within the face recognition domain, perhaps due to its potential legal and courtroom applications (for a review, see Meissner and Brigham, 2001). However, verbal overshadowing has been found to occur for memory tasks involving other difficult-to-describe visual stimuli, such as the recognition of colours (Schooler and Engstler-Schooler, 1990) and mushrooms (Melcher and Schooler, 2004). For example, Schooler and Engstler-Schooler (1990) found participants, describing the colour of a presented card in as much detail as possible, were subsequently less able to identify the original colour when it was presented along with five visually similar distracter colours (e.g., when the target and distracters could all have been described as army green).

Verbal overshadowing has also been observed in non-visual domains, such as the recognition of voices (Perfect, Hunt and Harris, 2002) and tastes (Melcher and Schooler, 1996). Perfect et al. (2002) presented participants with a recording of a voice which said "Just follow the instructions, don't press the alarm, and no one will get hurt'. Participants then either described the voice or engaged in a control activity. They then heard an audio-lineup consisting of the target and five distracter voices. A reliable effect of verbal overshadowing was found: only 21% of participants describing the voice correctly identified the target voice from the lineup compared to 50% of no description controls. In addition, other domains involving non-verbal cognition, such as insight problem solving (i.e., the sudden and unexpected solving of a problem following an impasse) and affective decision-making also have been found to be vulnerable to interference from verbalisation. For example, Schooler, Ohlsson and Brooks (1993) asked participants to "think-aloud" while working on a series of insight and non-insight problems (i.e., analytic problems which can be solved using a logical, step by step method). Those participants who described their thought processes correctly solved substantially fewer insight problems than participants providing no description. In contrast, for non-insight problems the performance of description and no description participants was similar. Similarly, Wilson and Schooler (1991) have shown verbalisation to affect the quality of participants' affective preferences. They asked participants to taste a number of different brands of strawberry jam and to rate their liking for each one. Description participants were further asked to list their reasons for liking or disliking each jam. These participants produced "non-optimal" jam preferences. That is, unlike no description participants, description participants' jam preferences did not correlate well with the rankings given by taste experts (taken from a consumer reports magazine). In a further study, Wilson, Lisle, Schooler, Hodges, Klaaren and La Fleur (1993) asked participants to evaluate two different posters with the option of taking one of these posters home. Those participants who were asked to introspect about their reasons for liking their chosen poster were less satisfied with the choice they had made three weeks later compared to control participants who did not analyse their reasons. Thus effects of verbal overshadowing have been documented across several different perceptual and non-cognitive domains and it appears that verbal overshadowing arises when non-verbal knowledge is essential for performance.

Verbal Overshadowing and the Role of Perceptual Expertise

The generalisation of verbal overshadowing to other visual, sensory and affective domains has led researchers to propose that susceptibility to verbal overshadowing occurs when non-verbal expertise with a particular stimulus substantially outweighs verbal ability. Evidence consistent with this notion comes from studies which have compared the extent to which participants with varying levels of perceptual expertise are susceptible to the effects of verbal overshadowing. For example, Melcher and Schooler (1996) recruited participants with varying levels of wine tasting proficiency. Wine tasting is a domain within which both perceptual and verbal expertise can be developed over time. Expert wine tasters, in addition to perceptual expertise, are in possession of an extensive descriptive vocabulary which can be applied to wines. Three levels of wine-tasting expertise were considered: non-wine drinkers (drank wine less than once a month), untrained wine drinkers (drank wine regularly but had no formal training in wine-tasting) and expert wine drinkers (professional wine drinkers or individuals who had undertaken several wine-tasting courses).

Participants either described or did not describe a tasted target wine, following which they were asked to rate the similarity in taste of 4 wines (the target plus 3 distracters) to the target. Verbal overshadowing was not evident for non-wine drinkers (assumed to have low levels of both perceptual and verbal expertise) or expert wine drinkers (assumed to have high levels of both perceptual and verbal expertise). However, verbal overshadowing was evident for untrained wine drinkers: description participants exhibited poorer recognition performance than their counterparts in the no description condition. Melcher and Schooler (1996) proposed that untrained wine drinkers were susceptible to verbal overshadowing due to a disparity between their perceptual knowledge of wines and their limited ability to verbally describe these complex stimuli.

More recently, Melcher and Schooler (2004) examined the relationship between expertise and verbal overshadowing by manipulating the training participants received in a previously unfamiliar domain; mushroom recognition. Participants either received perceptual training (i.e., learning to categorise mushrooms in a perceptual learning task), conceptual training (i.e., receiving a lecture about mushrooms which emphasised verbal knowledge, including information about the characteristics used by mushroom experts to classify mushrooms), or no training. Compared to those who had received no training, participants receiving perceptual training showed negative effects of describing a target mushroom on a subsequent recognition task. This was presumably due to the perceptual expertise they had developed through training now outweighing their verbal ability. In contrast, for those exposed to conceptual training providing a description numerically enhanced their recognition performance as compared to a no description condition. This apparent beneficial effect of verbalisation suggests that newly acquired conceptual/verbal information can under certain circumstances be useful, or at least not harmful, for recognition. It may be that conceptual training encouraged participants to make use of conceptual/verbal information when initially encoding the stimuli.

Accounts of verbal overshadowing can be broadly separated into those which emphasise either specific memory representations or processing styles. Meissner, Brigham and Kelley (2001) proposed a *misinformation* account of verbal interference whereby verbalisation gives rise to a novel distorted verbal memory representation of the described stimulus which then serves to interfere with the original perceptual memory representation (see also the recoding interference account, Schooler and Engstler-Schooler, 1990). According to this account, individuals with verbal expertise should be able to use their verbal/conceptual knowledge effectively to describe their perceptual experiences. Hence verbal/conceptual expertise protects against verbal interference because the newly generated verbal representation is less likely to be contaminated with self-generated misinformation (Melcher and Schooler, 2004).

Alternatively, Schooler and colleagues have proposed a *transfer-inappropriate processing* account (cf., Schooler, 2002). In essence, engaging in verbalisation leads to a general shift in participants 'processing style' from a predominantly perceptual/global to verbal/local processing style (see Melcher and Schooler, 2004, for a discussion of alternative conceptualisations of this processing shift). This shift in processing gives rise to the disruptive effects of verbalisation on recognition memory as the perceptual processes engaged in at encoding are no longer applied at recognition. On this account, verbal/conceptual expertise within a domain would allow participants to more readily engage in verbal/local processing of the perceptual stimulus which is more commensurate with the process of verbalisation. Importantly, these two accounts make different predictions concerning the effects of verbalisation upon recognition memory. If verbalisation gives rise to a novel verbal representation of the described stimulus then any negative effects of verbalisation should be restricted to recognition of the stimulus that is initially described. On the other hand, if verbalisation gives rise to a more general processing shift then we would expect the interference from verbalisation to extend to other stimuli in the recognition test which have not previously been verbalised (cf., Schooler, 2002; Brown and Lloyd-Jones, 2002, 2003).

Several studies within the domain of face recognition have shown that verbal overshadowing can extend beyond the particular stimulus that is described. For example, Dodson, Johnson and Schooler (1997) presented participants with both a male face and female face and asked participants to describe one of these faces or to engage in a no description control activity. Providing a description of one of the faces interfered with participants' ability to recognise both the described and *non-described* face. More recently, in a novel paradigm involving the presentation of multiple stimuli, Brown and Lloyd-Jones (2003) have demonstrated that describing a *single* face can lead to impaired recognition of a *number of different* faces, which have not previously been verbalised. They argued that their findings were consistent with a transfer-inappropriate processing account. That is, effects of verbal interference in their paradigm reflected a general shift in processing style rather than any alteration to a particular memory representation.

The Music Domain

Music is an alternative non-verbal domain which encompasses both non-verbal/perceptual and verbal/conceptual knowledge. Verbal/conceptual knowledge can convey musical properties such as musical notation, pitch sequence, key, mode (major or minor), harmony and temporal structure, which includes rhythm (tempo and meter) and event duration. A number of studies have shown that skilled musicians (as compared to novices) make use of auditory-based conceptual attributes, such as pitch and temporal structure, in their music learning (e.g., Palmer and Meyer, 2000; Drake and Palmer, 2000). It seems that musicians are able to form more highly structured representations of musical stimuli than nonmusicians. For instance, Mikumo (1997) found that musicians were able to rehearse effectively pitch information presented either in the auditory (humming or whistling), visual (presented as notes on a musical staff) or verbal (presented as a series of musical note names) domain during the encoding of tonal musical segments. However, the most effective encoding strategy for musicians was to make combined use of information from all three domains. This presumably allowed for a more elaborated representation to be formed in memory.

More generally, musical expertise has been found to correlate with superior performance on tests of verbal ability, in particular, verbal memory tasks (Brandler and Rammsayer, 2003; Chan, Ho, and Cheung, 1998). This finding has been attributed to a left-hemisphere preference which musicians' have been shown to exhibit in the processing of musical information (cf., Schuppert, Münte, Wieringa, and Altenmüller, 2000). For example, compared to non-musicians, musicians show more left-lateralized representations of musical stimuli (e.g., as indicated by a right ear advantage) which may arise as a result of changes in cortical organization as a consequence of their musical training. The left hemisphere is functionally linked with both language-related auditory processing and verbal memory (e.g., Morris, Abrahams and Polkey, 1995) and so the left-hemisphere dominance exhibited by musicians may relate to an ability to make efficient use of verbal/conceptual knowledge when forming representations of musical stimuli.

Alternatively, it has been suggested that musicians' assumed left-hemisphere dominance is associated with an increased reliance upon an analytical or local processing style (Bever and Chiarello, 1974). Both local and global processing distinctions have been implicated in music perception (e.g., Sanders and Poeppel, 2007). Evidence from behavioural studies with healthy non-musicians indicates that musical attributes apparent at a local level, such as rhythm, temporal structure and local pitch intervals (i.e., the size of the pitch interval between two notes) show a left hemisphere processing advantage (i.e., a right ear advantage, e.g.,

Peretz, 1990; Peretz and Morais, 1987). In contrast, the processing of more global properties of a melodic sequence, such as contour information (i.e., an up/down pattern of pitch changes which span several notes) is thought to be more right hemisphere dominant. Peretz (1990), for example, found that patients with right hemisphere damage failed to discriminate effectively between melodies differing in contour information. In particular, the processing of global musical properties has been found to be beneficial for melody discrimination (e.g., Schulkind, Posner and Rubin, 2003). Nevertheless, musicians have been shown to demonstrate flexibility in their usage of global versus local processing when appropriate task demands are evident (Peretz and Babai, 1992).

More generally, the right hemisphere is assumed to possess a significant role in music perception. In particular, music appears to activate the right hemisphere more than the left (e.g., Zatorre, Evans and Meyer, 1994; Schiavetto, Cortese and Alain, 1999). In addition, damage to the right hemisphere can give rise to impairments in the processing of local as well as global aspects of melodies (Peretz, 1990). These findings have led some researchers to suggest that a global processing system is a necessary prerequisite for the processing of local musical information (cf., Schuppert et al., 2000).

The Present Experiment: Verbal Overshadowing in Music Memory

Here, we focus upon establishing the effects of verbal overshadowing within a specific domain of auditory memory, namely music recognition. Musical expertise likely determines the extent to which perceptual and verbal knowledge or processes are relied upon when encoding and subsequently recognising musical segments. Thus, non-musicians memory for musical segments may be vulnerable to verbal overshadowing as a result of a disparity between their perceptual and verbal expertise. Consistent with this, Schooler and colleagues have reported an unpublished study in which describing a previously heard musical segment impaired non-musicians ability to distinguish that same musical segment from a number of similar distracters (Houser, Fiore, and Schooler, 1997).

In previous studies which have examined the role of perceptual versus verbal expertise in determining effects of verbal overshadowing a verbal description has been requested of the *same* stimulus that is later to be recognised (e.g., Melcher and Schooler, 1996; Ryan and Schooler, 1998; Melcher and Schooler, 2004). However, as outlined previously, research focusing specifically upon faces has found that verbal overshadowing is not always restricted to the described stimulus (cf. Brown and Lloyd-Jones, 2002, 2003).

The following experiment examined the generality of a processing account of verbal overshadowing by applying the Brown and Lloyd-Jones (2002, 2003) multiple presentation paradigm in an alternative perceptual domain. In their paradigm, participants were exposed to 12 to-be-remembered faces and then described (or not, in the control condition) an additional (13th) face. Subsequently, participants had to discriminate the original 12 faces from 12 distracters (in a 'yes/no' recognition task). We closely followed the original Brown and Lloyd-Jones design. We do note however, that effects of verbal overshadowing in this paradigm were moderated by task-order effects which can be attributed to a repeated measures design. In particular, verbal overshadowing was only apparent when the description task was undertaken after the no description control condition. Brown and Lloyd-Jones (2002, 2003) argued that when the no description task followed the description task carry-over effects from the description onto the control condition attenuated any observation of verbal overshadowing. That is, when participants verbally describe the face in the first block, they will then be more likely to covertly describe the face when encountering the second block: there is no reason for them to change their mental set. In contrast, when encountering the face for the first time in the no description condition, there is no encouragement to verbally describe it until the second block. Therefore, we closely examined the influence of any carry-over effects on verbal overshadowing in the present experiment.

In the present experiment, participants were presented with a block of 12 musical segments in a study phase. These were followed by a 13th musical segment which participants described from memory (or ignored and completed a filler task). Participants were then presented with a 'yes/no' recognition task which included the 12 (old) segments from the study phase and 12 (new) previously unheard segments. We assessed whether the verbal interference arising from describing a single musical segment extended to the recognition of other previously heard but non-described musical segments. On the basis that global processing of musical stimuli has been implicated in successful melody discrimination and that the act of describing may induce a shift from global to local processing, we would expect verbal overshadowing to occur within the present paradigm. In addition, we examine the role of musical expertise by assessing the vulnerability of musicians to verbal overshadowing. We predicted that verbal overshadowing would be either less evident or not apparent at all for musicians because they possess both perceptual and verbal/conceptual expertise within the musical domain.

Method

Participants. There were 32 male and female participants. All were University of Leeds undergraduate students. All were native English speakers, with normal hearing. Participants were naïve as to the purpose of the experiment. Musical ability was assessed via a short questionnaire. Participants were allocated to the musicians group if they had played an instrument for more than 10 years, and indicated one or more of the following: fluency in music notation; receiving musical training for at least 6 years; or practised playing an instrument for 15 hours or more a week. All other participants were assigned to the non-musicians group.

Materials and Apparatus. The musical segments presented at encoding and test were single note melodies of 48 Irish folk tunes taken from The Petrie Collection of the Ancient Music of Ireland website, University of Leeds (http://www.leeds.ac.uk/music/research/petrie/home.htm). Melodies were computer-generated MIDI files with the timbre approximation of a piano. The stimuli were converted into WAV files and edited to be between 8 and 16 seconds in length, based on the ending of the fourth bar of the piece. The musical segments had a mean duration of 12 seconds with an average tempo of 87 and contained between 11 and 48 notes (mean number of notes = 25). Half the musical segments were in a major key and half in a minor key. The 48 musical segments were divided into two stimulus sets, each containing 24 segments. One stimulus set consisted of segments with a metre of 3/4 and the other stimulus set consisted of segments with a metre of 6/8. Presentation of stimulus sets was counterbalanced across conditions. Within each stimulus set, items were randomly divided into two sets of 12 study items. These were counterbalanced as targets and distracters throughout the experiment.

At test, the 12 study items were mixed with 12 unheard items from the same stimulus set. The description stimuli were two additional musical segments different from those appearing as encoding and test materials. These included one segment belonging to a minor key with a metre of ¾, and the other belonging to a major key with a metre of 6/8. The two description stimuli were presented with the stimulus group that possessed the same metre. Stimuli were presented using a stand-alone PC using Superlab 1.4 (General Purpose Psychology Testing Software, Cedrus Corporation, USA). Participants listened to melodies through headphones at a comfortable listening level.

Design. A mixed factorial design was employed with verbalization condition (description vs. no description) as a within-participants factor and musical expertise (musician vs. non-musician) and condition order (description condition first vs. description condition second) as between-participants factors. The dependent measures were taken from signal detection theory and were recognition accuracy (d') and response bias (C) (e.g., Macmillan and Creelman, 2005; Snodgrass and Corwin, 1988; Wickens, 2002).

Participants were assigned to either the musician or non-musician group on the basis of their responses to the musical expertise questionnaire. All participants took part in both a description and no description condition. Thus, each participant undertook two separate stimulus blocks, one after the other, with each block containing 12 target stimuli in a study phase followed by the same 12 targets plus 12 distracters in a test phase. The two description stimuli (A and B) were rotated so that for an equal number of musicians and non-musicians each appeared as the last item in both the description and no description condition. Hence, half the participants heard description stimulus A in the description condition and description stimulus B in the no description condition, whilst the remaining participants heard description stimulus A in the no description condition and description stimulus B in the description condition. The description stimulus was presented as the last item in the study phase, whether or not it was to be described, and did not occur in the recognition test.

In addition, the order in which the description and no description conditions were undertaken was counterbalanced. Half the musicians and half the non-musicians undertook the description condition first followed by the no description condition, whilst the remaining musicians and non-musicians undertook the no description condition first followed by the description condition.

Procedure. Participants were tested individually and completed the following procedure twice, once for each of the two verbalization conditions. During a study phase participants heard 12 later to-be-recognised unfamiliar melodies, followed by a 13th melody. Melodies were separated by a 5 second inter-stimulus interval. Prior to beginning the study phase participants were informed that they would be asked to attempt to recognize the melodies in a later recognition test. Following the study phase participants were asked either to describe the last melody they had heard (the description condition) or to engage in a no description task (no description condition).

In the description condition, participants were given 5 minutes in which to provide a detailed description of the last melody they had heard. To help them formulate a description they were provided with a list of possible melodic features that could be used to describe the stimulus. These were; rhythm (beat); pitch; mode (feeling of the piece); key; and tempo (speed). The following instructions were provided: 'Please try to describe as fully as possible the last excerpt of music you heard. You have been provided with a list of possible melodic features you could use to describe it, but you do not have to use them all. Please try to be as complete as possible in your account and use the entire 5 minutes provided for your description'. In the no description condition, participants were provided with a filler activity: a random number was presented by the experimenter and participants were given 30 seconds in which to count backwards from this number in threes. At the end of the 30 seconds the experimenter provided a new number. In all 10 numbers were presented and the total time of the filler activity was 5 minutes.

Immediately following the experimental manipulation participants undertook the music recognition task. This involved the presentation of 24 musical segments, including 12 target (old) items and 12 distracter (new) items. Participants were informed that they would hear a series of musical segments and that following each segment they must indicate, as quickly and accurately as possible, whether they had heard the melody in the previous study phase (old) or whether it was new (new). Participants made their recognition decision by pressing one of two keys on the computer keyboard. Following the completion of the recognition test, participants immediately began the second part of the experiment. They were informed that they would hear a completely new set of musical segments and that the task between the study phase and recognition phase in the second part of the experiment would be different.

Data Analysis. Analyses of accuracy were carried out to assess whether expertise or verbalization influenced discrimination (d') or response-bias (C). Statistical analyses of discrimination and response bias were calculated following the prescriptions set out by Snodgrass and Corwin (1988). That is difficulties arise for the signal detection theory model at hit and false alarm rates of 1 or 0, therefore we transformed accuracy data by adding 0.5 to each frequency and dividing by N+1 (where N is the number of old or new items in the recognition test). Note, there were no significant results for the response-bias measure and so they are not reported.

A 2 x 2 x 2 mixed design analyses of variance (ANOVA) was carried out on the discrimination data with verbalisation (description vs. no description) as a within-participants factor, and expertise (musician vs. non-musician) and condition order (description condition first vs. description condition second) as between-participants factors. Main effects or interactions that failed to reach significance at a level of $p=0.05$, are not reported. Follow-up post-hoc tests (Bonferroni's t, $p <. 025$) were carried out on significant interactions. Table 1 shows discrimination, hits and false alarms as a function of expertise, description and condition order.

We also present post hoc analyses of description quality. Here, we examined the proportion of accurate musical descriptors produced by musicians and non-musicians, respectively.

Results

Discrimination (d'). There was a significant main effect of expertise, $F(1,28) = 9.29$, $p < 0.01$, with musicians showing overall better recognition performance than non-musicians. There was also a significant verbalisation x condition order interaction, $F(1,28) = 5.15$, $p < .03$.

Table 1. Means (standard deviations in brackets) for discrimination, hits and false alarms as a function of description, musical expertise and condition order

		Description	No Description
Description First			
Musicians	d'	1.44 (.60)	1.41 (.66)
	Hits	.74 (.11)	.71 (.08)
	FA	.25 (.15)	.23 (.17)
Non-Musicians			
	d'	.89 (.77)	.57 (.65)
	Hits	.66 (.15)	.61 (.16)
	FA	.35 (.19)	.41 (.18)
Description Second			
Musicians	d'	.97 (.35)	1.17 (.61)
	Hits	.68 (.07)	.66 (.13)
	FA	.32 (.09)	.26 (.17)
Non-Musicians			
	d'	.50 (.40)	.89 (.45)
	Hits	.59 (.08)	.63 (.10)
	FA	.40 (.09)	.30 (.08)

Note: For d' larger values indicate a greater ability to discriminate between old and new items.

Post-hoc comparisons revealed that when participants undertook the description condition as the second experimental block, discrimination was significantly poorer in the description than no description condition (a no description – description d' difference of .30, t (15) = –2.84, p =0.01). When participants undertook the description condition as the first experimental block, there was no significant difference between the description and no description condition (a no description – description d' difference of -.18, t (15) = 0.99, p=ns). Note, there was no verbalisation x expertise x condition order interaction, F(1,28) = 1.40, p =ns.

Description quality. To assess whether musical expertise influenced the quality of participants descriptions, descriptions were examined for the proportion of correct and incorrect music descriptors. We divided the music descriptors into technical descriptors (i.e., descriptors demonstrating musical knowledge, such as key, time signature) and non-technical descriptors (i.e., descriptors not requiring musical knowledge, such as identifying the instrument, quick or slow etc). Separate measures of description accuracy were calculated for technical and non-technical descriptors by dividing the number of correct descriptors in each category by the sum of all correct and incorrect descriptors. Subjective descriptors were those which could not be coded as correct or incorrect (e.g, judgements about the emotion of the musical segment).

The mean total number of descriptors (i.e., correct, incorrect and subjective) generated by musicians and non-musicians was 5.44 (SD = 2.03) and 4.94 (SD = 1.69) descriptors, respectively. Musicians generated overall more accurate technical music descriptors than non-musicians, $t(30) = 2.37$, $p < .05$. The mean proportion of accurate technical music descriptors was .43 (SD = .24) for musicians and .19 (SD = .30) for non-musicians. In contrast, non-musicians generated more accurate non-technical music descriptors than musicians, $t(30) = -3.58$, $p = .001$. The mean proportion of accurate non-technical music descriptors was .60 (SD = .27) for non-musicians and .29 (SD = .20) for musicians.

We also examined whether there was a correlation between participants' description quality (i.e., mean proportion of accurate technical or non-technical descriptors or total number of descriptors) and recognition performance. For musicians, the mean proportion of accurate non-technical descriptors was positively correlated with discrimination performance ($r = .56$, $p < .05$). For non-musicians no aspect of description quality was correlated with discrimination performance.

CONCLUSION

The present experiment has shown that verbal overshadowing occurs for the recognition of multiple musical segments following a single musical segment description. In this respect, we have extended the findings of Brown and Lloyd-Jones (2002, 2003) beyond the domain of face recognition to a new perceptual domain, namely auditory memory for musical segments. In addition, we found that verbal overshadowing influenced auditory discrimination in the same way for both musicians and non-musicians. This was despite overall better recognition performance and more accurate technical descriptions by musicians than non-musicians.

As was the case with Brown and Lloyd-Jones (2002, 2003; see also Lloyd-Jones and Brown, 2008) there is a caveat to these findings. Verbal overshadowing was only evident when the verbal description followed the control task. Therefore, a concern is that the effects on performance observed here are not the result of verbal overshadowing. Instead, they may reflect a general decline in performance in the second compared to first experimental block due to a build-up of proactive and retroactive interference arising with exposure to an increasing number of stimuli over time (e.g., Davies, Shepherd and Ellis, 1979; Deffenbacher, Carr and Leu, 1981). However, if the effects observed here were due solely to a build-up of such interference then performance should have been statistically significantly poorer in the control condition when it followed the verbal description. This was not the case. We found no significant difference in performance between the description condition presented first (d' = 1.17) and the no description condition presented second (d' = .99). In addition, we would have expected better performance in both the description and control conditions when they were presented first compared to second. This was also not the case. We found no significant difference in performance between the no description condition presented first (d' = 1.03) and second (d' = .99, $t(30) = .18$, p = ns) or between the description condition presented first (d' = 1.17) and second (d' = .74, $t(30) = 2.04$, p = ns).

Nevertheless, we do note that for the non-musician group in particular, when the description condition was presented first, discrimination was substantially poorer for the no description condition as compared to the description condition (d' values of .57 and .89, for no description and description conditions, respectively). However, this result may be spurious given both the large variability among scores in the description condition (a standard deviation of .77, with d' scores ranging from 1.81 to -.62; note the negative d' value reflects the fact that this particular participant's false alarm rate exceeded their hit rate; see Wickens, 2002, p.80, for further discussion) and the fact that musical expertise did not significantly contribute to our interpretation of the effects of description upon recognition memory (i.e., there was no three-way interaction between verbalisation, expertise and condition order variables)

Verbal overshadowing is a fragile phenomenon and there are a number of studies which have failed to replicate the effect (Davies and Thasen, 2000; Yu and Geiselman, 1993). There may be critical boundary conditions necessary for obtaining the effect. One critical determinant of verbal overshadowing appears to be the nature of the description (e.g., Meissner and Brigham, 2001). Brown and Lloyd-Jones (2002) found that directing participants to consider particular facial features (such as the eyes, nose, ears, and so on) elicited verbal overshadowing, whereas instructions which encouraged the recall of more global aspects of the face (e.g., attributions about personality) did not. Effects of verbal overshadowing have also been found to be alleviated under some conditions. Interestingly, Finger (2002) found that listening to instrumental music following the act of describing a face, but prior to undertaking the face recognition task produced a release from verbal overshadowing. This finding indicates that reinstating perceptual/non-verbal processing operations can allow the negative effects of verbalisation upon memory to be overcome. Indeed, verbal overshadowing is often found to attenuate over study and recognition test trials (e.g., Fallshore and Schooler, 1995; Melcher and Schooler, 1996) and it has been suggested that across trials participants become practiced at switching between verbal and non-verbal processing (Schooler, Fiore, and Brandimonte, 1997). Brown and Lloyd-Jones (2002, 2003, see also Lloyd-Jones and Brown, 2008) have similarly proposed that within their multiple stimuli presentation paradigm carry-over effects from the description onto the control condition attenuate the observation of verbal interference when the description condition is undertaken as the first block.

Let us now interpret the verbal interference observed here more fully. In the present experiment describing a single musical segment interfered with the recognition of multiple, but previously non-described, musical segments. This is consistent with an account of verbal overshadowing which involves a shift in 'processing style' rather than an over-reliance upon a verbal representation specific to the described stimulus (Brown and Lloyd-Jones, 2002, 2003, Lloyd-Jones and Brown, 2008; for a recent review, see Schooler, 2002). Previous research has found global music processing, that is extracting information about the overall temporal shape and contour of a melody rather than the properties of its individual notes or intervals, to be beneficial for melody discrimination (e.g., Schulkind et al., 2003). Thus, we propose that the processing of global properties of the musical segments would have been beneficial to recognition in the present paradigm given that participants were required to differentiate between large numbers of highly similar musical segments. However, providing a description invoked a general shift towards greater verbal/local processing at the expense of more beneficial perceptual/global processing. In turn, this led to less efficient music recognition.

Verbal overshadowing influenced the performance of non-musicians and musicians in the same way. Previously, we had predicted that verbal overshadowing would be less apparent for musicians as, unlike non-musicians, they possess both perceptual and verbal musical expertise. Consistent with this assumption, musicians exhibited better recognition overall and they also provided more accurate technical detail about the musical segment as compared to non-musicians. In addition, unlike non-musicians, musicians exhibited a relationship between description quality and recognition performance; those musicians providing more accurate non-technical descriptors were more likely to recognise the music later on. This suggests that musicians at recognition may have been relying to some extent upon a verbal representation of the previously heard musical stimuli. However, access to an accurate verbal description did not protect participants against effects of verbal overshadowing. Nevertheless, we cannot rule out the possibility that not all the musicians tested here held sufficient verbal expertise to protect against the detrimental effects of verbalisation (e.g. Bigand and Poulin-Charronnat, 2006).

The findings observed here suggest that global processing in musical perception may be of central importance for both experts and non-experts. Indeed, some researchers have argued that music perception is based on a hierarchical system with right-hemisphere global processing preceding any local analysis undertaken by a left-hemisphere sub-system (e.g., Schuppert et al., 2000). Consistent with this notion, Schiavetto et al. (1999) have reported a pattern of reaction time data and ERP activity whereby global changes in melody are detected at an earlier perceptual stage than local changes. They presented participants with a standard melody followed by repetitions of the same melody or a changed version. The changed versions deviated from the standard in terms of a single note which either violated the global contour of the melody (i.e., reversed pitch direction) or violated a local property of the melody (i.e., changed the interval between two notes whilst maintaining the global pitch direction). The participants' task was to indicate when they detected a change in the standard melody. The detection of global as compared to local violations was associated with faster reaction times and a larger early N2 deflection which has previously been associated with the processing of mismatches between stimuli (Näätänen, 1992). These findings have been interpreted as indicating a global precedence effect for melody perception.

In conclusion, the present findings have shown that verbal overshadowing can occur within an auditory domain, in particular the domain of music recognition. The findings are consistent with an account in which verbalisation induces the application of a processing style which is not optimal for music recognition. Global and local auditory processing has been implicated in musical perception and we propose therefore that verbalization can induce a shift from global to local auditory processing. The vulnerability of both musicians and non-musicians to verbal overshadowing in the present paradigm is consistent with accounts of music perception which propose that global processing is a necessary and perhaps automatic aspect of music perception (e.g., Schuppert et al., 2000).

REFERENCES

Bever, T. G. and Chiarello, R. J. (1974). Cerebral dominance in musicians and nonmusicians. *Science, 185*, 537-539.

Bigand, E., and Poulin-Charronnat, B. (2006). Are we "experienced listeners"? A review of the musical capacities that do not depend on formal musical training. *Cognition, 100*, 100-130.

Brandler, S., and Rammsayer, T. H. (2003). Differences in mental abilities between musicians and non-musicians. *Psychology of Music, 31*(2), 123-138.

Brown, C., and Lloyd-Jones, T. J. (2002). Verbal overshadowing in a multiple face presentation paradigm: Effects of description instruction. *Applied Cognitive Psychology, 16*, 873-885.

Brown, C., and Lloyd-Jones, T. J. (2003). Verbal overshadowing of multiple face and car recognition: Effects of within- versus across- category verbal descriptions. *Applied Cognitive Psychology, 17*, 183-201.

Chan, A. S., Ho, Y.-C., and Cheung, M. C. (1998). Music training improves verbal memory. *Nature, 396*(6707), 128.

Davies, G., Shepherd, J., and Ellis, H. (1979). Effects of interpolated mugshot exposure on accuracy of eyewitness identification. *Journal of Applied Psychology, 64*, 96-101.

Davies, G., and Thasen, S. (2000). Closed-circuit television: How effective an identification aid? *British Journal of Psychology, 91*, 411-426.

Deffenbacher, K. A., Carr, T. H., and Leu, J. R. (1981). Memory for words, pictures and faces: Retroactive interference, forgetting and reminiscence. *Journal of Experimental Psychology: Human Learning and Memory, 7*, 299-305.

Dodson, C. S., Johnson, M. K., and Schooler, J. W. (1997). The verbal overshadowing effect: Why descriptions impair face recognition. *Memory and Cognition, 25*, 129-139

Drake, C., and Palmer, C. (2000). Skill acquisition in music performance: Relations between planning and temporal control. *Cognition, 74*, 1-32.

Ellis, H. D., Shepard, J. W., and Davies, G. M. (1980). The deterioration of verbal descriptions of faces over different delay intervals. *Journal of Police Science and Administration, 8*, 101-106.

Fallshore, M., and Schooler, J. W. (1995). The verbal vulnerability of perceptual expertise. *Journal of Experimental Psychology: Learning, Memory and Cognition, 21*, 1608-1623.

Finger, K. (2002). Mazes and music: Using perceptual processing to release verbal overshadowing. *Applied Cognitive Psychology, 16*, 887-896

Houser, T., Fiore, S. M., and Schooler, J. W. (1997). Verbal overshadowing of music memory: What happens when you describe that tune? Cited in Schooler, J. W., Fiore, S. M., and Brandimonte, M. A. (1997). At a loss from words: Verbal overshadowing of perceptual memories. In D. L. Medin (Ed.), *The psychology of learning and motivation* (pp. 291-340). San Diego, CA: Academic Press.

Lloyd-Jones, T. J., and Brown, C. (2008). Verbal overshadowing of multiple face recognition: Effects on remembering and knowing over time. *The European Journal of Cognitive Psychology, 20,* 456-477.

Macmillan, N. A., and Creelman, C. D. (2005). *Detection Theory: A User's Guide (2nd edition).* Mahwah, NJ: Erlbaum

Meissner, C. A., and Brigham, J. C. (2001). A meta-analysis of the verbal overshadowing effect in face identification. *Applied Cognitive Psychology, 15*, 603-616.

Meissner, C. A., Brigham, J. C., and Kelley, C. M. (2001). The influence of retrieval processes in verbal overshadowing. *Memory and Cognition, 29*, 176-186.

Melcher, J. M., and Schooler, J. W. (2004). Perceptual and conceptual training mediate verbal overshadowing effect in an unfamiliar domain. *Memory and Cognition, 32*(4), 618-631.

Melcher, J. M., and Schooler, J. W. (1996). The misremembrance of wines past: Verbal and perceptual expertise differentially mediate verbal overshadowing of taste memory. *Journal of Memory and Language, 35*, 231-245.

Mikumo, M. (1997). Multi-encoding for pitch information of tone sequences. *Japanese Psychological Research, 39*(4), 300-311.

Morris, R. G., Abrahams, S., and Polkey, C. E. (1995). Recognition memory for words and faces following unilateral temporal lobectomy. *British Journal of Clinical Psychology, 34*(4), 571-576.

Näätänen, R. (1992). *Attention and Brain Function*. Hillsdale, NJ: Erlbaum

Palmer, C., and Meyer, R. K. (2000). Conceptual and motor learning in music performance. *Psychological Science, 11*, 63-68.

Peretz, I. (1990). Processing of local and global musical information by unilateral brain-damaged patients. *Brain, 113*, 1185-1205.

Peretz, I., and Babai, M. (1992). The role of contour and intervals in the recognition of melody parts: Evidence from cerebral asymmetries in musicians. *Neuropsychologia, 30*, 277-292.

Peretz, I., and Morais, J. (1987). Analytic processing in the classification of melodies as same or different. *Neuropsychologia, 25*, 645-652.

Perfect, T. J., Hunt, L. J., and Harris, C. M. (2002). Verbal overshadowing in voice recognition. *Applied Cognitive Psychology, 16*, 973-980.

Ryan, R., and Schooler, J. W. (1998). Whom do words hurt? Individual differences in susceptibility to verbal overshadowing. *Applied Cognitive Psychology, 12*, 105-125.

Sanders, L. D., and Poeppel, D. (2007). Local and global auditory processing: Behavioral and ERP evidence. *Neuropsychologia, 45*, 1172-1186.

Schiavetto, A., Cortese, F., and Alain, C. (1999). Global and local processing of musical sequences: An event-related brain potential study. *NeuroReport, 10*, 2467-2472.

Schooler, J. W. (2002). Verbalization produces a transfer inappropriate processing shift. *Applied Cognitive Psychology, 16*, 989-997.

Schooler, J. W., and Engstler-Schooler, T. Y. (1990). Verbal overshadowing of visual memories: Some things are better left unsaid. *Cognitive Psychology, 22*, 36-71.

Schooler, J. W., Fiore, S. M., and Brandimonte, M. A. (1997). At a loss from words: Verbal overshadowing of perceptual memories. In D. L. Medin (Ed.), *The psychology of learning and motivation* (pp. 291-340). San Diego, CA: Academic Press.

Schooler, J. W., Ohlsson, S. and Brooks, K. (1993). Thoughts beyond words: When language overshadows insight. *Journal of Experimental Psychology: General, 122*, 166-183

Schulkind, M. D., Posner, R. J., and Rubin, D. C. (2003). Musical features that facilitate melody identification: How do you know it's "your" song when they finally play it? *Music Perception, 21*(2), 217-249.

Schuppert, M., Münte, T. F., Wieringa, B. M., and Altenmüller, E. (2000). Receptive amusia: Evidence for cross-hemispheric neural networks underlying music processing strategies. *Brain, 123*, 546-559.

Snodgrass, J. G., and Corwin, J. (1988). Pragmatics of measuring recognition memory: Applications to dementia and amnesia. *Journal of Experimental Psychology: General, 117*(1), 34-50.

Wickens, T. D. (2002). *Elementary Signal Detection Theory*. Oxford University Press.

Wilson, T. D., Lisle, D. J., Schooler, J. W., Hodges, S. D., Klaaren, K. J., and LaFleur, S. J. (1993). Introspecting about reasons can reduce post-choice satisfaction. *Personality and Social Psychology Bulletin, 19*, 331-339.

Wilson, T. D., and Schooler, J. W. (1991). Thinking too much: Introspection can reduce the quality of preferences and decisions. *Journal of Personality and Social Psychology, 60*, 181-192

Yu, C. J., and Geiselman, R. E. (1993). Effects of constructing identikit composites on photo-spread identification performance. *Criminal Justice and Behaviour, 20*, 280-292.

Zatorre, R. J., Evans, A. C., and Meyer, E. (1994). Neural mechanisms underlying melodic perception and memory for pitch. *Journal of Neuroscience, 14*(4), 1908-1919.

In: Applied Memory
Editor: Matthew R. Kelley

ISBN 978-1-60692-143-2

Chapter 4

THE ISOLATION EFFECT AND ADVERTISING: ARE UNUSUAL ADVERTISEMENTS REMEMBERED BETTER?

Tamra J. Bireta[1] and Brielle A. Simels
Department of Psychology ,The College of New Jersey, Ewing, NJ, USA

ABSTRACT

The isolation effect is the finding that memory is improved for items that are distinctive. The isolation effect has led advertisers to suggest that their advertisements should be designed to "stand out" from other advertisements. The current study examined semantic and physical isolation effects for print advertisements. Participants viewed a slideshow containing four advertisements for trashcans. Each advertisement contained a different brand name and feature for the trashcan pictured in the advertisement. In Experiment 1, one of the four advertisements included a product feature rated as highly distinctive (semantic isolate) relative to the product features appearing in the other advertisements. The isolated advertisement in Experiment 2 included a product feature of a different font size and color (physical isolate) than the product features appearing in the other advertisements. Participants were tested on the brand names and features from the advertisements. Unlike previous experiments on isolation effects in advertising, participants were required to remember which feature was presented with which brand. Participants demonstrated an isolation effect, with better recall of the features from the distinctive advertisements than the regular advertisements. This benefit, however, did not reliably extend to memory for the brand names associated with the isolate. These findings demonstrate that the robust nature of the isolation effect is not limited to laboratory settings; rather, the effect is more generalizable and occurs in real-world situations as well.

[1] Corresponding author.

INTRODUCTION

Imagine you are at a department store trying to select a vacuum cleaner. You scan across the various brands of vacuum cleaners and try to remember what you know about each of these brands. When you see the Dyson™ brand, will you remember "*Lightweight that doesn't lose suction*"™ as Dyson's™ claim for their vacuums? The goal of an advertiser is to present a product in such a way that consumers will either increase their general liking of the brand or will remember some specific feature about the brand's product. People are bombarded with numerous advertisements for a countless number of products. Exposure to these numerous advertisements come from a variety of media, including television, radio, billboards, and more. Some research estimates suggest that people are exposed to as many as 2,500 advertising messages per day (Craig, Sternthal, & Leavitt, 1976; Phillips & Rasberry, 2005). Given that it is nearly impossible to remember all of the information presented within every advertisement, what can an advertiser do to increase the likelihood that a consumer will remember information from a particular advertisement?

One potential answer to this question may lie in a memory phenomenon known as the isolation effect (also known as the von Restorff effect, after Hedwig von Restorff, 1933). The isolation effect is the finding that when one item is made unique or distinct from its surrounding context, memory for the distinctive item is improved. Typically, memory for the distinctive item is compared to a control item that is consistent with the background items. The isolation effect has been used as "the generic label for the effects of distinctiveness on memory" (Hunt, 1995, p. 105; see also Schmidt, 1991). The purpose of the current study was to examine isolation effects for a more realistic situation involving memory for print advertisements. Several advertisements containing multiple brands and features of a product were presented to participants. One of the advertisements contained a unique feature. A subsequent memory test examined whether participants were more likely to recall the distinct feature and whether that benefit would extend to the associated brands.

THE ISOLATION EFFECT

In von Restorff's first experiments (described in Hunt, 1995), she tested recall of paired-associate lists of nonsense words (e.g., dok - pir), symbols (# - +), numbers (89 – 46), colored shapes (red square – green square), and letters (S – B). Four of the pairs were from the same type of items (e.g., nonsense syllables; homogenous), and the other four pairs were one of each of the other types of items (isolated). She found that recall was better for the isolated pairs compared to the homogenous pairs. In a recognition experiment, she presented lists that contained one isolate in the middle of a list (19 syllables and 1 number or 19 numbers and 1 syllable). With this manipulation there was even higher recall for the isolate.

Numerous studies have demonstrated the robustness of the isolation effect using various stimuli and methodologies, and the effect is reliably obtained for younger adults (for a review, see Hunt, 1995) and children (e.g., Cimbalo, Nowak, & Soderstrom, 1981; Howe, Courage, Vernescu, & Hunt, 2000; Rabinowitz & Andrews, 1973; Winters & Hoats, 1989). Research on isolation effects with older adults is quite limited, with one study demonstrating clear isolation effects for older adults (Bireta, Surprenant, & Neath, 2008) and another failing to obtain isolation effects for older adults (Cimbalo & Brink, 1982). The isolation effect has been reliably demonstrated using lists of words, geometric forms, and line drawings (e.g., Pick, Sweeny & Clay, 1991; Harcum, 1968; Karis, Fabiani, & Domchin, 1984). Isolation effects can be achieved with both physical (e.g., size, color, or font type) and semantic (e.g., meaningfulness or category) manipulations. The size of the isolation effect depends upon several factors. One factor is the manner in which the isolate differs from the other items in a list. Large isolation effects are obtained using size, color, and spacing manipulations, and isolation effects increase in magnitude as the difference between the isolate and the surrounding context increases (Gardner, 1983; Gumenik & Levitt, 1968; Hunt, 1995). Isolation effects have also been studied in paired-associate paradigms, in which one item (the "stimulus") is used as a cue for recall of a second item (the "response"). In this paradigm, isolation effects are defined as faster learning of the pair with the isolated item compared to the other pairs without the isolated item. Such effects have been obtained when either the stimulus or the response is isolated (e.g., Huang & Fleming, 1976; Nachmias, Gleitman, & McKenna, 1961).

Several theories have been proposed to account for the isolation effect. The traditional explanation, originally proposed by Jenkins and Postman (1948), is that the perceptual salience of the distinctive item attracts additional attention or processing (for a review, see Hunt & Lamb, 2001). The items that precede the isolate establish a context, such as the size of the list items, and the distinctive item becomes salient because it deviates from the established context. The mechanism by which the additional attention aids memory is not clear. Rundus (1971) proposed that the additional attention aids memory through differential rehearsal; the isolate is remembered better because it is rehearsed more than other items. Two lines of data have argued against the differential attention view (for a more thorough discussion, see Dunlosky, Hunt, & Clark, 2000). First, increased processing of the isolate should reduce processing of the immediately surrounding items, resulting in impaired memory for those surrounding items. Memory impairment for the surrounding items is found in some studies (e.g., Hunt & Mitchell, 1982), but not in others (e.g., Bruce & Gaines, 1976; Fabiani & Donchin, 1995; Schmidt, 1985). Second, isolation effects are obtained when the isolate is placed first in the list (e.g., Bellezza & Cheney, 1973; Kelley & Nairne, 2001; Pillsbury & Rausch, 1943). In such instances, the isolate should not receive differential attention since no context has been established.

A more promising explanation of the isolation effect focuses on processing at retrieval, rather than only processing at encoding. One possibility is that the processing during encoding results in the isolate and the other items being placed in different categories (e.g., Hunt & Lamb, 2001). At recall, the isolate is the only item in its category, compared to the several items that are in the alternative category. This results in better recall for the isolate. Nairne (2006; Kelley & Nairne, 2001) proposes a different retrieval-based explanation of the isolation effect using his feature model of immediate memory (Nairne, 1990). According to this model, processing of the items results in residual traces in primary memory. These traces are used as cues to retrieve items from secondary memory. Memory performance is a function of how well the cues can access the appropriate target. This depends upon two factors: (1) the match between the current retrieval cue and the target trace, and (2) the match between the cue and the remaining members of the set (Nairne, 2006). In a list containing a distinctive item, the residual trace in primary memory will contain features unique to the isolated item. Therefore, at retrieval, the cues used to retrieve items from secondary memory will uniquely match the isolate, and the isolate will significantly differ from the other items in the list. This results in improved memory performance for the isolate relative to the other items in the list.

There are real-world phenomena that may be related to the isolation effect. First, individuals are more likely to remember a person's face if it is very different from the faces with which they are familiar. Studies have found that when a face is rated as highly distinctive, it is better recognized than faces that are more typical (e.g., Going & Read, 1974; Hosie & Milne, 1995). Interestingly, a face will also be recognized better if it differs from the other faces in the set, even if the isolated face is only rated as distinctive within the context of the set (rather than relative to all of the faces with which a person is familiar; e.g., Cohen & Carr, 1975). Santos and Young (2005) found that a person's face is better remembered if it differs from the others by age, gender, or perceived intelligence. Main, Leland, and Bartlett (1998) altered photographs of faces by placing a dot on some of the faces, and found that this dot later facilitated recognition (even when the dot was not on the face during the testing phase). This suggests that having a noticeable facial blemish when you meet people could be seen as an asset in that your new acquaintances will be more likely to remember your face!

The isolation effect may also be related to the memory phenomenon known as the reminiscence bump; middle-aged and older adult participants recall more memories from their youth (ages 10 to 30) than would be predicted by memory retention functions (e.g., Rubin, Wetzler, & Nebes, 1986). This phenomenon occurs using numerous methodologies, including asking participants to recall autobiographical memories in response to cue words or to recall their most important memories (e.g., Rubin & Schulkind, 1997). Rubin, Rahhal, and Poon (1998) have used a distinctiveness account to explain such findings. According to this explanation, many unique events occur during youth (e.g., graduation, getting married, or the birth of a child) followed by increased stability in adulthood. At recall, these distinctive events of youth are better recalled than the more ordinary events of middle adulthood. This view has been supported by findings of another reminiscence bump for individuals who experience significant life changes in middle adulthood (e.g., Conway & Haque, 1999).

The isolation effect may also be applicable in educational settings. The materials that are given to students could be designed to take advantage of this effect. For example, keywords on printed materials could have altered fonts (e.g., bolded or differing in color) to make them more distinctive. Important concepts could be placed in a different location than the other material, such as in a box next to the text, or they could be supplemented by unique illustrations. An examination of textbooks reveals that authors often use these techniques. Such methods could also be applied to materials prepared by lecturers, including PowerPoint™ presentations and handouts.

The Isolation Effect in Advertising

Intuitively speaking, advertisers may be able to take advantage of the memory benefit for isolated items by making their advertisements unique. According to Kessler (1985), distinctive advertising should be more memorable and, further, more effective. Lynch & Srull (1982) state that information that is unexpected and visually separated from the rest of the design elements in an advertisement not only captures more attention and is processed more extensively, but it is also better recalled than expected information. For example, if an advertisement for a Dyson™ brand vacuum contained an atypical or visually distinctive object or statement, a consumer's attention might be captured by the unexpected information, and therefore the consumer's recall for the unexpected information would be higher. Surprisingly, only two studies have examined the isolation effect in direct relation to advertising.

Gardner (1983) investigated the effects of attribute prominence on recall. Gardner designed two versions of a print advertisement for a single product. The advertisements contained "Brand R" in the heading and discussed four attributes within the copy. Physical attribute prominence (distinctiveness) was manipulated by displaying the target attribute, *Special Nylon Stitching*, in the headline and in a cartoon-type bubble in the middle of one of the advertisements. The non-distinctive version included the *Special Nylon Stitching* attribute in the copy, along with the other three attributes, but it was not displayed in the heading or in the cartoon-type bubble. Participants viewed one of the two versions of the advertisements. After viewing the advertisement, participants were asked to list the product characteristics that came to mind when they thought of the advertised brand. Gardner found that mean proportion recall of the target attribute was significantly higher for participants who viewed the distinctive version (0.78) compared to the non-distinctive version (0.55). Gardner also discussed how this type of manipulation could be used to divert attention from another component of the advertisement. Specifically, an advertiser may be able to make a desirable attribute more prominent, thus reducing attention and memory for less desirable information, such as the warning message in a cigarette advertisement. In Gardner's study, participants recalled fewer ordinary attributes after viewing the distinctive version (2.17) compared to the non-distinctive version (2.51) of the advertisement. Such findings support Gardner's speculation.

Isolation effects also have been obtained for advertising slogans. Pick, Sweeney and Clay (1991) created eleven advertising slogans for Heineken beer. They considered two of the eleven slogans to be distinctive and the remaining nine to be mundane. The distinctive slogans were *Heineken. The beer that made Milwaukee jealous* and *Heineken. Ya hoo, that's some brew*. An example of a slogan considered ordinary was *Heineken has great taste*. Participants viewed either a list of the nine ordinary slogans, or a list in which a middle slogan was replaced with one of the two distinctive slogans. Participants were asked to rate the slogans for distinctiveness on a four-point scale. After the rating task, participants completed a distractor task and were then given a surprise recall test. The slogans considered distinctive were rated highly on distinctiveness (3.3 to 3.5), as was another slogan, *Heineken. You'll like what we imported for you*. These highly distinctive slogans were recalled well, with means of 45 to 85 percent. Slogans with low distinctiveness ratings (1.6 to 2.7) ranged from 7 to 53 percent recalled. The authors obtained a statistically significant positive correlation ($r = 0.53$) between the distinctiveness ratings and recall. The results of the study confirm that distinctiveness is an important variable in memory for advertising material.

Since the isolation effect has led advertisers to suggest that their advertisements should be designed to "stand out" from other advertisements, the primary purpose of this project is to examine whether the isolation effect occurs for memory of print advertisements. Although Pick et al. (1991) demonstrated that a unique slogan is remembered better than a less distinctive slogan, real-world situations typically involve a variety of features and brands. Thus, consumers must not only remember brand names and product information, but also which information is associated with which brand. Two experiments were conducted in which participants viewed a series of four print advertisements for trashcans and were then tested on either their memory for the brands or their memory for the features. The test for brand recall is equivalent to the real-life situation in which one remembers that there is a product that has a certain feature, such as a vacuum that does not lose suction, and recall involves remembering the brand name that is associated with this particular feature. The test for feature recall is analogous to a situation in which one is viewing a series of brand names for a given product and needs to recall the features that are associated with a particular brand. The isolate was either an unusual feature (known as a semantic isolate, Experiment 1) or a feature that was visually distinct (known as a physical isolate, Experiment 2). The semantic isolate was a product feature ("remote controlled") that was rated in a pretest as being highly distinctive for a trashcan. The physical isolate was distinctive in that it was presented in a font that differed from the features in the other three advertisements.

Based upon previous research on the isolation effect (e.g., Hunt, 1995), we predicted that the isolated feature would be better recalled than the other features. Because the isolation effect is very robust in laboratory studies, we predicted that the recall benefit for the isolate would be obtained even with the requirement of recalling the feature with the correct brand. A different type of isolation effect may occur as well; the brand name that is paired with the isolate may also be recalled better in the brand recall test due to its association with the unique feature. However, it is unclear whether the improved memory for the isolated feature will result in higher recall of the brand name, as participants are not explicitly told to form associations between the brands and features (as they are instructed in paired associate learning). Existing studies on the isolation effect have not examined whether the isolation effect extends to information that is indirectly associated with the isolate. With two experiments in the current study examining two different isolation manipulations (semantic and physical), it becomes possible to compare the size of the two effects within the context of advertising. The physical manipulation should result in a larger isolation effect than the semantic manipulation, as this is the typical finding in laboratory research (e.g., Hunt, 1995).

EXPERIMENT 1

Method

Participants. Participants were 70 undergraduates from The College of New Jersey who participated in order to partially fulfill a psychology course requirement or for extra credit in a psychology course.

Materials. Participants viewed one of four slideshows using Microsoft PowerPoint™. Each slideshow consisted of four advertisements for trashcans (for an example, see Figure 1). The backdrop photographs for the advertisements were identical, with the only difference amongst the various advertisements being a slightly different trashcan photograph inserted along with the invented brand names and features. One of the four advertisements in each slideshow contained the feature that was rated as highly distinctive (*Remote Controlled: Never Take Out Your Trash Again*), and the other three advertisements contained the features that were rated to be less distinctive *(Foot Pedal: Makes for an Easy Open Lid; Lock Wheels: Keep Your Trash From Rolling;* and *Attached Lid: Won't Blow Away in the Wind*; see Table

1). Undergraduates, who did not participate in the main experiment, rated the distinctiveness of each brand name (n=36) and feature (n=21). The distinctiveness of each brand and feature was evaluated using a Likert scale, with 1 representing "not unique" and 5 representing "very unique." The semantic isolate was rated as highly distinctive (M = 4.43 out of 5) relative to the other features. A series of t-tests confirmed that the rating for the isolate was significantly higher than that for the *attached lid* (M = 2.48, t(20) = 5.12, $p < 0.05$), *foot pedal* (M = 2.81, t(20) = 6.93, $p < 0.05$), and *lock wheels* (M = 3.14, t(20) = 4.37, $p < 0.05$) features (see Tables 1 and 2). The created brand names for the trash advertisements were all rated similarly for distinctiveness: Rhino (M = 2.64), Canman (M = 2.78), Trashsense (M = 3.03), and Bauhaus (M = 3.06).

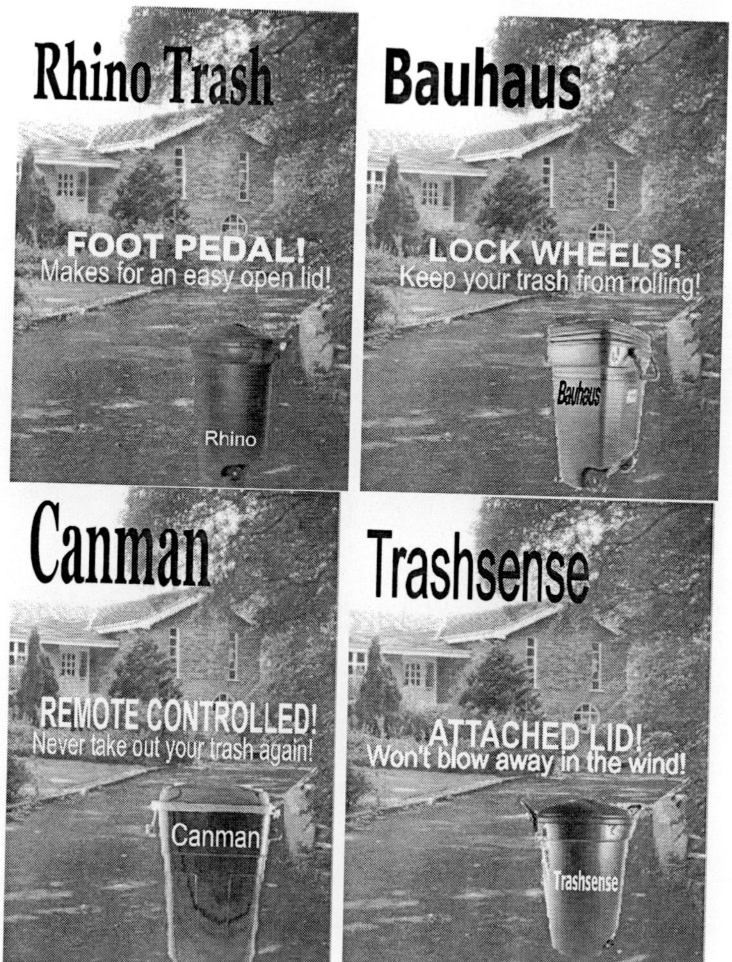

Figure 1. Sample stimuli from Experiment 1 containing the semantic isolate.

Each slideshow contained four advertisements, with the particular position (first advertisement, second advertisement, etc.) of each brand name and feature varying, with the constraint that the isolate occurred in all four positions across the four versions. This was done to reduce any confounds from primacy and recency effects. The particular brand name and feature pairings varied so that a particular feature did not consistently appear with a particular brand. As some brand names were rated marginally higher in their distinctiveness than others, the various versions of the advertisements contained different brand and feature pairings in order to prevent any brand recall advantage. The response sheets consisted of two versions: one version listing the brand names and participants were asked to recall the appropriate product features; and another version listing the product features and participants were asked to recall the appropriate brand names.

Design and Procedure. Participants first were instructed to sign in and read and sign a consent form. Participants were told that they were going to view a short PowerPoint™ slideshow containing advertisements and that after viewing the slideshow, they would be asked some questions. They then were presented with a series of four advertisements displayed for 20 seconds each, with the onset of the next advertisement immediately following the offset of the previous advertisement. Each participant saw one of the four versions of the slideshows. Immediately following the slideshow, participants were given either the feature or brand response sheet. Participants were told that they should try to recall the brand name with the feature it was originally paired with (or vice versa) and that they could guess if they were unsure. Recall was not timed. Participants were tested one at a time, and the experimenter remained in the room to ensure compliance with the instructions.

Results and Discussion

Memory for Features. A response for feature recall was scored as correct if the main meaning was retained (e.g., e.g., "trashcan won't roll" instead of *lock wheels: keep your trash from rolling* would be scored as correct) and the feature was written with the correct brand. As expected, recall of the isolate was very high (M = 0.83; see Table 1). In the subsequent analyses, alpha was set at 0.05. A series of t-tests confirmed that the recall for the isolate (*remote controlled*) was significantly higher than that for the *attached lid* (M = 0.67, t(35) = 2.24), *foot pedal* (M = 0.61, t(35) = 2.47) and *lock wheels* (M = 0.58, t(35) = 3.00) features. Thus, the semantic manipulation resulted in a clear isolation effect using print advertisements.

Memory for Brands. A response for the brand was scored as correct if the correct brand was recalled (correct spelling was not required) and the brand was written with the correct feature. The brand paired with the isolate (which varied across different versions) was not better recalled the brands paired with the other features (see Table 1). A series of t-tests confirmed that recall of the brand paired with the isolate (M = 0.65) was not significantly higher that of the brand paired with *attached lid* (M = 0.68, t(33) = -0.30), *foot pedal* (M = 0.62, t(33) = 0.33), or *lock wheels* (M = 0.59, t(33) = 0.57) features. Therefore, the benefit of the isolate appears to be limited to recall of the unique feature and does not extend to memory for the brand. This does not appear to be due to ceiling or floor effects, as performance ranged from a mean proportion recall of 0.59 to 0.68. Interestingly, recall levels for the brand names was very similar to recall levels for the features (range of 0.58 to 0.67 for the non-isolates). The lack of an isolation effect for the brand names also does not appear to be due to a lack of power, as the brand associated with the *attached lid* feature was recalled slightly better than the brand associated with the isolate.

The results of Experiment 1 are consistent with previous studies of the isolation effect in finding that distinctive advertisements are better recalled than non-distinctive advertisements. However, the benefit is limited to recall of the isolated features and does not extend to recall of the brands. This suggests that the brand name of a product serves as a sufficient cue to find improved recall of a distinctive feature, but that memory of a distinctive feature is not sufficient for better memory of the brand name. There is no evidence, therefore, that information indirectly associated with an isolate is afforded any recall advantage. Thus, creating a very unique and memorable feature does not appear to be a sufficient advertising strategy for creating high recall of a brand.

Table 1. Mean proportion recall of features and corresponding brands and distinctiveness ratings of features in Experiment 1

Feature	Mean Recall		Distinctiveness Rating
	Feature	Brand	
Remote Controlled: Never Take Out Your Trash Again (Semantic Isolate)	0.83	0.65	4.43
Foot Pedal: Makes for an Easy Open Lid	0.61	0.62	2.81
Lock Wheels: Keep Your Trash From Rolling	0.58	0.59	3.14
Attached Lid: Won't Blow Away in the Wind	0.67	0.68	2.48

EXPERIMENT 2

Experiment 1 was successful in obtaining a semantic isolation effect for a realistic advertising situation in which participants viewed multiple advertisements with varying brand names and features. The results of Experiment 1 also suggested that isolation effects do not extend to information associated with the isolate. Both types of isolation effects (improved memory for the feature and improved memory for the associated brand) might occur if a different type of distinctiveness manipulation was used. Laboratory studies typically find that physical isolation effects are larger than semantic isolation effects. A physical manipulation of distinctiveness might, then, also result in an isolation effect for the associated brand. To that end, there were three purposes of Experiment 2: to determine if a physical isolation effect would be obtained with print advertisements, if the effect would be larger than the semantic isolation effect obtained in Experiment 1, and if an isolation effect would be obtained for the associated brand.

Method

Participants. Participants were 122 undergraduates from The College of New Jersey who participated in order to partially fulfill a psychology course requirement or for extra credit in a psychology course. None of the participants had previously participated in Experiment 1.

Materials. The materials were identical to Experiment 1, with one exception; the isolated feature was physically different from the other advertisements, rather than semantically different (see Figure 2). The isolate (*Stronger Material: Means Less Dents*) was rated similarly in distinctiveness to the other items by the same raters used for Experiment 1.

A series of t-tests confirmed that the distinctiveness rating for this feature ($M = 2.57$) was not significantly different than that for the *foot pedal* ($M = 2.81$, $t(20) = -0.83$, $p = 0.21$) or *attached lid* feature ($M = 2.48$, $t(20) = 0.31$, $p = 0.38$) and was slightly lower than that for the *lock wheels* feature ($M = 3.14$, $t(20) = -2.03$, $p < 0.05$; see Table 2). The isolate was made physically distinctive by displaying it in bolded, yellow print with a font size of 66. The features for the other three advertisements were all displayed in non-bolded, black print with a font of size 36. Due to the multitude of visual elements inherent in a color print advertisement, we varied the isolate on three dimensions (size, bolding, and color) to ensure that the physical difference would be easily detected.

Design and Procedure. The design and procedure were identical to Experiment 1.

Table 2. Mean proportion recall of features and corresponding brands and distinctiveness ratings of features in Experiment 2

Feature	Mean Recall		Distinctiveness Rating
	Feature	Brand	
Stronger Material: Means Less Dents (Physical Isolate)	0.88	0.62	2.57
Foot Pedal: Makes for an Easy Open Lid	0.72	0.69	2.81
Lock Wheels: Keep Your Trash From Rolling	0.75	0.72	3.14
Attached Lid: Won't Blow Away in the Wind	0.61	0.69	2.48

Results and Discussion

Memory for Feature. As expected, the physical isolate was better recalled than the other features (see Table 2). The same scoring criteria were used in Experiment 2 as Experiment 1. A series of t-tests confirmed that the recall for the isolate ($M = 0.88$) was significantly higher than that for the *attached lid* (M = 0.61, t(63) = 2.56), *foot pedal* (M = 0.72, t(63) = 3.07) and *lock wheels* (M = 0.75, t(63) = 2.05) features. Thus, Experiment 2 replicated the isolation effect for advertisement features, but with a physical, rather than a semantic, isolate.

In order to compare the size of the physical isolation effect in Experiment 2 with the semantic isolation effect in Experiment 1, recall of the isolate was compared with the average of the other 3 features in each experiment. In Experiment 1, recall of the semantic isolate (0.83) was 0.21 higher than the mean recall of the other three features (0.62)

In Experiment 2, recall of the physical isolate (0.88), though slightly higher than recall of the semantic isolate in Experiment 1 (due to better overall performance in Experiment 2), was only 0.18 higher than the other three features (0.69). Therefore, unlike typical laboratory experiments, the current study did not obtain a larger physical than semantic isolation effect. This is somewhat surprising given that the physical isolate was made distinctive on three dimensions (size, color, and font).

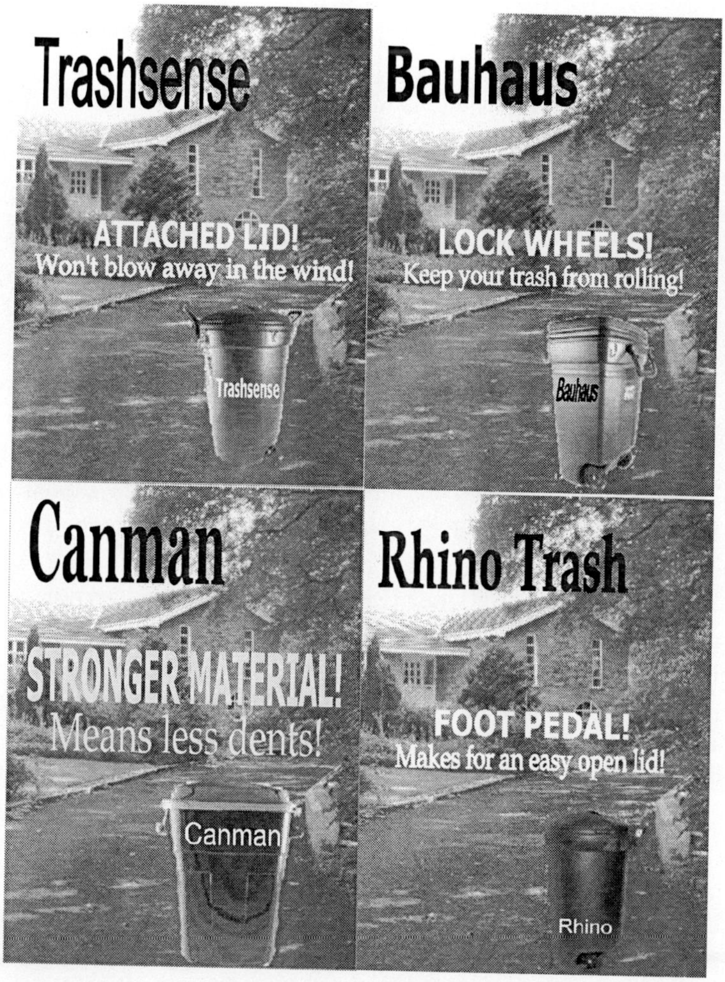
Trashsense
ATTACHED LID!
Won't blow away in the wind!
Trashsense
Bauhaus
LOCK WHEELS!
Keep your trash from rolling!
Bauhaus
Canman
STRONGER MATERIAL!
Means less dents!
Canman
Rhino Trash
FOOT PEDAL!
Makes for an easy open lid!
Rhino

Figure 2. Sample stimuli from Experiment 2 containing the physical isolate.

Memory for Brands. A series of t-tests confirmed that the recall for the brand paired with the isolate (M = 0.83) was significantly higher that for the brand paired with *attached lid* (M = 0.69, t(57) = 1.93) and *foot pedal* (M = 0.69, t(57) = 1.93) features, and there was a trend towards higher recall of the isolate's brand compared to the brand paired with *lock wheels* (M = 0.72, t(57) = 1.52). Unlike the semantic isolate in Experiment 1, the physical isolate generally afforded better recall of the brand compared to recall of the brands for the non-distinctive features. This does not appear to be due to lower recall of the brands for non-isolates in Experiment 2 (range of 0.69 to 0.72), as recall levels for the brands in Experiment 2 were actually slightly higher than those of Experiment 1 (0.59 to 0.68). The data suggest that the brand associated with a physical isolate (0.83) experiences a memory benefit that the brand associated with a semantic isolate (0.65) does not.

CONCLUSION

As predicted, isolation effects (or von Restorff effects, after von Restorff, 1933) were obtained for both the semantic (Experiment 1) and physical (Experiment 2) manipulations of distinctiveness. The results of this study demonstrate that product features displayed in print advertisements are better recalled if they are distinctive; this distinctiveness can come in the form of the feature being meaningfully different from features in other advertisements or physically (visually) different from other advertisements. These findings confirm Pick, Sweeney and Clay's (1991) finding of higher recall for features with higher ratings of distinctiveness. The obtained isolation effects are also consistent with Gardner's (1983) results revealing that participants exposed to the distinctive version of an advertisement were more likely to recall the distinctive attribute.

Contrary to our predictions, the physical isolation effect was not larger than the semantic isolation effect. The effect sizes were similar in both experiments despite the fact that the physical isolate was made distinctive on three dimensions (size, color, and font) rather than the traditional manipulation of just one dimension. One possible explanation is that the semantic manipulation in Experiment 1 was slightly different than traditional semantic manipulations. In a typical laboratory study of semantic isolation effects, participants view a list of words that all come from a single category, such as *types of flowers*. The semantic isolate is an item that comes from a different category, such as a *type of animal*. The semantic isolate is distinctive in that it comes from a different category. In Experiment 1, the semantic isolate was unique not only because it was different from the other features, but also because it was a feature that one would not expect to be associated with trashcans. One might even argue that the feature was bizarre or impossible. Thus, there may be an additional level of distinctiveness with a meaningful advertisement that is not present in a list of words.

The results of Experiments 1 and 2 did not provide evidence that isolation effects reliably extend to recall of the brand associated with the distinctive product features. Specifically, when given the list of features, participants did not show reliably better recall for the brand associated with the unique feature than the brand that was associated with the non-distinctive feature. This isolation effect for the corresponding brand name was obtained only in Experiment 2 with the physical isolation effect, and then only partially. The benefit for the brand name was not found in Experiment 1 with the semantic isolation effects. This implies that some, but not all, distinctiveness manipulations with product features will lead to increased memory for the brand name. One explanation for the lack of a benefit for information associated with the semantic isolate may come from Gardner (1983). She states that a distinctive feature of an advertisement can distract participants from another portion of the advertisement. In her study (discussed in the *Introduction*), participants who viewed a distinctive attribute in an advertisement were less likely to recall the other attributes compared to participants who viewed the non-distinctive version of the advertisement. The unusualness of the semantic isolate in the current study may have been somewhat distracting to participants, causing them to allocate fewer resources towards processing the brand name. If there were a slight benefit for information associated with an isolate, this benefit might be negated by the participant allocating fewer resources towards processing that information. Support for this possibility comes from studies in which memory is impaired for items surrounding the isolate (e.g., Hunt & Mitchell, 1982). However, many studies have found that neighboring items are not impaired (e.g., Bruce & Gaines, 1976; Fabiani & Donchin, 1995; Schmidt, 1985). Thus, the conditions under which memory for neighboring items is improved versus impaired are not clear.

The findings from these two experiments demonstrate that the robustness of the isolation effect is not limited to laboratory settings; rather, the effect is more generalizable and occurs in real-world situations as well. This study is consistent with earlier research findings in which distinctive aspects of advertisements were well remembered, and the results extend these findings to a more realistic situation in which participants see multiple advertisements with different features and varying brand names. The results of the current experiments lend further support for the hypothesis that distinctiveness plays a large role in the memorability of information, with the added support that information associated with the isolate can be better recalled as well. The fact that isolation effects were obtained in Experiment 1 and Experiment 2, even with the real-world requirement of associating brands with their corresponding features, suggests that consumers may make associations between distinctive aspects of an advertisement for a product and the brand of the product itself. As far as the authors are aware, the current study is the first to employ this method of recalling information associated with an isolate, both in the advertising literature and traditional laboratory studies. Since the current study found some evidence of isolation effects extending beyond the items themselves to associated items, this could prove to be a fruitful line of further research.

One might conclude from this study that an advertiser solely needs to make an advertisement different from the others for it to be well remembered. One important point made by von Restorff, however, is that making an item different from the background items is not sufficient to yield better memory for that item. That is, if the list contains all different types of items (symbol, word, digit, letter, etc.), the isolate will be different from the background items, but an isolation effect will not be obtained. In order for the isolate to be well remembered, von Restorff argued that the isolate needs to stand out "as figure against the ground of the homogenous items" (Hunt, 1995, p. 107). She explained that the isolate is better recalled than the background items not because recall of the isolate is exceptional, but because the similarity of the other items resulted in those items having poor recall. The implications of her findings are that an advertiser cannot simply make an advertisement different from the others and expect it to be well recalled. The research suggests that one must find a dimension in which all of the other advertisements are identical, and make the new advertisement unique on this dimension.

Further research needs to be conducted to determine the extent to which isolation effects for real-world situations differ from those obtained in the lab, such as the slightly smaller physical effect compared to the semantic isolation effect in the current set of experiments. In addition, it is unclear why some manipulations of distinctiveness result in better memory for items that are associated with the isolate (in this case, the associated item was the brand name) and exactly what the underlying mechanism is that affords isolation effects to associated items.

References

Bellezza, F. S., & Cheney, T. L. (1973). Isolation effect in immediate and delayed recall. *Journal of Experimental Psychology, 99*, 55-60.

Bireta, T. J., Surprenant, A. M., & Neath, I. (2008). Age-related differences in the von Restorff isolation effect. *The Quarterly Journal of Experimental Psychology, 61*, 345-352.

Bruce, D., & Gaines, M. T. (1976). Tests of an organizational hypothesis of isolation effects in free recall. *Journal of Verbal Learning and Verbal Behavior, 15*, 59-72.

Cimbalo, R. S., & Brink, L. (1982). Aging and the von Restorff isolation effect in short/term memory. *Journal of General Psychology, 106,* 69-76.

Cimbalo, R. S., Nowak, B. I., & Soderstrom, J. A. (1981). The isolation effect in children's short-term memory. *Journal of General Psychology, 105,* 215-223.

Cohen, M. E., & Carr, W. J. (1975). Facial recognition and the von Restorff effect. *Bulletin of the Psychonomic Society, 6,* 383-384.

Conway, M. A., & Haque, S. (1999). Overshadowing the reminiscence bump: Memories of a struggle for independence. *Journal of Adult Development, 6*, 35-44.

Craig, S. C., Sternthal, B., & Leavitt, C. (1976). Advertising wearout: An experimental analysis. *Journal of Marketing Research, 13*, 365-372.

Dunlosky, J., Hunt, R. R., & Clark, E. (2000). Is perceptual salience really needed in explanations of the isolation effect? *Journal of Experimental Psychology: Learning, Memory, and Cognition, 26*, 649-657.

Fabiani, M., & Donchin, E. (1995). Encoding processes and memory organization: A model of the von Restorff effect. *Journal of Experimental Psychology: Learning, Memory, and Cognition, 21*, 224-240.

Gardner, M. P. (1983). Advertising effects on attributes recalled and criteria used for brand evaluations. *The Journal of Consumer Research, 10,* 310-318.

Going, M., & Read, J. D. (1974). Effects of uniqueness, sex of subject, and sex of photograph on facial recognition. *Perceptual and Motor Skills, 39*, 109-110.

Gumenik, W. E., & Levitt, J. (1968). The von Restorff effect as a function of the difference of the isolated item. *American Journal of Psychology, 81,* 247-252.

Harcum, R. E. (1968). Perceptual serial position curves with a frequently isolated element. *American Journal of Psychology, 81,* 334-346.

Hosie, J. A., & Milne, A. B. (1995). Distinctiveness and memory for unfamiliar faces. In T. Valentine (Ed.), *Cognitive and computational aspects of face recognition – Explorations in face space* (pp. 95-112). London, Routledge.

Howe, M. L., Courage, M. L., Vernescu, R., & Hunt, M. (2000). Distinctiveness effects in children's long-term retention. *Developmental Psychology, 36,* 778-792.

Huang, I. N., & Fleming, J. (1977). Differential effects of stimulus and response isolation in paired-associate learning. *Journal of General Psychology, 95*, 187-191.

Hunt, R. R. (1995). The subtlety of distinctiveness: What von Restorff really did. *Psychonomic Bulletin & Review, 2,* 105-112.

Hunt, R. R., & Lamb, C. A. (2001). What causes the isolation effect? *Journal of Experimental Psychology: Learning, Memory, and Cognition, 27*, 1359-1366.

Hunt, R. R., & Mitchell, D. B. (1982). Independent effects of semantic and nonsemantic distinctiveness. *Journal of Experimental Psychology: Learning, Memory, and Cognition, 8*, 81-87.

Kelley, M. R., & Nairne, J. S. (2001). von Restorff Revisited: Isolation, generation, and memory for order. *Journal of Experimental Psychology: Learning, Memory, and Cognition, 27*, 54-66.

Jenkins, W. O., & Postman, L. (1948). Isolation and the spread of effect in serial learning. *American Journal of Psychology, 61*, 214-221.

Karis, D., Fabiani, M., & Donchin, E. (1984). "P300" and memory: Individual differences in the von Restorff effect. *Cognitive-Psychology, 16,* 177-216.

Kessler, F. (1985). Now we pause for a (very) brief message. *Fortune, 112,* 75.

Lynch, J. G., & Srull, T. K. (1982). Memory and attentional factors in consumer choice: Concepts and research methods. *The Journal of Consumer Research, 9,* 18-37.

Main, K. M., Leland, L. S., & Bartlett, G. (1998). The properties of one: Facial memory and the isolation effect. *Journal of General Psychology, 125,* 192-206.

Nairne, J. S. (1990). A feature model of immediate memory. *Memory & Cognition, 18*, 251-269.

Nairne, J. S. (2006). Modeling distinctiveness: Implications for general memory theory. In R. R. Hunt & J. B. Worthen (Eds.), *Distinctiveness and memory* (pp. 27-46). New York, NY: Oxford University Press.

Nachmias, J., Gleitman, H. & McKenna, V. (1961). The effect of isolation of stimulus and response in paired associates. *American Journal of Psychology, 74*, 452-456.

Pick, D. F., Sweeny, J., & Clay, J. A. (1991). Creative advertising and the von Restorff effect. *Psychological Reports, 69,* 923-926.

Pillsbury, W. B., & Rausch, H. L. (1943). An extension of the Kohler-Restorff inhibition phenomenon. *American Journal of Psychology, 56*, 293-298.

Phillips, M., & Rasberry, S. (2005). *Marketing Without Advertising: Inspire Customers to Rave about Your Business to Create Lasting Success*. San Francisco: NOLO publishing.

Rabinowitz, F. M., & Andrews, S. R. (1973). Intentional and incidental learning in children and the von restorff effect. *Journal of Experimental Psychology, 100,* 315-318.

Rubin, D. C., Rahhal, T. A., & Poon, L. W. (1998). Things learned in early adulthood are remembered best. *Memory & Cognition, 26*, 3-19.

Rubin, D. C., & Schulkind, M. D. (1997). Distribution of important and word-cued autobiographical memories in 20-, 35-, and 70-year old adults. Psychology and Aging, 12, 524-535.

Rubin, D. C., Wetzler, S. E., & Nebes, R. D. (1986). Autobiographical memory across the adult life span. In D. C. Rubin (Ed.) *Autobiographical memory* (pp. 202-221). New York: Cambridge University Press.

Rundus, D. (1971). Analysis of rehearsal processes in free recall. *Journal of Experimental Psychology, 89*, 63-77.

Santos, I. M., & Young, A. W. (2005). Exploring the perception of social characteristics in faces using the isolation effect. *Visual Cognition, 12,* 213-247.

Schmidt, S. R. (1985). Encoding and retrieval processes in the memory for conceptually distinctive events. *Journal of Experimental Psychology: Learning, Memory, and Cognition, 11,* 565-578.

Schmidt, S. R. (1991). Can we have a distinctive theory of memory? *Memory & Cognition, 19*, 523-542.

von Restorff, H. (1933). Analyse von Vorgangen in Spurenfeld. I. Über die Wirkung von Bereichsbildungen im Spurenfeld [Analysis of processes in the memory trace. I. On the effect of group formations on the memory trace]. *Psychologische Forschung, 18,* 299-342.

Winters, J. J., Hoats, D. L. (1989). On the development of the isolation effect in free recall: isolation by color. *Bulletin of the Psychonomic Society, 27,* 219-222.

In: Applied Memory
Editor: Matthew R. Kelley
ISBN 978-1-60692-143-2

Chapter 5

APPLIED PART-SET CUING

Joanna C. Bovee[1*], Caroline Fitz[2], Gretchen Yehl[3], Stacey Parrott[3], and Matthew R. Kelley[3]

[1] Department of Psychology, University of Illinois at Chicago, Chicago, IL, USA
[2] Department of Psychology, Northwestern University, Evanston, IL, USA
[3] Department of Psychology, Lake Forest College, Lake Forest, IL, USA

ABSTRACT

This chapter was designed to accomplish three main goals: (a) to review current theoretical explanations of part-set cuing phenomena, (b) to examine research of everyday applications of part-set cuing, and (c) to report the results of two new experiments that explore part-set cuing inhibition and facilitation in everyday memory contexts. In Experiment 1, participants compiled grocery lists as a confederate either physically walked them through a grocery store or showed a video of her recent store trip. At test, some participants were told that they lost the list (free recall—no cues), while others were told that a coffee spill made half the list illegible (free recall—part set cues). In Experiment 2, visiting high school students and their parents completed a campus tour and then were asked to complete a surprise reconstruction of order test. They were shown 12 pictures of campus buildings/names in a new random order. Half the tests comprised consistent part-set cues (6 buildings shown in proper positions) and half consisted of control cues (6 buildings and 6 positions eliminated from consideration). As expected, Experiment 1 (free recall) produced reliable part-set cuing inhibition and Experiment 2 (reconstruction) showed part-set cuing facilitation.

INTRODUCTION

Imagine that you are a student in a history course and you are asked to remember twenty key events that lead to World War I for a subsequent test. Just prior to the test, the instructor gives you a choice: (a) take a test with hints (i.e., a random half of the events are provided;

* Corresponding author.

recall remaining ten events), or (b) take a test without hints (i.e., recall all twenty events). In both cases, the proportion of correct responses will represent your test score. Which test would you choose? Most people would likely choose the test with hints, assuming that the retrieval cues would facilitate their performance. Contrary to popular belief, however, providing part of set of to-be-remembered (TBR) items at test typically inhibits free recall performance—a phenomenon known as *part-set cuing inhibition* (e.g., Nickerson, 1984; Slamecka, 1968).

Part-set cuing inhibition has proven robust in free recall, having been replicated under a wide variety of laboratory manipulations, including: episodic and semantic memory (e.g., Brown, 1968), categorized and uncategorized lists (e.g., Basden, 1973; Mueller & Watkins, 1977; Rundus, 1973; Watkins, 1975), nonlinguistic stimuli (e.g., Peynircioglu, 1987), intra- and extra-list cuing (e.g., Basden, Basden, & Galloway, 1977; Mueller & Watkins, 1977; Watkins, 1975), and varying numbers of cues (e.g., Roediger, 1973; Slamecka, 1972). Importantly, however, part-set cues do not always inhibit performance. Indeed, participants often show *part-set cuing facilitation* when they are asked to remember events in a temporal sequence using serial recall (Basden, Basden, & Stephens, 2002; Kelley & Bovee, 2007) or reconstruction of order measures (Serra & Nairne, 2000; Kelley & Bovee, 2007). Hence, in the previous example, choosing a test with hints would enhance performance if the twenty key events had to be recalled chronologically.

In the present chapter, we will begin by examining the leading explanations of these phenomena, including the strategy disruption hypothesis (e.g., Basden et al., 1977) and a dual-mechanism approach (Bauml & Aslan, 2006). Then, we will consider a relatively unexplored area of research—applications of part-set cuing. To date, the majority of part-set cuing studies have been employed in the lab with simple word stimuli (Nickerson, 1984). More recently, however, researchers have explored part-set cuing in broader contexts, such as examining these phenomena with social or collaborative memory tasks (e.g., Andersson, Hitch, & Meudell, 2006) and with false memory tasks (e.g., Reysen & Nairne, 2002). Still, applications of part-set cuing to real-world contexts are relatively sparse. We will address this final issue by exploring two new experimental applications of part-set cuing.

Explanations of the Part-Set Cuing Phenomena

Researchers have attempted to uncover the underlying causal mechanisms that drive these part-set cuing phenomena, however most theories have focused exclusively on explaining part-set cuing inhibition (e.g., see Nickerson, 1984 for an exhaustive review of part-set cuing theory and research from 1968-1983). Three explanations in particular—the *competition at retrieval hypothesis* (e.g., Rundus, 1973), the *cue overload hypothesis* (Mueller & Watkins, 1977), and the *editing task hypothesis* (Roediger & Tulving, 1974)—have been shown to provide incomplete accounts of how part-set cues influence retention. These hypotheses cannot account for the full range of inhibition effects (e.g., Basden et al., 1977; Peynircioglu, 1989; Nickerson, 1984; Raaijmakers & Shiffrin, 1981; Sloman, Bower, & Rohrer, 1991; Watkins; 1975), nor can they explain the facilitation effects with order retention (e.g., Serra & Nairne, 2000).

Strategy Disruption Hypothesis. In contrast, the *strategy disruption hypothesis* (e.g., Basden et al., 1977; Basden & Basden, 1995) suggests that when participants encode information, they typically employ a specific organizational strategy (e.g., temporal location, spatial location, mnemonic devices, interitem associations, etc.) that they believe will facilitate their subsequent recall. Consistent with the principle of transfer appropriate processing (e.g., Morris, Bransford, & Franks, 1977), retention is influenced by the degree of match between organizational strategies at encoding and the strategies employed at retrieval. Hence, part-set cuing inhibition will arise when the presence of cues at test promotes a retrieval strategy that is inconsistent with the participant's original encoded organization of the TBR events. On the other hand, facilitation will occur when the retrieval strategy is consistent with original encoding.

Over the past three decades, many studies have explored the strategy disruption hypothesis (e.g., Basden et al., 1977; Basden & Basden, 1995; Peynircioglu, 1989). For instance, Brown and Hall (1979) examined the influence of item strength and number of cues on semantic memory and showed that the strategy disruption hypothesis best accounted for their results. The experiment began with a free-association task in which participants generated four responses to 20 separate stimulus words (e.g., *bird* and the responses *canary, tree, chirp,* and *fly*). In a second session two days later, participants were given a surprise recall test in which they were asked to regenerate their responses, sometimes in the presence of cues and other times without cues. On cued trials, one-third of the participants received a single previous generated word from a set as cue, another third received two of the four previous answers as cues, and the last third received three of the four previous responses as cues. Additionally, strength of the cue item was manipulated by taking cues from varying output positions at the time of initial item generation, assuming that earlier output reflects stronger association.

Brown and Hall (1979) reasoned that, if part-set cuing disrupts participants' recall strategies, then the main effects of number of cues and strength of cues should not be significant. That is, the presence of any cue of any strength should be sufficient to disrupt participants' intended recall strategies. If, however, the results indicated that stronger cue items produced greater inhibition, then Rundus' (1973) competition at retrieval theory would be supported. Alternatively, if performance decreased as the number of cues increased, results would be in favor of the cue-overload hypothesis (Mueller & Watkins, 1977). Consistent solely with the strategy disruption hypothesis, Brown and Hall reported the classic part-set cuing inhibition effect, with no main effects for cue number or item strength.

The strategy disruption hypothesis can also account for facilitation effects with order retention (e.g., Kelley & Bovee, 2007). For instance, Basden et al. (2002) showed that participations regularly used seriation as a strategy for serial recall tests. In their study, participants showed part-set cuing facilitation when they were provided with cues consistent with a serial (or chaining) strategy—that is, when cued items were shown in their original positions, performance was enhanced relative to a control cue condition. Accordingly, they showed part-set cuing inhibition when the cues were inconsistent with a serial strategy (i.e., cued items in incorrect positions).

In general, the strategy disruption hypothesis has enjoyed a great deal of success accounting for a wide range of empirical findings. However, there have been occasional challenges to the hypothesis (e.g., see Peynircioglu, 1989; but see Basden, Basden, Church, & Beaupre, 1991 for a rebuttal). Indeed, recent evidence by Serra and Oswald (2006) has proven problematic for a strict interpretation of the strategy disruption hypothesis. They noted an important shortcoming in the strategy disruption literature, namely, that past research routinely failed to measure the "strategy" being employed by participants. To gain a better understanding of the underpinnings of strategy disruption, Serra and Oswald measured the degree to which a particular strategy was used, the amount of strategy disruption, and the impact of that disruption on recall in a series of three experiments.

In their first two experiments, Serra and Oswald (2006) used 12-item lists that they developed in such a way as to make the participants adopt a forward-associative seriation recall strategy. List structures were based on the idea that people form interitem associations based on serial position (i.e., chaining) and that people are more likely to form associations between semantically related items. In the developed set of lists, each item was semantically associated with the following list item (e.g., earth-ground-beef-cow-milk, etc.). Although participants were not informed of the nature of the lists, Serra and Oswald clearly expected that many participants would implicitly self-adopt the seriation strategy. Following each list presentation, participants either completed free recall test with either no cues or part-set cues.

To determine whether participants self-adopted the forward-associative seriation strategy and if it was disrupted by the presence of cues, Serra and Oswald examined the output order of the recalled items relative to the original presentation order. For both cued and uncued trials, participants appeared to self-adopt the researchers' intended recall strategy. However, the output order more closely resembled the original order on uncued trials than on cued trials. This was taken as evidence that cues had disrupted the participants' recall strategy. Importantly, however, although the cues had disrupted recall strategy, they did not significantly impair recall performance. In both experiments, participants recalled an equal or greater proportion of the TBR items in the cued condition than in the uncued condition.

In their third experiment, Serra and Oswald used the same list items, but presented the words in a random order—that is, the forward semantic relations between items were removed from the list structures. Interestingly, participants' recall order (or strategy) did not differ significantly across cue conditions—they recalled the list items in a manner consistent with the original presentation order, at a rate slightly above chance. This time, however, recall performance resembled traditional part-set cuing inhibition with higher recall accuracy of TBR items on uncued trials than cued trials. Clearly, the lack of part-set cuing inhibition in the first two experiments was not an artifact of the list items or of the procedure. Instead, the absence of part-set cuing inhibition likely reflects that the semantic associations between items in the first two experiments were stronger recall aids than the forward chaining associations alone.

Serra and Oswald's findings pose a serious challenge to a strict view of the strategy disruption hypothesis as an explanation of the part set cuing. Under certain conditions, such as when list items are highly semantic related, the strategy can be disrupted by the presence of cues without impairing recall. Additionally, the traditional part-set cuing effect can occur without a large disruption of the recall strategy, as seen in Experiment 3. In an attempt to reconcile these findings with the previous literature, Bauml and Aslan (2006) proposed a dual mechanism account of part-set cuing.

Dual Mechanism Account. According to Bauml and Aslan (2006), the detrimental effect of part-set cuing can be caused by either strategy disruption or retrieval inhibition with encoding as a mediating factor. In situations wherein participants are likely to form a high number of interitem associations between list items (e.g., instructed to encode serially, multiple study sessions), recall will be based primarily on these associations. The presence of part-set cues, then, might disrupt the participants' rigid recall strategy and decrease the number of TBR items recalled. The associations between items remain intact, however, and may be used again once cues are removed to recall the items in a 'chained' fashion. This transient nature of the PSC has been confirmed in several of the studies mentioned above (e.g., Basden et al, 1977; Mueller & Watkins, 1977; Watkins; 1975). However, when participants form a low number of interitem associations between items or fail to find distinct relations between items, the mechanism responsible for the traditional part set cuing effect is different.

This alternative mechanism, according to Bauml and Aslan (2006), may involve retrieval-induced forgetting (Anderson, 1994), in which retrieving an item from memory inhibits the representations of competing responses. Whereas retrieval-induced forgetting has typically focused on overt item retrieval, Bauml and Aslan extended it to covert retrieval as well. In a part-set cuing paradigm when participants do not form interitem associations (e.g., categorized lists), re-exposure of list items as cues causes covert retrieval of these nontarget items, consequently inhibiting target items' representations in memory and making them less likely to be recalled. Because a person will eventually self-terminate retrieval after a number of retrieval failures, the search of memory will likely stop before all the target items are recalled. Retrieval inhibition differs from Rundus's competition-at-retrieval hypothesis (1973) or Mueller and Watkin's (1978) cue overload hypothesis. In these accounts, the cuing impairment is produced by changes to the association strengths between items. By using a retrieval-induced forgetting approach, Bauml and Aslan emphasized that the part-set cuing effect is due to representational-based changes to the items, which should provide longer-lasting inhibition.

Bauml and Aslan (2006) explored these ideas across a series of three experiments designed to identify the contexts in which strategy disruption was the mediating mechanism (i.e., high associative encoding conditions) and the contexts in which retrieval inhibition was the mediating mechanism (i.e., low associative encoding conditions). Following high associative encoding, strategy disruption should produce part-set inhibition on an initial cued test but not on a later test when part-set cues are removed. In contrast, following low associative encoding, retrieval inhibition should yield part-set inhibition on an initial test and this inhibition should remain even when cues are removed on a later test.

In their first experiment, Bauml and Aslan manipulated interitem associations formed between subjects and retrieval cues at test within subjects. Lists were composed of 16-items each and an equal number of items in a list from two categories. Items were presented individually in a random order. In the low associative condition, participants saw a list once during the study phase. In the high associative condition, participants had successive study-test trials of each list so that they would be more likely to form interitem associations. Items were presented in the same order on each trial. Following the study phase, participants completed a critical recall test with half the trials cued and the other half uncued. On the cued critical recall tests, participants were given half the items from each category and instructed to use them as cues to recall the remaining items. On free recall critical tests, participants were given the category names and instructed to recall all of the list items. After a short distractor task, everyone completed a free recall test in which they were told recall all of the items by category.

As predicted, in the high associative condition, participants showed part-set cuing inhibition—they recalled more target items on uncued trials than cued trials during the critical test. However, performance between cued and uncued groups was equivalent on the final free recall test, reflecting that part-set cuing inhibition was transient and was released once cues removed. In the low associative condition, participants again recalled more target items on uncued than cued trials on the critical test. Although, this part-set cuing inhibition remained for the final free recall test—there still was a decrement in recall performance for those who has received cues during the critical phase of the experiment. This longer-lasting inhibition was consistent with Bauml and Aslan's retrieval inhibition mechanism account for situations with a low number of interitem associations.

Experiment 2 followed-up Experiment 1 by determining if re-exposure to cue items in the critical test created output interference on the final test. If it had, then it is possible that the re-exposure to cue items during the critical test strengthened their representations in memory, rather than suppressing the target item representations, and made them more likely to be recalled first in the final test before the target items. To resolve whether differences in the first experiment were due to long-lasting inhibition by part-set cues or due to output interference, Bauml and Aslan controlled for participants output order. They repeated the low-associative condition from Experiment 1, but controlled for output order by using category-plus-first-letter-recall tests. During the critical tests, participants in the cued condition were given whole nontarget items as cues and letter cues to test their memory for the target items only. Participants in the uncued condition were given letters cues in a random order for the target items only. For the final test, all participants received letter cues for target and nontarget items. Target items were tested before nontarget items to control for output order interference. In all tests, items were blocked by category. During the critical test, performance on cued trials was again less than on uncued trial. This pattern remained the same in the final test. Thus, the detrimental effects in these first two experiments appear not to be due to output order inference, but are due, instead, to retrieval inhibition of target items.

In their final experiment, Bauml and Aslan attempted to replicate their prior findings using different materials and a different procedure. In this three-factor mixed design, participants were tested on their memory for two 24-item non-categorized lists. High and low associative encoding was manipulated between-subjects—the low associative group was not given specific instructions during the study phase, except to the read the words aloud as they were individually presented, whereas the high associative group was instructed to make a meaningful sentence for each list item and to interrelate these sentences to form a story. As in the first two experiments, cuing during the critical test was manipulated within-subjects. On cued trials, participants read the nontarget items aloud and wrote the target items below them. On uncued trials, participants freely recalled as many items as they could. All participants then completed a final free recall test. As expected, part-set cuing inhibition was transient in the high association condition, but long-lasting in the low association condition.

Across their three experiments, Bauml and Aslan (2006) demonstrated that the mediating mechanism behind PSC-inhibition can differ across encoding contexts. When a person is able to create associations between the items and reduce interitem interference, part-set cuing inhibition is released once cues are removed and a person can return to his or her original recall strategy. However, when items are encoded with a relatively few interitem associations, part-set cuing inhibition is not as transient. Presumably, this long-term suppression of target item representations is caused by covert retrieval in nontarget cue items and is very similar to what occurs in retrieval-induced forgetting. To date, this dual-mechanism hypothesis appears to provide the most complete account of extant data.

Given that the effects of part-set cuing can be sometimes detrimental and sometimes beneficial, one may wonder whether these findings extend beyond traditional laboratory settings and stimuli to more applied settings. Indeed, by understanding the influences of strategy disruption and retrieval inhibition, people potentially may avoid real-world situations that are ripe for inhibition or reconfigure those situations to promote better memory performance. In the next sections, we will consider broader applications of the part-set cuing phenomena.

Applications of Part Set Cuing

As implied in the opening of this chapter, part-set cuing appears to have a natural application to the field of education. Teachers should find part-set research particularly relevant as they construct exams, whereas students would do well to keep these phenomena in mind as they study for and complete their exams. Surprisingly, researchers have neglected to explore this application in any systematic way. Moreover, any applications of part-set cuing research are difficult to find, as the literature is dominated by basic research. Indeed, we found only two 'applications' of part-set cuing—within the contexts of collaborative inhibition and false memory—and whether these are true applications is a matter of debate. Regardless, the research is interesting and relevant to everyday life, and is reviewed below.

Collaborative Inhibition. Collaborative inhibition refers to a decline in recall performance as a result of cross-cuing, or the information exchange that takes place between two or more individuals during the discussion of a memory event (e.g., Basden, Basden, Bryner, & Thomas, 1997; Weldon & Bellinger, 1997). Items recalled by group members appear to undermine the many benefits to group collaboration, in that such recall acts as part-set cues for others in the group, which disrupts their retrieval strategies. For instance, Andersson, Hitch, and Meudell (2006) found that after studying a word list, participants who were given spoken cues during recall remembered fewer words than participants in the free recall condition. Notably, participants whose spoken cues were distributed throughout the recall period (i.e., cues consistent with participants' retrieval strategies) remembered more target words as compared to participants who were given spoken cues only at the beginning of the recall period (i.e., cues inconsistent with participants' retrieval strategies).

Dagnall, Parker, and Munley (2007) provided further evidence of this common strategy-disruption mechanism between cross-cuing and part-set cuing that led to inhibited recall of information. Participants solved anagrams either independently or in pairs, and afterwards were asked (either independently or with a partner) to remember the words presented as anagrams. Beyond the finding that individuals who encoded independently (i.e., solved anagrams individually) and recalled with a partner forgot more items than those who encoded and recalled anagrams individually, results indicated that pairs who encoded collaboratively forgot fewer items than those who encoded individually and then worked collaboratively on the recall task. Dagnall et al. concluded that just as the part-set cuing effect can be reduced through the use of consistent cues, collaborative inhibition can be limited through joint encoding, which leads to similar retrieval strategies and thus, less strategy disruption during recall. Overall, cross-cuing and part-set cuing appear to operate similarly, as they both disrupt retrieval strategies. Perhaps individuals should attempt to limit their social interactions when they try to remember an event, because two heads aren't always better than one, at least when it comes to the recall of information.

Part-Set Cuing of False Memories. In two experiments, Reysen and Nairne (2002) demonstrated the effects of part-set cuing on false memories. Specifically, Reysen and Nairne assessed the proportion of nonpresented critical items (e.g., list items: bed, rest, nap; critical non-presented item: sleep) recalled during free recall and cued recall tasks. In their first experiment, after studying a word list, participants recalled a higher proportion of critical words on the free recall test than on the cued recall test. Put another way, retrieval cues inhibited the recall of nonpresented words that were falsely remembered during the memory task. As an extension of this finding, their second experiment explored the effects of different memory test conditions upon item recall. In particular, Reysen and Nairne compared the influences of random cues and consistent cues on the recall of nonpresented critical words. In contrast to the finding that participants recalled a greater proportion of studied words (i.e., words that were correctly remembered, that actually appeared on the list) in the consistent cue condition than in the random cue condition, there were no significant differences between the recall of critical words in the consistent and random cue conditions; consistent and random cues equally inhibited participants' false memories.

Taken together, Reysen and Nairne's (2002) experiments highlight the robust part-set cuing effects that apply to false memories, as measured by the recall of nonpresented critical words. Critical items appear to operate similarly to studied items in that the recall of both becomes hampered in the presence of retrieval cues. However, in regards to the finding that the presentation of consistent cues reduced the part-set cuing effect for the studied items but not for the critical items, critical words may function somewhat differently as compared to studied words, at least in terms of their recall.

Given the paucity of applied research on the part-set cuing phenomena, one is left to speculate about the situations in which part set cues might influence memory. Any setting in which a person is working with partial information (e.g., using an old or corrupted computer file; listening to a closing argument or summary) could potentially disrupt a person's recall strategy, actively inhibit retrieval, or in certain circumstance, even facilitate recall of desired information. In the following experiments, we consider two common real-world scenarios which demonstrate the applicability of part-set cuing inhibition and facilitation.

EXPERIMENT 1

Experiment 1 was designed to explore the generality of part-set cuing inhibition to the ability to remember items on a grocery list. Specifically, participants were given a scenario in which their friend's grandmother needed help grocery shopping. The friend then takes the participants on either a real or a virtual trip to the grocery store while the participant views and writes down the grocery items. On a subsequent memory test, participants were either informed that they lost the grocery list (free recall condition) or that there was a coffee spill and only half of the items were legible (part-set cue condition). Participants attempted to recall as many items as possible. In both the applied (real-world) and lab-analog scenarios, we expected that participants in the part-set condition would recall fewer items than participants in the free recall (no cue) condition

Method

Participants. Forty-eight Lake Forest College psychology students earned extra credit in exchange for participation in experiment. In the applied condition, groups of five or fewer individuals were transported to a local grocery store for experimental sessions lasting about 20 minutes. In the lab analog condition, groups of up to four individuals were tested at a time. Seated in separate cubicles, each participant completed the task on an IBM-compatible computer in sessions lasting approximately 15 minutes.

Materials. One grocery list was created and used for both the applied and lab analog conditions. The list contained 20 items, each consisting of two words (e.g. seedless grapes, kosher franks, curry powder). Three tests were constructed: one version of a free recall test and two counterbalanced versions of a part-set test. The free recall test sheet consisted of 20 rows and two columns of blank lines. On the part-set tests, half of the items (every other item; odd/even counterbalanced) were displayed at the top of the test sheet, in a random order, and 10 blank rows with 2 columns appeared at the bottom of the sheet. For each test, participants were instructed to recall the items in any order. In addition to the test sheets, one blank grocery list (20 rows of 2 columns) was created and employed in the presentation phase.

Separate orders of the grocery list items were constructed for the applied and lab-analog conditions. Both orders, however, were consistent with how a person might encounter the items while shopping at a store (i.e., items in the same aisle would follow each other on the list). For the lab analog condition, a short video was created which displayed each item for 12 seconds—four seconds showing a person's hand taking the grocery item and 8 seconds displaying the item's name (white letters on black background; 36-pt Times New Roman font; centered). A two second inter-stimulus-interval followed presentation of each item.

Procedure. All participants were given the same scenario: they were told that they were going to grocery shop for their friend's grandmother while the friend was out of town. They were instructed that they would visit the grocery store with the friend (in person or virtually) and that they should take careful notes on the list because grandmother has very particular tastes. In the applied condition, participants were transported to a local grocery store where they were given blank grocery lists and pens. Participants were then led around the store, in an efficient and logical route, as the experimenter showed and named 20 grocery items. Participants were asked to write the item names on the blank grocery list as they were shown. Following the last item, the grocery lists were collected and the tests were administered.

In the lab analog condition, participants were given similar instructions as in the applied condition except they were told that they would see a short video depicting the friend shopping for the items instead of visiting the grocery store in person. After viewing each item, participants were instructed to write down the item name on a blank grocery list. Following presentation in both conditions, participants were randomly given either a part-set cued or free recall test. Participants completed the tests at their own pace and were debriefed upon test completion.

Results and Discussion

Figure 1 displays the proportion of correct responses as a function of setting and cue condition. A 2 (Setting: Lab Analog vs. Real World) x 2 (Cue Condition vs. No Cues) between-subjects ANOVA revealed that neither the main effect of setting nor the interaction were statistical significant (both F's < 1). However, there was a significant main effect of cue condition, $F(1,44) = 10.729$, $p < .001$. Overall, participants remembered more items in the absence of cues (free recall) than with part-set cues, which reflects traditional *part-set cuing inhibition.* Planned comparisons revealed significant part-set cuing inhibition across both settings. Specifically, in the applied condition, participants remembered a significantly greater proportion of grocery items on the free recall test (0.72) than on the cued recall test (0.54). Similar results were found in the lab analog as free recall performance (0.67) exceeded cued recall performance (0.49).

As expected, regardless of setting, participants remembered more items in the free recall condition as compared to participants in the part-set cue condition. Hence, real-world scenarios appear to elicit the same part-set cuing inhibition effect that occurs in laboratory settings. When individuals are given cues to help facilitate their memory performance, those cues tend to hinder recall performance.

EXPERIMENT 2

Experiment 2 was designed to explore the generality of part-set cuing facilitation using an everyday task in which sequential information is particularly important. The motivation for the study came from the following rather common scenario. Imagine that after a busy day of running errands around town, you arrive home and realize that your driver's license (or any card or key) is no longer in your wallet. You cannot recall the last time you remember seeing it because you did not have any use for it during the day, but you did use your wallet quite often. With all the places you stopped, you may have difficulty remembering where you went. In an attempt to retrace your steps, you might use receipts to piece the day's journey back together. However, the receipts would offer an incomplete representation of the day because not every location you visited would yield a receipt. Will looking at these clues help you to remember the order of the day's events? Or, will they interfere with your recall of the remaining locations?

Conducting this exact study in the real world would be particularly challenging, but one can easily imagine how part-set cuing might influence memory in this situation. The present experiment attempted to maintain the spirit of the scenario—by having participants visit several locations and then give them a surprise memory test—while using a more feasible and controlled design. We used prospective students and parents who were visiting Lake Forest College as participants in this study. These first-time visitors completed a standardized tour of 12 campus buildings and were surprised with an incidental reconstruction of order in which they were asked to identify the sequence of buildings that they had just seen. Half the participants were provided with 6 consistent part-set cues (even or odd half of items) while the remaining participants were given 6 control cues (half items/positions eliminated from test).

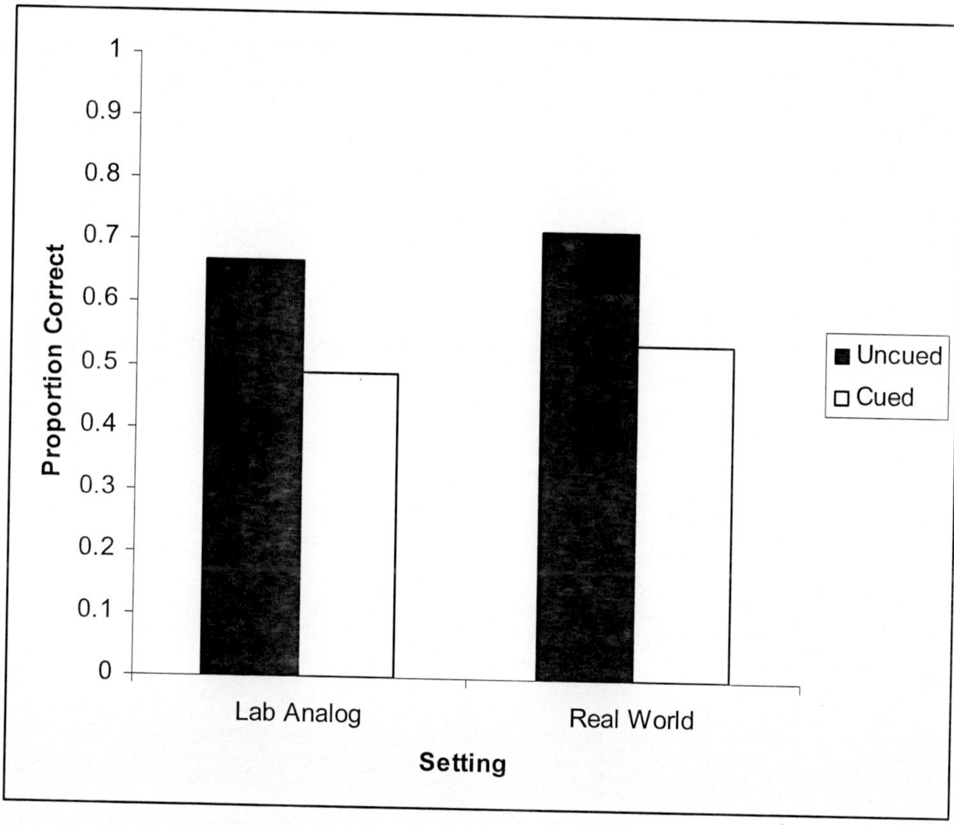

Figure 1. Proportion correct as a function of setting and cue condition.

Consistent with past research (e.g., Serra and Nairne, 2000), we expected part-set cuing facilitation with performance in the consistent condition exceeding that of the control condition.

Method

Participants. Upon completion of a tour of the Lake Forest College campus, 87 campus visitors (prospective students; parents; siblings) were asked whether they would take a brief memory test, about three minutes in length, about the buildings they viewed on the tour. Sixty-eight participants agreed to complete the memory test. In all, 64% of the sample was female. The majority of the participants were in the 15-24 yr (55%) and 45-54 yr (29%) age ranges. The remaining 16% of participants were distributed rather evenly across the 25-34, 35-44, and 55-64 age ranges—a few participants in each category.

Materials. We created a standard tour of twelve campus buildings that was implemented in the same order by a variety student tour guides. Test sheets consisted of the names and thumbnail photographs of each campus, presented in a random order, each with its own corresponding letter (see Appendix). The numbers 1-12, representing the sequential order of the buildings, appears on the bottom the test sheet. Four versions of the test were created—two that provided *consistent part-set cues* where half of the letters of proper buildings were placed in proper serial positions, and two that provided *control cues* where half of the buildings and serial positions were eliminated from the test (X's appeared in the eliminated positions). In both cases, participants were asked to reconstruct the order of the remaining buildings (highlighted by a box around the name/photograph). Test sheets were printed in color on standard 8" x 11" paper; writing utensils were provided.

Procedure. Upon arriving to the Admissions Office at Lake Forest College, campus visitors were taken on a standard walking tour in which 12 campus buildings were introduced and described in a standard sequential order. Following the tour, visitors were asked if they would be interested in participating in a psychology research project in which their memories for the tour would be tested. Upon reading and signing an informed consent form, participants were given a test sheet and were asked to reconstruct the sequence of buildings they visited on their campus tour by writing the letters associated with the buildings in their appropriate serial positions. Participants were randomly assigned to the consistent cue and control cue conditions and were instructed to use all the letters (reconstruct all six building positions) even if they had to guess. When the test was complete, participants returned the sheets to the tour guide and were thanked for their participation.

Results and Discussion

Figure 2 displays the proportion of correctly reconstructed items at each serial position pair for the consistent and control cue conditions, respectively. A 2 (cue condition: consistent vs. control) x 6 (serial position pair: 1-2, 3-4, 5-6, 7-8, 9-10, 11-12) mixed factor analysis of variance (ANOVA) revealed a significant main effect of cue condition, $F(1,66) = 10.644$; $p < .01$. Overall, participants were able reconstruct the order of the campus buildings more effectively with consistent part-set cues (0.63) than with control cues (0.46). The main effect of serial position also was reliable, $F(5,330) = 19.244$; $p < .001$, which reflects that the serial position curve was generally bow-shaped, with pronounced primacy and recency effects. Finally, cue condition and serial position did not interact, $F < 1$. As predicted, consistent part-set cues facilitated reconstruction performance in an incidental, everyday memory task.

CONCLUSION

The present chapter was designed to explore the theoretical accounts and everyday applications of part-set cuing inhibition and facilitation. Basic research suggests that two processes—strategy disruption and retrieval inhibition—are particularly important for these phenomena (e.g., Bauml & Aslan, 2006). However, more research is needed to further elucidate these processes and to determine whether other factors might also influence retention in the part-set paradigm. Moreover, additional research is needed to explore how part-set cuing might affect retention in real world settings, especially given that only a few, loosely-defined, applications of part-set cuing have been examined thus far (e.g., Reysen & Nairne, 2002; Weldon & Bellinger, 1997).

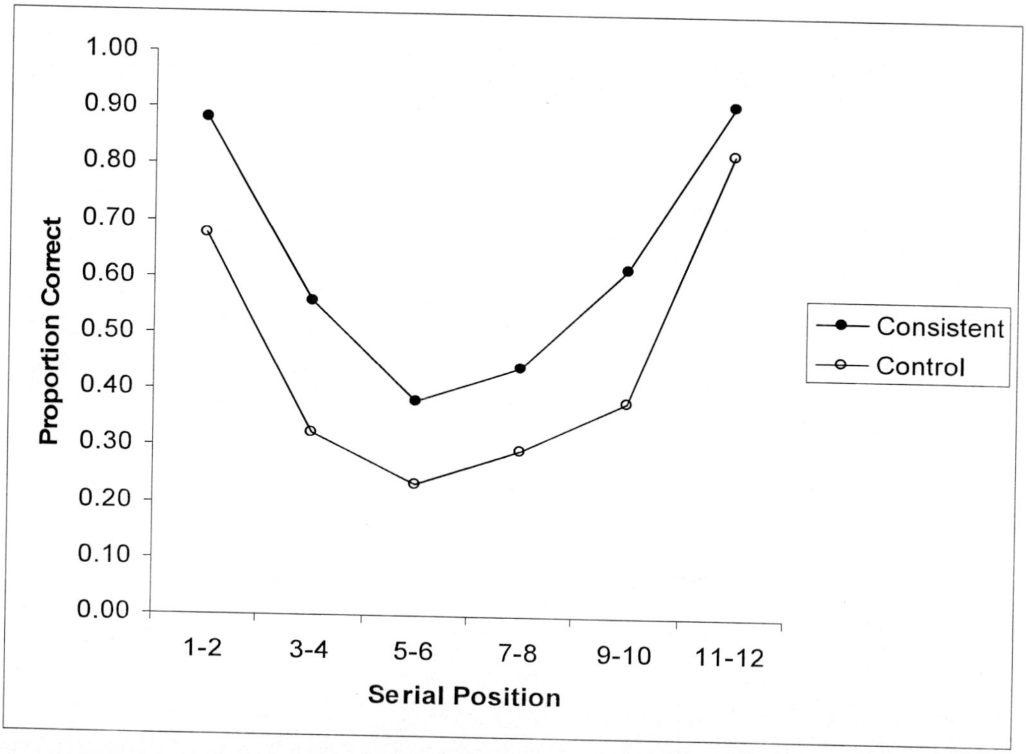

Figure 2. Proportion of correctly reconstructed items as a function of cue condition and serial position.

To this end, Experiments 1 and 2 served as initial forays into applied part-set research and they suggest that part-set cuing influences everyday retention outside the laboratory in very predictable ways. In the first experiment, whether participants learned a grocery list while visiting or viewing a grocery store, part-set cues (in the form of an incomplete grocery list) impaired their recall performance. These findings are consistent with much basic research showing that part-set cuing inhibition is the norm for free recall tasks (e.g., Nickerson, 1984). In the second experiment, first-time campus visitors showed a mnemonic benefit when remembering the sequence of buildings on their campus tour when they were provided with consistent part-set cues as compared to control cues. Such part-set cuing facilitation in the presence of consistent part-set cues is the norm when examining participants order retention (e.g., Serra & Nairne, 2000). Clearly, part-set cuing can influence memory in everyday settings but much more research is needed before we can comment on the ultimate scope and generality of these phenomena.

References

Anderson, M. C. (2003). Rethinking interference theory: Executive control and the mechanism of forgetting. *Journal of Memory and Language, 49,* 415–445.

Andersson, J., Hitch, G., and Meudell, P. (2006). Effects of the timing and identity of retrieval cues in individual recall: An attempt to mimic cross-cuing in collaborative recall. *Memory*, *14*(1), 94-103.

Basden, B. H., Basden, D. R., Bryner, S., and Thomas, R. L. (1997). A comparison of group and individual remembering: Does collaboration disrupt retrieval strategies? *Journal of Experimental Psychology: Learning, Memory, and Cognition, 23,* 1176-1191.

Basden, B. H., Basden, D. R., Church, B. A., and Beaupre, P. (1991). Setting boundary conditions on the part-set cuing effect. *Bulletin of the Psychonomic Society, 29*(3), 213-216.

Basden, B. H., Basden, D. R., and Stephens, J. P. (2002). Part-set cuing of order information in recall tests. *Journal of Memory and Language, 47*, 517-529.

Basden, D. R. (1973). Cued and uncued recall of unrelated words following interpolated learning. *Journal of Experimental Psychology, 98*, 429-431.

Basden, D. R., and Basden, B. H. (1995). Some tests of the strategy disruption interpretation of part-list cuing inhibition. *Journal of Experimental Psychology: Learning, Memory, and Cognition, 21*(6), 1656-1669.

Basden, D. R., Basden, B. H., and Galloway, B. C. (1977). Inhibition with part-list cuing: Some tests of the item strength hypothesis. *Journal of Experimental Psychology: Learning, Memory, and Cognition, 3*(1), 100-109.

Bauml, K. and Aslan, A. (2006). Part-list cuing can be transient and lasting: The role of encoding. *Journal of Experimental Psychology: Learning, Memory, and Cognition, 32*(1), 33-43.

Brown, A. S., and Hall, L. A. (1979). Part-list cueing inhibition in semantic memory structures. *American Journal of Psychology, 92*, 351-362.

Brown, J. (1968). Reciprocal facilitation and impairment in free recall. *Psychonomic Science, 10*, 41-42.

Dagnall, N., Parker, A., and Mulney, G. (2007). Social collaboration, inhibition, and context. *Psychological Reports, 100*, 691-699.

Kelley, M. R., and Bovee, J. C. (2007). Part-set cuing and memory for order. In A. Columbus (Ed.), *Advances in Psychology Research*. (Vol. 51, pp. 133-148). Hauppauge, NY: Nova Science.

Morris, C. D., Bransford, J. D., and Franks, J. J. (1977). Levels of processing versus transfer appropriate processing. *Journal of Verbal Learning and Verbal Behavior, 16*, 519-533.

Mueller, C. W., and Watkins, M. J. (1977). Inhibition from part-set cuing: A cue-overload interpretation. *Journal of Verbal Learning and Verbal Behavior, 16*, 699-709.

Nickerson, R. S. (1984). Retrieval inhibition from part-set cuing: A persisting enigma in memory research. *Memory and Cognition, 12*(6), 531-552.

Peynircioglu, Z. F. (1987). On the generality of the part-set cuing effect: Evidence from nonmemory tasks. *Journal of Experimental Psychology: Learning, Memory, and Cognition, 13*(3), 437-442.

Peynircioglu, Z. F. (1989). Part-set cuing effect with word-fragment cuing: Evidence against the strategy disruption and increased-list-length explanations. *Journal of Experimental Psychology: Learning, Memory, and Cognition, 15*(1), 147-152.

Raaijmakers, J. G. W., and Shiffrin, R. M. (1981). Search of associative memory. *Psychological Review, 88*(2), 93-134.

Reysen and Nairne (2002). Part-set cuing of false memories. *Psychonomic Bulletin and Review, 9*(2), 383-393.

Roediger, H. L. III. (1973). Inhibition in recall from cueing with recall targets. *Journal of Verbal Learning and Verbal Behavior, 12*(6), 644-657.

Roediger, H. L. III., and Tulving, E. (1974, May). Part-list cuing and directed forgetting. Paper presented at the meeting of the Midwestern Psychological Association, Chicago.

Rundus, D. (1973). Negative effects of using list items as recall cues. *Journal of Verbal Learning and Verbal Behavior, 12*, 43-50.

Serra, M., and Nairne, J. S. (2000). Part-set cuing of order information: Implication for associative theories of serial order memory. *Memory and Cognition, 28*(5), 847-855.

Serra, M. and Oswald, K. M. (2006). Part-list cuing of associative chains: Tests of strategy disruption. *Journal of General Psychology, 133*(3), 301-317.

Slamecka, N. J. (1968). An examination of trace storage in free recall. *Journal of Experimental Psychology, 76*(4), 504-513.

Slamecka, N. J. (1972). The question of associative growth in the learning of categorized material. *Journal of Verbal Learning and Verbal Behavior, 11*, 324-332.

Sloman, S. A., Bower, G. H., and Rohrer, D. (1991). Congruency effects in part-list cuing inhibition. *Journal of Experimental Psychology: Learning, Memory, and Cognition, 17*(5), 974-982.

Watkins, M. J. (1975). Inhibition in recall with extralist 'cues'. *Journal of Verbal Learning and Verbal Behavior, 14*, 294-303.

Weldon, M. S., and Bellinger, K. D. (1997). Collective memory: Collaborative and individual process in remembering. *Journal of Experimental Psychology: Learning, Memory, and Cognition, 23,* 1160-1175.

In: Applied Memory
Editor: Matthew R. Kelley
ISBN 978-1-60692-143-2

Chapter 6

HYPERMNESIA, REMINISCENCE, AND REPEATED TESTING

***Hajime Otani**[1], *Nicholas R. Von Glahn*[2], *Phillip N. Goenert*[3], *Mai Migita*[1], and *Robert L. Widner, Jr.*[1]**

[1] Department of Psychology, Central Michigan University, Mount Pleasant, MI, USA
[2] Department of Psychology and Sociology, California State Polytechnic University, Pomona, CA, USA
[3] Department of Psychology, Brandon University, Brandon, MB, Canada

ABSTRACT

Hypermnesia is a phenomenon in which memory performance improves across repeated tests even though no new exposure to the study material occurs between tests. Hypermnesia is a combined effect of reminiscence (item gains) and intertest forgetting (item losses). When reminiscence exceeds intertest forgetting, memory performance increases across repeated tests to produce hypermnesia. In this chapter, we review basic findings and theories and explore possible applications of hypermnesia. Based upon the review, we propose the following. In education, repeated testing can be used to maximize students' recall and promote long-term retention. In forensic settings, repeated testing can be used to uncover new information but repeated testing can also increase incorrect recall and distort source information. For older adults, we propose that a decline in reminiscence may indicate abnormal aging process. In clinical psychology, hypnotic hypermnesia is not a special case of hypermnesia but hypnosis can increase false confidence by highly hypnotizable individuals. Finally, we propose that hypermnesia is a normal memory phenomenon that should be included in a standardized memory scale to measure the level of memory functioning. We conclude the chapter by suggesting that the practitioners of repeated testing must be aware of the benefits and costs of repeating a test.

---

* Corresponding author.

Introduction

Hypermnesia is a term coined by Erdelyi and Becker (1974) to describe the finding that memory performance improves across repeated tests, even though participants are not re-exposed to the study material between tests. This phenomenon was first described by Ballard (1913). In his study, Ballard asked children to remember lines of a poem and tested their memory by repeating a test twice: immediately after studying the poem and two days later. The results showed that performance was better on the second day than on the first day. Ballard coined the term reminiscence to describe "the remembering again of the forgotten without re-learning" (p. 1). Interestingly, Ballard's finding did not ignite the interest of other researchers, mainly because there was confusion between reminiscence and hypermnesia. The former represents recovery of previously unrecalled items, whereas the latter represents improvement in performance across repeated tests. These two concepts are different because the latter includes intertest forgetting or forgetting of previously recalled items. That is, as a test is repeated, reminiscence may occur, but reminiscence does not guarantee hypermnesia because performance would not improve across tests if more items are lost (intertest forgetting) than are gained (reminiscence) on a repeated test. Because some experiments failed to find improvement across tests (hypermnesia), Ballard's finding was regarded as a "now you see it, now you don't" phenomenon (Buxton, 1943) and was neglected until the 1970's when Erdelyi and colleagues began their systematic investigation.

Basic Findings and Theories

In their pioneering study, Erdelyi and Becker (1974) asked participants to study words or pictures followed by a forced free recall test that was repeated three times. Between tests, participants were asked to either think quietly about the study items or to write any words that came to mind for 7 minutes. There was also a control group where the tests were repeated without an interval between tests. Erdelyi and Becker administered forced recall tests to control for a possible shift in response criterion. That is, participants may loosen their response criterion on a later test (i.e., start to output the items they withheld on a previous test), which may give an appearance of memory improvement. To control for this possibility, Erdelyi and Becker required participants to write a specific number of items (40 items) on each test. The results showed that memory performance improved as much as 20 percent across tests for pictures, whereas memory performance remained the same across tests for words. Two aspects of their results are notable. First, their results provided convincing evidence that memory can improve across tests even though participants are not re-exposed to the study material between tests. It is convincing because improvement in performance was not contaminated by a possible shift in response criterion. Second, improvement occurred only for pictures, indicating that whatever the reason, hypermnesia is material specific. It is important to note, however, that both of these points were later questioned. For instance, some researchers questioned whether forced tests are necessary (Otani and Whiteman, 1994; Roediger and Payne, 1985; but see Erdelyi, Finks, and Feigin-Pfau, 1989). Further, numerous studies have shown that verbal materials also produce hypermnesia, even though hypermnesia is more easily obtained with pictures than words (see Payne, 1987, for an extensive review).

Nevertheless, there is no doubt that these two points launched a new era in hypermnesia research.

Following Erdelyi and Becker (1974), numerous studies showed hypermnesia to be a robust phenomenon (but see Izawa, Hayden, and Franklin, 2005, for a possible objection to this statement). Most of these studies were conducted to test the theories of hypermnesia. The first theory was *the imagery hypothesis*, proposed by Erdelyi and Becker. Because hypermnesia occurred only with pictures, these researchers proposed that hypermnesia requires pictorial input. This hypothesis was later modified to include pictorial encoding because verbal materials processed pictorially also produced hypermnesia (e.g., Erdelyi, Finkelstein, Herrell, Miller, and Thomas, 1976). The imagery hypothesis was based on the Generate-Recognize model of memory (Hogan and Kintsch, 1974; Kintsch, 1970). This model assumes that recall requires generation of possible target items followed by the recognition of actual targets among the generated items. Erdelyi and Becker assumed that because pictures are more easily recognized than words, participants would have more time generating other targets on a repeated test if they were recalling pictures instead of words. A number of studies have supported this hypothesis (Erdelyi and Becker, 1974; Erdelyi et al., 1976; Erdelyi and Kleinbard, 1978; Madigan, 1976; Popkin and Small, 1979; Shapiro and Erdelyi, 1974; Yarmey, 1976). The problem with this hypothesis, however, is that a number of other studies showed that imagery is not necessary for hypermnesia to occur. For instance, Roediger and Thorpe (1978) asked participants to encode low and high imagery words by either creating visual images (imagery condition) or by thinking about the meaning of each word and its associates (semantic condition). The results showed that hypermnesia was present in both the imagery and semantic conditions, indicating that visual encoding is not necessary. However, hypermnesia was greater for high imagery words than for low imagery words, indicating that visual encoding may still play an important role.

By now, researchers generally agree that the imagery hypothesis is not a viable hypothesis. However, the literature does indicate that it is easier to find hypermnesia with pictures than with words. In an extensive review of the literature, Payne (1987) found that 90% of the studies that used pictures showed hypermnesia whereas only 50% of the studies that used words showed hypermnesia. Mandler (1994) reclassified these studies and showed that the common factor among the studies showing hypermnesia was elaborative encoding. Elaborative encoding was present in 86% of the studies that showed hypermnesia whereas elaborative encoding was present in only 9% of the studies that did not show hypermnesia. Accordingly, pictorial representation per se may not be important. Nevertheless, it would be useful to pursue further why the difference exists between pictures and words.

An alternative to the imagery hypothesis was proposed by Roediger and colleagues. This hypothesis, referred to as *the level of recall hypothesis*, was based on the observation that cumulative recall across each successive minute of testing was similar between a single 21-minute test and three 7-minute tests (Roediger and Thorpe, 1978). Two aspects of this observation are important. First, if cumulative recall (i.e., the number of unique items recalled so far) reaches asymptote at the end of the first test, recall performance would not improve across repeated tests because no new items would be added no matter how many times a test is repeated. Second, how quickly cumulative recall reaches asymptote is determined by the level of asymptote. It was observed that more time is needed for cumulative recall to reach asymptote when asymptote is higher. An implication of this observation is that if the asymptotic level is high enough, cumulative recall would continue to rise beyond the first test.

In other words, given that two conditions produce a different level of asymptotic recall, hypermnesia is more likely to occur in the condition that produces a higher level of asymptotic recall.

Roediger, Payne, Gillespie, and Lean (1982) tested this assumption in three experiments. In Experiment 1, encoding condition was manipulated as participants were asked to answer one of three questions (semantic, rhyme, or letter) about the study items. All three conditions produced hypermnesia using both net recall (the number of items correctly recalled on each test) and cumulative recall (the number of unique items recalled so far on each successive minute of testing). Further, consistent with the level of recall hypothesis, a positive relationship was found between the level of recall and the amount of hypermnesia. In Experiment 2, participants were presented with nonsense syllables that were either presented once or three times. Again, consistent with the level of recall hypothesis, hypermnesia was found with the condition that produced the highest recall level. In Experiment 3, Roediger et al. tested the notion that the level of recall, as opposed to the type of encoding, is responsible for hypermnesia. To eliminate the possible difference in encoding, semantic recall was examined. Participants were asked to recall from categories of different sizes (presidents = 39, birds = 75, sports = 96). The results confirmed the level of recall hypothesis by showing that hypermnesia was positively related to category size and the level of recall.

Initially, the level of recall hypothesis was regarded as more successful than the imagery hypothesis. However, soon it became apparent that this hypothesis needed further elaboration and modification. One reason is that the hypothesis failed to predict the results obtained by Payne (1986). In this study, Payne equated the recall level between pictures and words by presenting each item once, twice, or three times. He then examined cumulative recall to find the conditions that produced similar cumulative recall levels between words and pictures. The results showed that cumulative recall performance was similar between words and pictures when words were presented three times and pictures were presented twice, as well as when words were presented twice and pictures were presented once. However, despite the fact that cumulative recall was similar between words and pictures, hypermnesia was greater with pictures than with words. This finding revealed an important omission of the level of recall hypothesis. Because the hypothesis was based on cumulative recall, it did not take into account intertest forgetting. That is, even though two conditions may produce similar item gains, as shown by cumulative recall, the amount of improvement across tests would not be the same if intertest forgetting is different. The level of recall hypothesis does not have anything to say about intertest forgetting. The second weakness of the level of recall hypothesis was that the hypothesis itself was descriptive at best. Roediger and Challis (1989) agreed that the hypothesis was "a functional account of the phenomenon" (p. 192) and did not propose any "molecular theoretical mechanisms" (p. 192) that would explain the underlying processes of memory improvement.

Currently, two accounts provide alternatives to the level of recall hypothesis. One is a further elaboration of the level of recall hypothesis, which is based on two notions embedded in the Search of Associative Memory (SAM) model (Raaijmakers and Shiffrin, 1980, 1981; see Payne, Hembrooke, and Anastasi, 1993): *incrementing* and *alternative retrieval routes*. The notion of incrementing implies that as an item is repeatedly retrieved, it becomes progressively easier to retrieve because the strength of association between the stored image of the item and its retrieval cues become stronger. According to Payne et al. (1993), this notion would explain intertest forgetting in hypermnesia because as an item is repeatedly recalled across tests, this item becomes more resistant to forgetting. Reminiscence requires both notions of incrementing and alternative retrieval routes. As an item becomes easier to retrieve, more time would become available to search for previously unrecalled items. However, actually finding previously unrecalled items requires finding alternative retrieval routes. The notion of alternative retrieval routes is based on the idea that previously inaccessible items become accessible when new retrieval cues become available. The roles of incrementing and alternative retrieval routes have been documented in hypermnesia studies. For instance, the results of Roediger and Payne (1982) showed that the speed of retrieval increased as a test was repeated, indicating that recalling previously recalled items became progressively easier (incrementing). Further, Otani, Widner, Whiteman, and St. Louis (1999) reported that reminiscence was increased when additional cues were presented at encoding. Otani et al. assumed that extra cues provided at encoding acted as extra retrieval cues during retrieval, which enabled participants to find alternative retrieval routes. However, these notions do not account for the patterns of results that were observed when the type of processing was manipulated at encoding, as described below.

The alternative to the SAM-inspired account is the account based on notions of relational and item-specific processing proposed by Hunt and colleagues (Einstein and Hunt, 1980; Hunt and Einstein, 1981; Hunt and McDaniel, 1993). According to these researchers, relational processing emphasizes similarity among to-be-remembered items, whereas item-specific processing increases distinctness of each item. Based on this explanation, hypermnesia is a combined effect of relational and item-specific processing. In particular, Hunt and McDaniel (1993) proposed that relational processing reduces intertest forgetting, whereas item-specific processing increases reminiscence. One of the advantages of this account is its ability to explain the patterns of results that were observed when relational and item-specific processing were manipulated at encoding. When participants were asked to perform relational processing, hypermnesic improvement was greater between test 1 and test 2 than between test 2 and test 3 (early improvement). In contrast, when participants were asked to perform item-specific processing, improvement was greater between test 2 and test 3 than between test 1 and test 2 (late improvement). Hunt and colleagues offered the following explanation. Given that relational processing reduces intertest forgetting, improvement becomes visible early because item gains (i.e., reminiscence) exceed item losses (i.e., intertest forgetting). However, on subsequent tests, level of improvement declines because reminiscence approaches asymptote in a negatively accelerating fashion. The pattern is reversed for item-specific processing because, unlike relational processing, it does not reduce intertest forgetting. That is, even though item-specific processing facilitates reminiscence, improvement does not become apparent early on because item gains are masked by intertest forgetting. However, as intertest forgetting approaches asymptote on subsequent tests, improvement becomes more visible.

These patterns have been observed across several studies (e.g., Burns, 1993; Burns and Schoff, 1998; Klein, Loftus, Kihlstrom, and Aseron, 1989; McDaniel, Moore, and Whiteman, 1998), and as a result, a number of researchers have used these patterns to identify the presence or absence of item-specific processing (e.g., Burns and Gold, 1999; Burns, Jenkins, and Dean, 2007; Burns, Martens, Bertoni, Sweeney, and Lividini, 2006; Engelkamp and Seiler, 2003; Mulligan, 2002; Olofsson, 1997). However, despite its success in explaining these patterns, the exact mechanisms underlying the effect of relational and item-specific processing are still not clear. McDaniel et al. (1998) proposed that relational processing reduces intertest forgetting by promoting a consistent retrieval plan across tests, whereas item-specific processing facilitates reminiscence either via fluctuating retrieval cues during tests or by creating a richer memory representation at encoding. Although these proposals are reasonable, there have not been direct tests of these ideas.

Current State of the Literature. Based on research so far, the following conclusions seem warranted. First, hypermnesia is not an artifact, even though some studies in the past have failed to observe it (see Erdelyi, 1996; Izawa et al., 2005; Payne, 1987). Second, for whatever the reason, hypermnesia is easier to obtain with pictures than with words (see Erdelyi, 1996; Payne, 1987). Third, forced tests are not necessary (Otani and Whiteman, 1994; Roediger and Payne, 1985), yet researchers need to be aware of potential threats posed by shifting response criterion (Erdelyi et al., 1989; see also Erdelyi, 1996)—especially when samples from different populations, such as young versus older adults, are compared (e.g., Widner, Otani, and Smith, 2000). Fouth, hypermnesia is difficult to obtain in recognition (Otani and Hodge, 1991; Otani and Stimson, 1994; Payne and Roediger, 1987; also see Otani, Kato, and Widner, 2005), unless a non-standard method of testing is adopted to emphasize active retrieval during tests (Erdelyi and Stein, 1981; Groninger and Murray, 2004; Kazén and Solís-Macías, 1999). Fifth, repeatedly recalling items make these items more resistant to forgetting; that is, repeating a test three times is not the same as administering a single test with the same duration (Mulligan, 2005). Sixth, hypermnesia is difficult to observe with older adults (Finkel, Fox, and McGue, 1995; Otani, Kato, Von Glahn, Nelson, Widner, and Goernert, 2008; Widner et al., 2000) unless memory being tested is autobiographical in nature (Bluck, Levine, and Laulhere, 1999). Seventh, hypermnesia has also been demonstrated with collective recall; that is, when multiple individuals recall information together (e.g., Weldon and Bellinger, 1997). In the following section, we will describe possible applications of hypermnesia and repeated testing.

EDUCATION

Two aspects of hypermnesia are well suited for application in educational settings. One is that memory retrieval can be maximized through repeated testing, which allows teachers to assess students' memory of the material more accurately. Besides, differences in test scores by as little as 10% can make a substantial difference in a student's final grade (e.g., an "A" instead of a "B"). Unfortunately, none of our students would embrace the idea that they have to take the same test multiple times, especially when there is no study period between tests. Still, research suggests that repeating tests does improve memory scores for educationally relevant materials, as shown by Otani and Griffith (1998). These researchers used two types of prose material: fairy tale and expository passage. They also manipulated encoding strategies, relational and item-specific processing, which were adopted from Einstein, McDaniel, Owen, and Cote (1990). Participants in the relational processing condition were asked to order the sentences that were presented on cards to create a coherent story, whereas participants in the item-specific processing condition were asked to fill in blanks with letters to make the paragraph comprehensible. There was also a control condition where participants were asked to read the paragraph. Three free recall tests were administered with a 2-minute "think" interval between tests during which participants were asked to think about the passage silently. The results were as expected; significant improvement in performance (i.e., hypermnesia) was observed in both the relational and item-specific processing conditions, with as much as 33% improvement across three tests. Other studies have also shown hypermnesia with prose materials—Ballard (1913) using a poem and Wheeler and Roediger (1992) using Bartlett's (1932) "War of Ghosts." It is, therefore, safe to conclude that hypermnesia can be obtained with educationally relevant materials. The question is how to convince teachers and students that repeating the same tests multiple times, without a study period between tests, is beneficial.

The second aspect of hypermnesia, which is suited for educational application, is that by repeating a test, one can promote long term retention. Perhaps, this would convince teachers and students that repeating a test is not a waste of time. Roediger and Karpicke (2006a) recently published a thorough review of this phenomenon, referred to as the testing effect. In essence, this effect shows that a test is more than an assessment tool; it can be used to enhance long-term retention. For instance, Roediger and Karpicke (2006b) showed the effect using educationally relevant material (i.e., prose). In Experiment 1, they asked participants to study a passage followed by another study period (Study-Study or SS) or a test (Study-Test or ST). Participants then took a final test after a 5-minute, 2-day, or 1-week delay. The results indicated that the SS condition outperformed the ST condition at the 5-minute interval. However, for the 2-day and 1-week intervals, the ST condition showed better performance than the SS condition. Thus, taking a test enhanced the long-term retention of the material. In Experiment 2, Roediger and Karpicke compared the efficacy of taking a single test and multiple tests before the final test. In the STTT condition, participants took three tests after studying a passage, whereas in the SSST condition, participants studied the passage three times and took a single test. In a control condition, participants studied the passage four times without a test (SSSS condition). The final retention test occurred either after 5 minutes or one week later for all conditions. The results indicated that, at the short retention interval, performance was better with more study periods (i.e., SSSS > SSST > STTT). However, following a one-week retention interval, the pattern was reversed; taking more tests was better. The advantage of the STTT condition relative to the other conditions makes sense based on hypermnesia research. As mentioned earlier, repeatedly retrieving items makes those items more resistant to forgetting (Mulligan, 2005). Consistent with such an observation, Roediger and Karpicke found that forgetting over a one-week period was inversely related to the amount of testing (i.e., STTT < SSST < SSSS). The testing effect is a robust effect that occurs with both recall and recognition (see Roediger and Karpicke, 2006a). In light of such findings, telling students to study more may not be appropriate; instead, students should be told to spend more time testing what they have studied.

Eyewitness Memory

Eyewitness memory is another obvious application of hypermnesia. The goal of interviewing eyewitnesses is to obtain as much information as possible about the witnessed event, and therefore, anything that increases memory for the to-be-remembered event, including repeated testing, should be helpful to crime investigators. In fact, several studies have supported this claim. For instance, Scrivner and Safer (1988) asked participants to watch a two-minute video clip of a staged crime and then tested participants over four consecutive tests to examine how many forensically relevant details they could remember. Scrivner and Safer found that participants continued to remember more information across all four repeated tests; thus, finding hypermnesia for eyewitness materials. Interestingly, this increase in memory performance was not restricted to the first three tests, which were administered with only a short-interval between tests, but instead, memory performance continued to improve between the third and fourth test, which were separated by 48 hours.

Similar effects of repeated testing have been reported with children. La Rooy, Pipe and Murray (2005) asked children (approximately 5 to 6 years of age) to interact with a "friendly-pirate" who engaged in 20 event-activities with the children. These children were interviewed immediately after their interaction with the pirate and then again 24 hours later (Experiment 1). During the interview, children were asked to recall everything they could recall about the visit with the pirate, followed by four open-ended questions asking about some specific aspects of the visit. Their recall protocol was scored for 55 actions and objects that were associated with the 20 event-activities. The results showed that correctly recalled details increased across the repeated interviews, showing hypermnesia. However, when these children were interviewed after a 6-month delay (without the four specific questions), no hypermnesia was observed across three free recall tests that were separated by 5-minute intervals (Experiment 2). In Experiment 3, participants were interviewed once immediately after the visit and twice after a 6-month delay, with 24 hours separating the latter two interviews. The results showed that correctly recalled details decreased from the first (immediate) to the second interview (the initial interview after 6 months) and stayed the same from the second to the third interview (the second interview after 6 months)—that is, no hypermnesia. But, what was remarkable was that in both Experiments 2 and 3, the cumulative recall (i.e., reminiscence) increased across interviews. Apparently, these children could recall new details even after a 6-month retention interval. However, repeating interviews did come with costs; errors increased across repeated interviews in all three experiments. In terms of percentage, errors were much greater when the retention interval was 6 months (Experiments 2 and 3: 30% and 44%, respectively) than when the retention interval was short (Experiment 1: 8%). La Rooy et al., therefore, recommended that repeated interviews with children should be conducted when their memories are still "fresh" (p. 250).

One of the key differences between eyewitness events and other types of to-be-remembered materials is the emotionality of the event. That is, in a forensic setting, the witnessed event is often a crime and tends to be emotionally arousing (e.g., seeing someone wielding a gun). Fortunately, hypermnesia was reported with emotionally arousing materials. Bornstein, Liebel, and Scarberry (1998) asked participants to watch either a short film that contained a violent event or the same film with the violent event being edited out. The film had three segments: the initial scene showing the events prior to the violent event, the violent event, and the follow-up scene showing the events after the violence. After viewing the film, participants completed three forced recall tests that were separated by 5-minute "think" intervals during which participants were asked to think about the film they viewed. The results showed that recall performance increased across three tests, for all three segments of the film, and for both the violent and non-violent films. Interestingly, the initial and the last segments showed an advantage for the non-violent film, despite the fact that these two segments were identical for both versions of the film. These results were consistent with the notion that emotional arousal creates anterograde and retrograde amnesia. In contrast, for the middle segment, participants recalled more details from the violent film than from the non-violent film, showing what is referred to as, *emotionally enhanced memory* (Talmi, Schimmack, Paterson, and Moscovitch, 2007). With regard to errors, Bornstein et al. found that errors increased across three tests for both the violent and non-violent films. However, Bornstein et al. also noted that the number of errors was low (M = 1.5 and 1.6 for the third test, for the violent and the non-violent film, respectively), supporting La Rooy et al.'s (2005) conclusion that the increased error rate associated with repeated testing is not a serious problem when the retention interval is relatively short.

In our own laboratory, we (Kern, Libkuman, and Otani, 2002) used pictures from the International Affective Picture System (IAPS: Lang, Bradley, and Cuthbert, 1999) to manipulate arousal. We asked participants to view 23 slides that were either emotionally arousing or emotionally neutral. Because witnessing a crime often involves negative emotion, we used arousing pictures with negative valance (i.e., unpleasant). Three free recall tests were administered with a 5-minute think interval between tests. On these tests, participants were asked to write one word or a short phrase that described each recalled picture. The results were consistent with Bornstein et al. (1998) with one exception: recall performance did not increase across tests for neutral pictures. In contrast, arousing pictures produced hypermnesia. We are still not sure why we failed to observe hypermnesia with neutral pictures. At least, we know that the results were unlikely to be a Type II error because using the same pictures, Migita (2007) obtained the same results. We are currently pursuing the possibility that, just like words, pictures differ in multiple dimensions, in addition to arousal and valence, and that these additional dimensions may also influence whether memory increases across repeated tests (see Libkuman, Otani, Kern, Viger, and Novak, 2007, for the norms that include more than arousal and valence). In terms of the number of errors, we also observed an increase in errors across three tests.

Based on these studies, it seems clear that repeatedly interviewing eyewitnesses would yield additional information. However, some researchers are still not convinced of the benefit of repeated interviews because, although all studies have shown reminiscence across repeated tests, there have been cases where researchers have failed to find hypermnesia due to increased intrusions and intertest forgetting (Eugenio, Buckhout, Kostes, and Ellison, 1982; Turtle and Yuille, 1994). In particular, Turtle and Yuille (1994) called into question the results of Scrivner and Safer (1988) by arguing that their procedure was not ecologically valid because they used too short of a retention interval and that in a real forensic situation, eyewitnesses are not given a timed recall test (e.g., 7 minutes to complete the test). Therefore, Turtle and Yuille told their participants that the memory task should take approximately 20 minutes, but in practice they gave participants as much time as they wanted to recall all relevant information about the to-be-remembered event. Afterwards, these researchers asked participants to complete the recall task again after a one, two, and three-week delay. The results indicated that there was reminiscence across the tests, but not hypermnesia. To further demonstrate their point, Turtle and Yuille demonstrated hypermnesia with their to-be-remembered event using procedures more similar to Scrivner and Safer (i.e., three consecutive 7-minute tests with a 5-minute delay interval between tests).

There are also other factors that determine how effectively repeated tests would improve memory for an eyewitness event. For instance, Dunning and Stern (1992) found that participants showed an increase in memory across repeated tests (i.e., hypermnesia) when a free-recall test was used, but when the subjects were asked to complete a multiple-choice test about the event, participants neither displayed hypermnesia nor an increase in incorrect recall across tests. Therefore, this study showed that even for eyewitness memory, it is difficult to show hypermnesia with repeated recognition tests.

In sum, it appears that using forensically relevant materials, repeated testing would produce hypermnesia when the retention interval is relatively short and when free recall is used. Further, repeated testing would yield new details (i.e., reminiscence) even after a long delay. However, with long delays, increased error rates would become a concern. Therefore, caution needs to be exercised when using repeated interviews. The same point will be made in the next section regarding the effect of repeated testing on source memory. Thus, in a forensic setting, repeatedly interviewing witnesses may yield benefits (i.e., reminiscence) but one needs to be concerned about the costs (i.e., increased errors).

SOURCE MEMORY

In a forensic setting, remembering relevant information is obviously very important; however, oftentimes, remembering where the information came from is equally important. For instance, you may vaguely remember that someone said, "I will kill you." But, did you actually hear it or imagine hearing it? Was it a man's voice or a woman's voice? Where did you hear it? In the memory literature, the former type of information (i.e., what it was) is known as item memory, whereas the latter type (i.e., where it came from) is known as source memory (Johnson, Hashtroudi, and Lindsay, 1993). The majority of studies investigated hypermnesia with item memory; however, a few studies investigated hypermnesia with source memory. For instance, Henkel (2004) asked participants to view pictures or imagine viewing pictures. Their memory was tested by either item recall or source recall. On item recall tests, participants were asked to recall presented items, whereas on source recall tests, participants were asked to recall presented items and indicate whether each recalled item was presented as a picture or an imagined item. Each type of test was repeated three times without study periods between tests. The results indicated that item recall increased across tests, showing a typical hypermnesic effect. However, source errors, defined by claiming imagined items as seen items, also increased as the test was repeated. Further, source errors were greater when imagined items were conceptually or physically similar to the seen items relative to when imagined items were not similar to the seen items. Henkel (2007) recently reported that source errors were more pronounced for older adults than younger adults, especially when the imagined items were similar to the seen items. These results revealed yet another peril of repeating a test—namely, it can distort one's source memory.

Using a different paradigm, we also found similar results (Goernert, 2005; Goernert, Widner, and Otani, 2006; 2007). The paradigm we used was referred to as *directed forgetting*, where participants were asked to remember some items and to forget other items, even though after the presentation, memory of both to-be-remembered and to-be-forgotten items was tested. We repeated tests three times without study periods between tests to investigate hypermnesia of both *remember* and *forget* items. The results indicated that recall of both remember and forget items increased across tests for words (Goernert, 2005) and pictures (Goernert et al., 2006; 2007) using a list method, where remember and forget instructions were provided for different lists (Goernert, 2005) as well as using an item method, where remember and forget instructions were provided after each item (Goernert et al., 2006; 2007). What was interesting was that even though item memory increased across tests, source memory apparently declined across tests. When we asked participants to classify the recalled items into remember and forget items, participants misclassified some items, and these classification errors increased across tests.

Kelley and Nairne (2003) used yet another paradigm showing the difficulty of obtaining hypermnesia with source memory. In this paradigm, these researchers investigated the effect of repeated testing on memory for order. Participants were asked to study five lists of five items (words or pictures). Following presentation, participants were asked to take either three recall tests or three reconstruction tests without study periods between tests. On reconstruction tests, participants were given all the items they studied (in a new order) and were asked to reconstruct the lists by putting the items in the correct lists in the correct order within the list. Three experiments showed that recall performance increased across tests, whereas reconstruction performance declined across tests. It is interesting to note that Kelley and Nairne observed reminiscence with reconstruction tests; however, overall performance of reconstruction tests declined across tests because more order information was lost, relative to what was gained, as the test was repeated.

Similar findings were reported by Kelley and Lehman (2006) using naturalistic material. In this study, Kelley and Lehman presented a series of images that depicted the events that are associated with going to a cafeteria. Two different orders were used to present the images: logical and random. In the logical order condition, the images were arranged in a natural order of going to cafeteria (i.e., arrive at the cafeteria, take a tray, wait in line, etc), whereas in the random condition, the images were randomly ordered. On a reconstruction test, participants were asked to arrange the images, which were presented in a new random order, in the order of presentation by writing the letter assigned to each image (A-T). The reconstruction test, which lasted 7 minutes, was repeated twice without a study period between tests. The results indicated that performance declined across tests for the random order condition, whereas performance stayed the same across tests for the logical order condition. The random order condition also showed reminiscence and intertest forgetting, whereas the logical order condition did not. Kelley and Lehman attributed the lack of change in scores across tests in the logical order condition to a ceiling effect. It appears that participants could take advantage of their script knowledge (e.g., Schank and Abelson, 1977) of going to a cafeteria to reconstruct the order quite well in the logical order condition. However, in the random order condition, repeated testing distorted order information because participants could not use their script knowledge.

As shown, all three paradigms have produced consistent results; item memory increased across tests, whereas source memory decreased across tests. In terms of practical applications, probing one's memory multiple times, as is routinely done in forensic settings, would risk distorting source information. Although repeated interviewing would yield additional information, it may be wise not to rely too much on repeated testing for source information.

Aging

As mentioned earlier, studies have shown that hypermnesia is difficult to obtain with older adults. Widner et al. (2000) tested young and older adults using monosyllabic words (Experiment 1) and line drawings (Experiment 2). Participants were asked to study a stimulus list, which was followed by three free recall tests. The results showed that recall performance improved across tests only for young adults in both experiments. Interestingly, reminiscence was similar between young and older adults, indicating that their ability to recover previously unrecalled items was still intact. However, older adults showed greater intertest forgetting than young adults, indicating that their ability to maintain what they recalled on previous tests was deficient. Similar findings were reported by Finkel et al. (1995), who asked young and older adults to study pairs of high imagery words along with line drawings of these words. Two free recall tests were administered. The results indicated that although more young adults showed hypermnesia than older adults, reminiscence was similar between the groups. In contrast, intertest forgetting was greater for older adults than for young adults. Finkel et al.'s explanation was based on the notions of relational and item-specific processing—presumably, older adults showed intact reminiscence because their ability to process item-specific information was intact (Luszcz, Roberts, and Mattiske, 1990), whereas older adults showed greater intertest forgetting because their ability to process relational information was deficient (Luszcz et al., 1990). The results of these studies were contrasted by the results reported by Bluck et al. (1999), which indicated that hypermnesia is similar between young and older adults. In this study, Bluck et al. investigated the memory of the television coverage of the reading of O. J. Simpson's verdict. Three interviews were administered, one after the other, approximately eight months after the televised verdict. The results showed that both young and older adults produced similar improvement in memory performance across the three interviews.

One obvious difference between Bluck et al. (1999) and the other two studies was that Bluck et al. used a video material, instead of words and pictures. Because in the past, hypermnesia was shown to be material specific (e.g., it is easier to obtain hypermnesia with pictures than words), Otani et al. (2008) suspected that hypermnesia in older adults was also material specific (i.e., only occurs with video materials). These researchers, therefore, used a 3-minute video clip, which was followed by two free recall tests. The results indicated that young adults showed improvement across two tests and older adults did not. However, when each age group was divided into low and high memory groups based on their scores on the first test, the older high memory group showed hypermnesia, whereas the older low memory group did not. In contrast, for young adults, both the low and high memory groups showed hypermnesia. Interestingly, the mean age of the participants in the older low memory group was significantly older than the mean age of the participants in the older high memory group. Hypermnesia, therefore, was inversely related to age. Further, reminiscence was similar between young and older adults in both the low and high memory groups, whereas intertest forgetting was greater for older adults, than young adults, in the low memory group but was similar between young and older adults in the high memory group.

Based on these results, it is clear that the ability to recover previously unrecalled items is intact in older adults. We propose that this aspect of aging memory can be used to detect abnormal aging processes. Perhaps, a decline in one's ability to recover previously unrecalled items (i.e., deficiency in reminiscence) may be diagnostic that something is amiss. We are currently trying to compare reminiscence between normal older adults and those who are suspected of having cognitive impairments.

Clinical Psychology

It is important to note that the term hypermnesia is sometimes used differently in clinical psychology. For instance, on the editorial of a special issue on learning, memory, and psychopathology, Elzinga and van den Hout (2008) wrote that hypermnesia and hypomnesia are two instances of "memory peculiarities" (p. 511) that are exhibited by clinical populations. In this paper, they defined hypermnesia as "intrusions, flashbacks, as in Posttraumatic Stress Disorder (PTSD)" (p. 511). Similarly, Linscott and Knight (2001) examined automatic hypermnesia or "exaggerated influence of automatic memory processes" (p. 577) in schizophrenia. As such, in clinical psychology, the term hypermnesia does not always imply the same phenomenon as the one presented in this book chapter.

As far as we are aware, clinical applications of hypermnesia, as Erdelyi and Becker (1974) defined it, have not been explored. However, as Erdelyi (1996) describes it in his book, hypermnesia and reminiscence have been routinely observed in the clinics of dynamic psychologists, including Janet, Breuer, and Freud. Perhaps, a notable exception to this lack of attention to hypermnesia and reminiscence in clinical psychology is in the area of hypnosis, a technique used by various psychologists since late 19th century to bring back lost memories into consciousness. In particular, researchers have been investigating whether hypnotic hypermnesia—enhanced recall under hypnosis—is the same hypermnesia phenomenon that is observed while people are awake, or whether it is actually induced by the hypnotic state. In a typical experiment, a memory test (R1) is administered prior to putting participants under hypnosis, and another test is administered while participants are under hypnotic state (R2). Using this paradigm, it would be difficult to determine whether the improvement across R1 to R2 simply reflects the effect of repeated testing (i.e., hypermnesia) or the effect of hypnosis (i.e., hypnotic hypermnesia). Based on an extensive review of the literature, Erdelyi (1994; 1996) concluded that hypnotic hypermnesia is not a special case of hypermnesia because improvement in memory across repeated tests occurs to the same degree, regardless of whether one is under hypnosis or being wake. Furthermore, laboratory-based hypermnesia and hypnotic hypermnesia show a striking family resemblance. That is, just like regular hypermnesia, hypnotic hypermnesia is material specific, being more likely to occur with meaningful materials, such as prose, pictures, and words, than with meaningless materials, such as nonsense syllables (see Erdelyi, 1994; 1996). Furthermore, just like regular hypermnesia, researchers have failed to find hypnotic hypermnesia with recognition (see Erdelyi, 1994; 1996). Therefore, it seems safe to conclude that hypnotic hypermnesia is nothing more than regular hypermnesia. Importantly, however, there may be a cost associated with recalling under hypnosis, namely, inflated confidence that incorrect items are correct.

For instance, Nogrady, McConkey, and Perry (1985) administered six recall tests, which were divided into three phases. During Phase I, participants took two free recall tests (recalling the names of the studied line drawings) under normal waking state. During Phase II, participants were divided into three conditions: hypnosis, imagination, and control.

Participants in the hypnosis condition received hypnosis induction; participants in the imagination condition received "imagination enhancement" exercise (i.e., solving a puzzle using imagery strategies); and participants in the control condition were simply told to solve a puzzle. After these procedures, participants took two free recall tests. Phase III was the post-hypnotic period during which the effect of post-hypnotic suggestion was examined. Participants from all three conditions took two tests, with participants in the hypnotic condition being told that they would experience post-hypnotic hypermnesia. The results showed that regardless of the conditions, the number of correctly and incorrectly recalled items increased across tests. What differed among the conditions was the number of incorrect items that participants rated as "very sure." A significant three-way interaction involving condition, hypnotizability, and tests indicated that, relative to any other conditions, highly hypnotizable participants in the hypnosis condition had a stronger tendency to rate incorrect items as "very sure" on the last three tests.

Similar findings were reported by Whitehouse, Dinges, Orne, and Orne (1988). These researchers asked high and low hypnotizable participants to take two forced cued-recall tests, with half the participants in both groups taking the second test (R2) under hypnosis. The results indicated that all groups showed a similar increase in performance from R1 to R2. Further, the number of new items recalled (i.e., reminiscence) on R2 was similar across the conditions. However, an increase in confidence ratings from R1 to R2 for incorrectly recalled items was greater for highly hypnotizable participants in the hypnosis condition relative to the other conditions. Based on these results, it appears that under hypnosis, highly hypnotizable individuals have a tendency to inflate confidence that incorrect items are correct. Practitioners of hypnosis, therefore, must keep this tendency in mind.

Aside from the area of hypnosis, we are not aware of any other specific applications of hypermnesia in clinical psychology (other than the regular practice of repeatedly interviewing clients). However, we wish to emphasize that hypermnesia is a reliable phenomenon and therefore, it could be incorporated in a memory scale as a measure of normally functioning memory. In particular, reminiscence and intertest forgetting might be used to index the level of memory functioning. As mentioned earlier, three studies (Finkel et al., 1995; Otani et al. 2008; Widner et al., 2000) reported that reminiscence is similar between young and older adults, whereas older adults show greater intertest forgetting than young adults. Our current goal is to extend our investigation into other populations, such as Parkinson's patients, whose symptoms include memory impairment, to determine whether reminiscence and intertest forgetting can be diagnostic of their level of memory functioning.

CONCLUSION

Hypermnesia is the basic finding that memory performance improves across repeated tests, even though participants are not exposed to the study material between tests. As shown, the phenomenon has potential applications in education, eyewitness memory, aging, and clinical psychology. However, as mentioned, when applying this phenomenon to the real world, one needs to be aware of the benefits as well as the costs of repeating a test. The first, and obvious, benefit of repeated testing is that, as a test is repeated, new information (i.e., reminiscence) often emerges. Clearly, this would be beneficial when one's goal is to access information that may be available in memory but is difficult to retrieve—as in educational settings when teachers are trying to assess students' true knowledge or in forensic settings when investigators are trying to uncover what witnesses can remember about a crime. Another benefit of repeated testing is that repeatedly retrieved information becomes more resistant to forgetting. This would be beneficial when one's goal is to facilitate long-term retention. Apparently, repeated testing is a more effective method of promoting long-term retention than repeated studying.

Importantly, however, one needs keep in mind the costs of repeated testing. As mentioned earlier, studies have shown that incorrect recall can increase as a test is repeated for both item and source memory. In a laboratory, it is easy to differentiate between correct and incorrect recall because the to-be-remembered materials are controlled by the experimenters. However, in some applied settings (e.g., forensic) it is often difficult, if not impossible, to know whether a given piece of information represents correct or incorrect recall because verifying the information against the original event is almost impossible. Unfortunately, based on hypermnesia research, consistency across repeated tests is not diagnostic of correct recall because incorrect recall can be repeated across tests as much as correct recall can be repeated. Further, correct recall can emerge as a test is repeated as much as incorrect recall can. In addition, correct recall can be lost as a test is repeated as much as incorrect recall can be lost. Based on these considerations, practitioners, particularly in the forensic area, must strike a balance between the benefits and costs of repeated testing. In other areas, where the practitioners have the control over to-be-remembered materials, as in the area of detecting memory impairment, one may not need to be concerned about the costs associate with repeated testing. And, this is where we see the greatest potential of applying repeated testing. For instance, repeated testing can be used to assess the level of memory functioning by clinical patients. Because to-be-remembered materials are controlled by the testers, increased errors would not be a problem. Perhaps, the error rate can also indicate the level of memory functioning along with reminiscence and intertest forgetting.

In conclusion, there is a need to further explore the application of hypermnesia and repeated testing. In the real world, repeatedly probing memory is more of a norm than simply probing memory once. For instance, if one is unable to remember a piece of information, he/she would keep on trying to remember rather than to give up after a single retrieval attempt. As such, in our opinion, studying memory using repeated testing would have more potential for real world applications than studying memory using only a single test.

References

Ballard, P. B. (1913). Oblivescence and reminiscence. *British Journal of Psychology Monograph Supplements, 1*, 1-82.

Bartlett, F. C. (1932). *Remembering*. Cambridge: Cambridge University Press.

Bluck, S., Levine, L. J., and Laulhere, T. M. (1999). Autobiographical remembering and hypermnesia: A comparison of older and younger adults. *Psychology and Aging, 14*, 671-682.

Bornstein, B. H., Liebel, L. M., and Scarberry, N. C. (1998). Repeated testing in eyewitness memory: A means to improve recall of a negative emotional event. *Applied Cognitive Psychology, 12,* 119-131.

Burns, D. J. (1993). Item gains and losses during hypermnesic recall: Implications for the item-specific-relational information distinction. *Journal of Experimental Psychology: Learning, Memory, and Cognition, 19*, 163-173.

Burns, D. J., and Gold, D. (1999). An analysis of item gains and losses in retroactive interference. *Journal of Experimental Psychology: Learning, Memory, and Cognition, 25*, 978-985.

Burns, D. J., Jenkins, C. L., and Dean, E. E. (2007). Falsely recalled items are rick in item-specific information. *Memory & Cognition, 35*, 1630-1640.

Burns, D. J., Martens, N. J., Bertoni, A. A., Sweeney, E. J., and Lividini, M. D. (2006). An item gains and losses analysis of false memories suggests critical items receive more item-specific processing than list items. *Journal of Experimental Psychology: Learning, Memory, and Cognition, 32*, 277-289.

Burns, D. J., and Schoff, K. M. (1998). Slow and steady often ties the race: Effects of item-specific and relational processing on cumulative recall. *Journal of Experimental Psychology: Learning, Memory, and Cognition, 24*, 1041-1051.

Buxton, C. E. (1943). The status of research in reminiscence. *Psychological Bulletin, 40*, 313-340.

Dunning, D., and Stern, L. B. (1992). Examining the generality of eyewitness hypermnesia: A close look at time delay and question type. *Applied Cognitive Psychology, 6,* 643-657.

Einstein, G. O., and Hunt, R. R. (1980). Levels of processing and organization: Additive effects of individual-item and relational processing. *Journal of Experimental Psychology: Human Learning and Memory, 6*, 588-598.

Einstein, G. O., McDaniel, M. A., Owen, P. D., and Cote, N. C. (1990). Encoding and recall of texts: The importance of material appropriate processing. *Journal of Memory and Language, 29*, 566-581.

Elzinga, B. M., and van den Hout, M. (2008). Special issue: Learning, memory, and psychopathology. *Acta Psychologica, 127*, 511-512.

Engelkamp, J., and Seiler, K. H. (2003). Gains and losses in action memory. *Quarterly Journal of Experimental Psychology A: Human Experimental Psychology, 56A*, 829-848.

Erdelyi, M. H. (1994). Hypnotic hypermnesia: The empty set of hypermnesia. International *Journal of Clinical and Experimental Hypnosis, 42*, 379-390.

Erdelyi, M. H. (1996). *The recovery of unconscious memories: Hypermnesia and reminiscence.* Chicago: University of Chicago Press.

Erdelyi, M. H., and Becker, J. (1974). Hypermnesia for pictures: Incremental memory for pictures but not for words in multiple recall trials. *Cognitive Psychology, 6*, 159-171.

Erdelyi, M. H., Finks, J., and Feigin-Pfau, M. B. (1989). The effect of response bias on recall performance, with some observations on processing bias. *Journal of Experimental Psychology: General, 118*, 245-254.

Erdelyi, M. H., Finkelstein, N., Herrell, B., Miller, B. and Thomas, J. (1976). Coding modality vs. input modality in hypermnesia: Is a rose a rose a rose? *Cognition, 4*, 311-319.

Erdelyi, M. H., and Kleinbard, J. (1978). Has Ebbinghaus decayed with time? The growth of recall over days. *Journal of Experimental Psychology: Human Learning and Memory, 4,* 275-289.

Erdelyi, M. H., and Stein, J. B. (1981). Recognition hypermnesia: The growth of recognition memory (*d'*) over time with repeated testing. *Cognition, 9*, 23-33.

Eugenio, P., Buckhout, R., Kostes, S., and Ellison, K. W. (1982). Hypermnesia in the eyewitness to a crime. *Bulletin of the Psychonomic Society, 19,* 83-86.

Finkel, D., Fox, P. W., and McGue, M. (1995). Age differences in hypermnesia: Word gain versus word loss. *Experimental Aging Research, 21*, 33-46.

Goernert, P. N. (2005). Source monitoring accuracy across repeated tests following directed forgetting. *British Journal of Psychology*, *96*, 231-247

Goernert, P. N., Widner, R. L., Jr., and Otani, H. (2006). Segregation accuracy in item-method directed forgetting across multiple tests. *British Journal of Psychology, 97,* 245-258.

Goernert, P. N., Widner, R. L., Jr., and Otani, H. (2007). Classification accuracy across multiple tests following item-method directed forgetting. *Quarterly Journal of Experimental Psychology, 60, 1178-1186.*

Groninger, L. D., and Murray, K. N. (2004). Reminiscence, forgetting, hypermnesia using face-name learning: Isolating the effects using recall and recognition memory measures. *Memory, 12*, 351-365.

Henkel, L. A. (2004). Erroneous memories arising from repeated attempts to remember. *Journal of Memory and Language*, *50*, 26–46

Henkel, L. A. (2007). The benefits and costs of repeated memory tests for young and older adults. *Psychology and Aging*, *22*, 580-595.

Hogan, R. M., and Kintsch, W. (1974). Differential effects of study and test trials in long-term recognition and recall. *Journal of Verbal Learning and Verbal Behavior, 10*, 562-567.

Hunt, R. R., and Einstein, R. R. (1981). Relational and item-specific information in memory. *Journal of Verbal Learning and Verbal Behavior, 19*, 497-514.

Hunt, R. R., and McDaniel, M. A. (1993). The enigma of organization and distinctiveness. *Journal of Memory and Language, 32*, 421-445.

Johnson, M. K., Hashtroudi, S., and Lindsay, D. S. (1993). Source monitoring. *Psychological Bulletin*, *114*, 3-28

Izawa, C., Hayden, R. G., and Franklin, M. (2005). Newly uncovered psychophysiological processes and Study-Test-Rest (S-T-R) presentation program effects for optimal learning: Empirical and theoretical investigations. In C. Izawa and Ohta, N. (Eds.), *Human learning and memory: Advances in theory and application: The 4th Tsukuba International Conference on Memory*. (pp. 27-59). Mahwah, NJ: Lawrence Erlbaum

Kazén, M., and Solís-Macías, V. M. (1999). Recognition hypermnesia with repeated trials: Initial evidence for the alternative retrieval pathways hypothesis. *British Journal of Psychology, 90*, 405-424.

Kelley, M. R. and Lehman, M. S. (2006). Repeated questioning for order of events: Disparate effects following logical versus random presentation. *Psychological Reports, 98*, 419-426.

Kelley, M. R. and Nairne, J. S. (2003). Remembering the forgotten? Reminiscence, hypermnesia and memory for order. *Quarterly Journal of Experimental Psychology A: Human Experimental Psychology, 56A*, 577-599.

Kintsch, W. (1970). Models for free recall and recognition. In D. A. Norman (Ed.), *Models of human memory* (pp. 331-373). New York: Academic Press.

Kern, R. P., Libkuman, T. M., and Otani, H. (2002). Memory for negatively arousing and neutral pictorial stimuli using a repeated testing paradigm. *Cognition and Emotion, 16*, 749-767.

Klein, S. B., Loftus, J., Kihlstrom, J. F., and Aseron, R. (1989). Effects of item-specific and relational information on hypermnesic recall. *Journal of Experimental Psychology: Learning, Memory, and Cognition, 15*, 1192-1197.

Lang, P. J., Bradley, M. M., and Cuthbert, B. N. (1999). International affective picture system (IAPS): Technical manual and affective ratings. Gainsville, FL. The Center for Research in Psychophysiology, University of Florida.

La Rooy, D., Pipe, M., and Murray, J. E. (2005). Reminiscence and hypermnesia in children's eyewitness memory. *Journal of Experimental Child Psychology, 90*, 235-254.

Libkuman, T. M., Otani, H., Kern, R. P., Viger, S. G., and Novak, N. (2007). Multidimensional normative ratings for the International Affective Picture System. *Behavior Research Methods, 39, 326-334*.

Linscott, R. J., and Knight, R. G. (2001). Automatic hypermnesia and impaired recollection in schizophrenia. *Neuropsychology, 15*, 576-585.

Luszcz, M. A., Roberts, T. H., and Mattiske, J. (1990). Use of relational and item-specific information in remembering by older and younger adults. *Psychology and Aging, 5*, 242-249.

Madigan, S. (1976). Reminiscence and item recovery in free recall. *Memory & Cognition, 93*, 489-504.

Mandler, G. (1994). Hypermnesia, incubation, and mind popping: On remembering without really trying. In C. Umilta and M. Moscovitch (Eds.), *Attention and performance XV: Conscious and nonconscious information processing* (pp. 3-33). Cambridge, MA: MIT Press.

McDaniel, M. A., Moore, B. A., and Whiteman, H. L. (1998). Dynamic changes in hypermnesia across early and late tests: A relational/item-specific account. *Journal of Experimental Psychology: Learning, Memory, and Cognition, 24*, 173-185.

Migita, M. (2007). *Effect of retrieval-induced forgetting on emotional memory*. Unpublished master's thesis, Central Michigan University, Mt. Pleasant, MI.

Mulligan, N. W. (2002). The emergence of item-specific encoding effects in between-subjects designs: Perceptual interference and multiple recall tests. *Psychonomic Bulletin and Review, 9*, 375-382.

Mulligan, N. W. (2005). Total recall time and hypermnesia: Investigating the benefits of multiple recall. *Psychological Research/Psychologische Forschung, 69*, 272-284.

Nogrady, H., McConkey, K. M., and Perry, C. (1985). Enhancing visual memory: Trying hypnosis, trying imagination, and trying again. *Journal of Abnormal Psychology, 94*, 195-204.

Olofsson, U. (1997). Win some, lose some: Hypermnesia for actions reflects item-specific processing. *Memory & Cognition, 25*, 797-800.

Otani, H., and Griffith, J. D. (1998). Hypermnesia for prose. *Journal of General Psychology, 125*, 147-155.

Otani, H., and Hodge, M. H. (1991). Does hypermnesia occur in recognition and cued recall? *American Journal of Psychology*, *104*, 101-116.

Otani, H., Kato, K., Von Glahn, N. R., Nelson, M. E., Widner, R. L., Jr., and Goernert, P. N. (2008). Hypermnesia: A further examination of age differences between young and older adults. *British Journal of Psychology, 99,* 265-278.

Otani, H., Kato, K., and Widner, R. L., Jr. (2005). Conscious and unconscious processes in hypermnesia. In N. Ohta, C. M. McLeod, and B. Uttl (Eds.) *Dynamic cognitive processes* (pp. 249-271). Tokyo: Springer-Verlag.

Otani, H., and Stimson, M. J. (1994). A further attempt to demonstrate hypermnesia in recognition. *The Psychological Record*, *44*, 25-34.

Otani, H., and Whiteman, H. L. (1994). Cued recall hypermnesia is not an artifact of response bias. *American Journal of Psychology*, *107*, 401-421.

Otani, H., Widner, R. L. Jr., Whiteman, H. L., and St. Louis, J. P. (1999). Hypermnesia: The role of multiple retrieval cues. *Memory & Cognition, 27*, 928-934.

Payne, D. G. (1986). Hypermnesia for pictures and words: Testing the recall level hypothesis. *Journal of Experimental Psychology: Learning, Memory, and Cognition, 12*, 16-29.

Payne, D. G. (1987). Hypermnesia and reminiscence in recall: A historical and empirical review. *Psychological Bulletin, 101*, 5-27.

Payne, D. G., Hembrooke, H. A., and Anastasi, J. S. (1993). Hypermnesia in free recall and cued recall. *Memory & Cognition, 21*, 48-62.

Payne, D. G., and Roediger, H. L., III (1987). Hypermnesia occurs in recall but not in recognition. *American Journal of Psychology, 100*, 145-165.

Popkin, S. J., and Small, M. Y. (1979). Hypermnesia and the role of imagery. *Bulletin of the Psychonomic Society, 13*, 378-380.

Raaijmakers, J. G. W., and Shiffrin, R. M. (1980). SAM: A theory of probabilistic search of associative memory. In G. H. Bower (Ed.), *The psychology of learning and motivation: Advances in research and theory* (Vol. 14, pp. 207-262). New York: Academic Press.

Raaijmakers, J. G., and Shiffrin, R. M. (1981). Search of associative memory. *Psychological Review, 88*, 93-134.

Roediger, H. L. III., and Challis, B. H. (1989). Hypermnesia: Improvements in recall with repeated testing. In C. Izawa (Ed.), *Current issues in cognitive processes: The Tulane Floweree Symposium on cognition* (pp. 175-199). Hillsdale, NJ: Lawrence Erlbaum Associates.

Roediger, H. L. III., and Karpicke, J. D. (2006a). The power of testing memory: Basic research and implications for educational practice. *Perspectives on Psychological Science,1,*181-210.

Roediger, H. L. III., and Karpicke, J. D. (2006b). Test-enhanced learning: Taking memory tests improves long-term retention. *Psychological Science, 17*, 249-255.

Roediger, H. L. III., and Payne, D. G. (1982). Hypermnesia: The role of repeated testing. *Journal of Experimental Psychology: Learning, Memory, and Cognition, 8*, 66-72.

Roediger, H. L. III., and Payne, D. G. (1985). Recall criterion does not affect recall level or hypermnesia: A puzzle for generate/recognize theories. *Memory & Cognition, 13*, 1–7.

Roediger, H. L. III., Payne, D. G., Gillespie, G. L., and Lean, D. S. (1982). Hypermnesia as determined by level of recall. *Journal of Verbal Learning and Verbal Behavior, 21*, 635-655.

Roediger, H. L. III., and Thorpe, L. A. (1978). The role of recall time in producing hypermnesia. *Memory & Cognition, 6*, 296-305.

Scrivner, E., and Safer, M. A. (1988). Eyewitnesses show hypermnesia for details about a violent event. *Journal of Applied Psychology, 73,* 371-377.

Schank, R. C., and Abelson, R. P. (1977). *Scripts, plans, goals, and understanding: An inquiry into human knowledge structures*. Oxford, England: Erlbaum.

Shapiro, S. R., and Erdelyi, M. H. (1974). Hypermnesia for pictures but not for words. *Journal of Experimental Psychology, 103*, 1218-1219.

Talmi, D., Schimmack, U., Paterson, T., and Moscovitch, M. (2007). The role of attention and relatedness in emotionally enhanced memory, *Emotion, 7*, 89-102.

Turtle, J. W., and Yuille, J. C. (1994). Lost but not forgotten details: Repeated eyewitness recall leads to reminiscence but not hypermnesia. *Journal of Applied Psychology, 79,* 260-271.

Weldon, M. S., and Bellinger, K. D. (1997). Collective memory: Collaborative and individual processes in remembering. *Journal of Experimental Psychology: Learning, Memory, and Cognition, 23,* 1160-1175.

Wheeler, M. A., and Roediger, H. L. (1992). Disparate effects of repeated testing: Reconciling Ballard's (1913) and Bartlett's (1932) results. *Psychological Science, 3*, 240-245.

Whitehouse, W. G., Dinges, D. R., Orne, E. C., and Orne, M. T. (1988). Hypnotic hypermnesia: Enhanced memory accessibility or report bias? *Journal of Abnormal Psychology, 97*, 289-295.

Widner, R. L., Jr., Otani, H., and Smith, A. (2000). Hypermnesia: Age-related differences between young and older adults. *Memory & Cognition, 28*, 556-564.

Yarmey, A. D. (1976). Hypermnesia for pictures but not for concrete and abstract words. *Bulletin of the Psychonomic Society, 8*, 115-117.

In: Applied Memory
Editor: Matthew R. Kelley

ISBN 978-1-60692-143-2

Chapter 7

PLACEBOS AND MEMORY

***Seema L. Clifasefi*[*1], *and Sophie Parker*[2]**

[1] Addictive Behaviors Research Center, University of Washington, Seattle, WA, USA
[2] Department of Psychology, Victoria University of Wellington, Wellington, New Zealand

ABSTRACT

There is a common belief that 'pill popping' is the solution to a better memory. Is this the case? In this chapter, we consider the role of placebo substances in memory research, examine existing theory and data on the topic, and discuss how beliefs play a large and predictive role in whether a particular behavior is displayed under a placebo administration of the "said" substance. More specifically, we consider two diverging lines of placebo and memory research: (a) research that focuses purely on the cognitive aspects of memory; and (b) research that focuses on the social aspects of memory (memory distortions and false memories). We highlight the differences between cognitive and social aspects of memory and delve into why placebos seem to affect certain types of cognitive faculties and not others. The chapter concludes by addressing some practical applications for this new area of research and by describing a novel study evaluating the effects of ginkgo biloba, a popular supplement purported to improve memory, in the context of eyewitness memory. Finally, we address the growing need for research of this type in the face of a worldwide surge in sales of so-called 'smart pills'.

INTRODUCTION

They have names like RxMemory®, Memory Upgrade® and ThinkDrink®. They promise to sharpen your thinking, improve your mental clarity, and even help you remember where you put your keys. Although none of these claims have been supported by the scientific literature, consumers still turn to pill popping and quick fix solutions to combat memory loss,

---

* Corresponding author.

as evidenced by the high sales in "smart" supplements[2]. Do these supplements work? The research we present in this chapter suggests that the answer may be yes, but not because of any breakthrough physiological properties contained in these substances. Instead, these supplements may work their magic simply through the power of belief.

The power of belief has long been known to be a cure for many ailments and diseases. In fact, a review of the medical literature dating as far back as the 17th century reveals that the act of taking a substance intended for healing purposes can produce a psychological response (*feeling better)* even when the medicines contain ingredients that have no proven healing properties (see Shapiro and Morris, 1978; Shapiro and Shapiro, 1997, for a review). This effect, known as the *placebo effect,* is a robust phenomenon most commonly observed in the health domain.

A placebo is defined as an inactive substance – that is, a substance with no physiological or active ingredients contained within it - and can serve two different functions. First, a placebo may be used as a medicinal cure, prescribed for psychological reasons even though the substance has no physiological effect. Second, a placebo may be used in the testing of new drugs by acting as a control. While these two definitions are fundamentally different— a type of medicinal cure or what Marlatt and Rohsenow (1980) refer to as a "therapeutic strategy," versus a pharmacologically inert substance used in drug trials to serve as a control—both can cause a *placebo effect.* A good example of the placebo effect is portrayed in the tale of Harry Potter and the Half-Blood Prince (2005). In the sixth book of this J.K Rowling series, a professor awards Harry Potter with a magic potion called Felix Felicis that purportedly results in the drinker of the potion having a day filled with good fortune and success. Harry's friend Ron Weasley is having confidence problems regarding his performance in a sporting game called Quidditch so Harry tricks Ron into believing that Ron has drunk the potion. In the Quidditch game, Ron performs with confidence and leads his team to victory, even though he has had nothing more than pumpkin juice. This is a well-illustrated example of the placebo effect in action. Although this scenario comes from a fantasy novel, the situation itself is hardly fiction. In fact, the power of belief has been shown to be enough to induce people to endure more pain (Benedetti, Pollo and Colloca, 2007), feel happier (Kirsh and Sapirstein, 1999) and even reduce body fat (Crum and Langer, 2007).

WHY DO WE GET PLACEBO EFFECTS?

Why is it that ordinary, intelligent people can act or feel differently after consuming an inert substance? Although there are several theories accounting for how placebos work (see Stewart-Williams, 2004 for a review), one of the most prominent theories in the placebo literature is the theory of expectancy. According to an expectancy theory, the set of beliefs that a person holds about a particular substance actually predicts and drives the behavior (see Fillmore and Vogel-Sprott, 1992; Fillmore, Mulvihill and Vogel-Sprott, 1994; Kirsch, (1985, 1997). In other words, if people are led to expect a positive outcome as a result of taking a substance, it is more likely that they will have such an experience compared to those who are led to expect a negative outcome from the same substance. For instance, in one study,

---

[2] This statement is based on a report by Health Focus® International profiling marketing trends of health supplements in the United States (http://www.healthfocus.net/ supplement.htm)

participants drank decaffeinated coffee but were told it was the real thing. Those who were told that caffeine improves motor performance performed better on a motor task than those who were told that caffeine impairs motor performance (Fillmore and Vogel-Sprott, 1992). The results of this study showed that people tended to act in line with how they expected the drug to make them behave, not necessarily in line with the pharmacological effects of the drug.

To that end, a recent study conducted by Crum and Langer (2007) has shown that expectancy alone—even in the absence of any substance—can be enough to result in physical changes. Participants were a group of hotel room attendants who cleaned an average 15 to 20 rooms a day. The researchers were interested in whether people's beliefs about perceived levels of exercise could be manipulated in such a way as to result in measurable and positive health outcomes. Half of the attendants were informed that the type of work that they did satisfied a number of requirements for a healthy life style. Specifically, they were given examples of how their daily activities were good for their health and how many calories each activity burned. In the non-informed group, attendants were not given any specific information pertaining to the beneficial effects of their work on their health. During an initial information session both groups completed a number of self-report scales and corresponding physiological measures taken such as body mass index (BMI), waist-to-hip ratio and blood pressure. After four weeks, the group of attendants who thought of their daily work as exercise showed a significant reduction in body fat percentage, blood pressure, body weight and BMI. Specifically, the group of informed attendants lost an average of 2 pounds between their Time 1 and Time 2 weigh in and lowered their blood pressure by 10%. Simply believing that the work that they were undertaking was physical enough to burn calories and satisfy the requirements for a healthy lifestyle was enough to result in measurable objective health outcomes. Together, these studies show that what individuals are told about their condition is the single most important determinant in whether they display behaviors in line with their expectancies.

THE BALANCED PLACEBO DESIGN (BPD)

One of the methods that has been used to study individuals' expectancies has been the balanced placebo design (BPD; Marlatt and Rohsenow, 1980). This method allows for the independent examination of the psychological and physiological reactions to a given substance. In this 2 x 2 procedure, subjects are told that they will receive an active substance or a placebo, and what they are told is either true or false By examining the two cells in which people are given false information, researchers can distinguish between pure physiological reactions to the active agent and pure psychological responses.

Much of what we know about expectancies and placebo effects come from BPD studies with alcohol (Collins, Gollnisch and Izzo, 1996; George, Stoner, Norris, Lopez and Lehman, 2000; Lang, Goeckner, Adesso and Marlatt, 1975; Lansky and Wilson, 1981; Hull and Bond, 1986 Vuchinich, Tucker and Sobell, 1979). These studies show that wide ranges of behaviors are affected by the belief that one has received alcohol. For example, people become less inclined to suppress socially taboo behaviors that lead to: decreased sexual inhibition (Lansky and Wilson, 1981; George and Marlatt, 1986; George et al., 2000), increased risk taking

(McMillan, Smith, and Wells-Parker, 1989), and increased aggression (Cherek, Steinberg and Manno, 1985; Lang et al., 1975). Interestingly, these studies also show that behaviors that tend to fall outside the sphere of social influence, such as reaction time, memory for word lists, tests of general knowledge, or perceptual tasks do not seem to be affected by alcohol placebos (Clifasefi, Takarangi and Bergman, 2006 Hull and Bond, 1986; Maylor and Rabbitt, 1993, Nelson, McSpadden, Fromme and Marlatt, 1986).

Why is it that alcohol placebos affect some behaviors, while not affecting others? The widely held view as to why placebo alcohol affects social behaviors and not non-social ones is that alcohol provides individual's with an excuse to engage in social behaviors that are typically inhibited by societal constraints (Hull and Bond, 1986; Marlatt and Rohsenow, 1980). In other words, alcohol provides an external outlet of blame such that one can argue their behavior away by saying, "it wasn't me, it was the alcohol". To this end, memory is not typically thought of as a behavior that is inhibited in every day life, and is traditionally viewed in the cognitive domain. However, there is a growing awareness that memory has a social component (Gergen, 1994; Neisser, 1980; Neisser and Hyman, 2000). For example, whom would you be today without your memory for your past experiences? What role do memories play in shaping your identity? One arm of research purports that memory actually serves a social function in that it allows people to relate their own personal story to the bigger picture and form a self identity (Neisser, 1980, 1991; Neisser and Harsch, 1993; Neisser and Hyman, 2000). One of the central tenets of this research is that the accuracy of a memory does not matter as much as how we use that memory to define ourselves. Another arm of memory research has been to determine how external social influences affect how and what we remember (Dodd and Bradshaw, 1980; French, Garry and Mori, 2008; Loftus, Miller and Burns, 1978; Vornik, Sharman and Garry, 2003). Most of this research has been drawn out by the eyewitness and false memory literature. There is in fact, a distinct social component of memory that can be influenced and manipulated by external factors and suggestion, which is why we believe that using placebos as a tool to study this component of memory may illuminate some of the complexities of memory. One paradigm in particular that aptly demonstrates how memory contains both social and cognitive components is that of the misinformation effect.

The Misinformation Effect

The misinformation effect has been one of the most robust methods used to study eyewitness memory and memory suggestibility (Loftus et al., 1978; Tousignant, Hall and Loftus, 1986). The classic method for studying the misinformation effect consists of three critical stages. In the first stage subjects watch an event, in the second stage they are provided with postevent information (PEI) about the event. The PEI is specifically designed so that half the time subjects receive neutral or generic information about what they have previously witnessed in the event, referred to as control information and half the time the information is deliberately misleading, referred to as misleading information. The last phase of the paradigm comes in the form of a memory test where subjects are asked about the specific details of the original event. Time and time again, over a myriad of studies, it has been demonstrated that when people are provided with false and misleading information regarding an earlier encountered event or a scene, their ability to accurately remember details from that event declines (Loftus et al., 1978; Loftus, 1991; Sutherland and Hayne, 2001; Takarangi, Parker and Garry, 2006).

The uniqueness of the misinformation effect paradigm is that it allows researchers to tease apart the components of memory that are purely cognitive from those that are purely social and thus makes it an ideal vehicle for studying how placebos may or may not affect memory. Cognitive factors such as time delay between the original event and misleading PEI, and repetition are two factors that have been shown to affect both control and misled performance (Loftus et al., 1978). For example, in one of the original misinformation studies conducted by Loftus et al. (1978), the timing between the original event, PEI and memory test was varied. Loftus et al. showed that the misleading PEI was the most harmful to memory when subjects received misinformation right before the memory test – 48 hours after witnessing the original event – thus giving the original event time to fade and making it even more vulnerable to suggestion. Memory accuracy for the control items also decreased after a significant time delay between the original event and the memory test as it became harder for people to remember the original event.

Research demonstrates that the extent to which a person falls prey to the misinformation is this eyewitness paradigm is not only dependent on cognitive factors, such as the ones mentioned above, but social factors too. When subjects are provided with misleading information about the event, they must at some stage (either consciously or unconsciously), capitulate to the misinformation. However, there are a number of social factors that mitigate whether capitulation occurs. For example, the misinformation effect can vary depending on the status of what might be called the "misinformation messenger" (Ceci and Bruck, 1993; Dodd and Bradshaw, 1980; French, Garry and Mori, 2008; Lindsay, 1990; Loftus, Levidow and Duensing, 1992; Vornik, Sharman and Garry, 2003). Factors related to the status of the person delivering the misinformation, such as age, authority, profession, power and attractiveness, have all been shown to influence the extent to which one is misled. For example, Dodd and Bradshaw (1980) showed that the impact of misleading PEI varied with the credibility of the misinformation messenger. Subjects were more influenced by misleading PEI when misinformation was supposedly written by a neutral source rather than by a defence lawyer. In another study, Vornik et al. (2003) showed that when subjects rated a speaker high on a scale of power and attractiveness they were also more likely to be misled by that speaker, compared to their counterparts who did not rate the speaker highly on these dimensions. Further evidence that status matters comes from a recent study by French et al. (2008). Their study showed that individuals were more swayed by misleading PEI if it was delivered to them by their romantic partner versus delivered to them by a stranger.

Taken together, the evidence suggests that both cognitive and social factors influence eyewitness memory performance. That is, misled performance is driven by cognitive factors as well as social factors (e.g. status of the person delivering the external suggestion); whereas control performance is affected only by cognitive factors (i.e. time delay that makes memory susceptible to decay). This fact makes the three-stage eyewitness paradigm an ideal one by which to study both the social and the non-social influences affecting memory.

Alcohol and the Misinformation Effect

If memory does indeed contain a social component, then alcohol placebos should theoretically affect this aspect of memory in the misinformation paradigm, while leaving the cognitive component in tact. Assefi and Garry (2003) set out to test this assumption by marrying the balanced placebo design procedure with the misinformation effect to evaluate the extent to which placebos could affect memory distortions.

Assefi and Garry (2003) reasoned that subjects who believed that they had consumed alcohol would be more likely to be misled because they may go through a deliberation process that results in them having less trust in their own memory and more trust in the PEI. For example, an individual could make the following argument, "Well, I was drunk when I saw the event, so now that there is something different here, it is probably because I can't remember the event properly". On the other hand, placebo alcohol is exactly that—a placebo—so it should therefore not impact memory for the actual event. Thus, memory for control items should remain unaffected.

The researchers used half the balanced placebo design; half the participants thought that they were receiving a vodka drink mixed with tonic while the other half thought they were receiving only tonic. In reality, none of the participants received any alcohol. To enhance the likelihood that subjects really believed that they were drinking vodka, subjects drank from glasses that had had the rims rubbed with vodka soaked limes and lemons. This was so that their drink would give off the subtle aroma of alcohol and add to the authenticity of their cover story. The vodka was poured from liquor bottles that appeared to have not had their seals broken and in full view of the subjects. The vodka was actually nothing more than flat tonic water. After consuming their beverages, subjects then took part in a standard misinformation effect study.

The results of the study were in line with what the researchers had hypothesized. While there was a misinformation effect in both conditions, subjects who were told that they had consumed alcohol (Told Alcohol) were more likely to be misled than those subjects who were told that they consumed only tonic (Told Tonic). Specifically, Told Alcohol subjects accurately recalled an average of 1.64 misled items in contrast to the 2.42 misled items that Told Tonic subjects recalled correctly. There was no placebo alcohol effect on memory for control items. That is, true and veridical memory for the original event was unaffected by the drink instruction with both groups performing equally on these test items. The overarching results from this study fit with the alcohol placebo literature. That is, in this study, the social component of memory—namely susceptibility to misinformation—was affected by an alcohol placebo, whereas, the cognitive component remained unaffected.

While Assefi and Garry were able to show that alcohol placebos negatively impacted memory, and these findings have theoretical implications for how memory is conceptualized, practically speaking, it would make more sense to use placebos to try and improve and enhance memory. First, as indicated by the high sales in herbal supplements that purport to improve and enhance cognitive functioning, there is a societal desire for people to want to make their memories better. Second, having accurate eyewitnesses would also benefit society since the effects of mistaken eyewitness testimony are seen all to often in real-world cases of wrongful conviction.

Studies that have evaluated whether drugs or herbal supplements can objectively improve memory have yielded inconclusive results (see McDaniel, Maier and Einstein, 2003 for a review). Likewise, prior to 2007, investigations that have attempted to improve memory with a placebo have also had a difficult time showing any objective positive memory effects. For example, in the seminal study investigating whether a placebo could improve memory, subjects were told that they would be receiving a drug that had memory enhancing qualities. After they took the supposed drug, all subjects were given a battery of tests, one of which was a free recall memory test. Although the false drug suggestion did improve subjects' self reports about their memory, it did not improve their actual memory performance (Kvavilashvili and Ellis, 1999).

Why is it that Kvavilashvili and Ellis (1999) were not able to observe an objective increase in memory performance? Kvavilashvili and Ellis's study used a dependent measure—a free recall test—on which performance is usually fixed. The fact that the cognitive component of memory (i.e. working memory capacity) is more or less stable suggests that it would be difficult to improve this particular component of memory. However, as we have previously argued, the eyewitness memory design not only includes this fixed type of memory performance, as demonstrated by performance on control items, but also captures the aspect of memory that is variable and influenced by social factors: performance on misled items. For this reason, we were interested in whether giving people a bogus cognitive enhancing supplement could positively affect their memories by increasing their resistance to false PEI information.

Clifasefi, Garry, Harper, Sharman, and Sutherland (2007) paired half the balanced placebo design with the misinformation effect and reasoned that if people were led to expect that a drug they had taken would increase their cognitive functioning, they may unconsciously adapt their behaviors to fall into line with these expectations. That is, if subjects expected that they would have more cognitive resources whilst watching the event, reading the PEI, and taking a memory test, they may in fact expend more cognitive effort during these phases.

To test their hypothesis, the researchers brought subjects to the laboratory under the guise that they were to take part in cutting edge research testing the effects of a new cognitive enhancing drug – R273 - on visual and verbal modes of learning. R273 was in fact nothing more than lime-flavoured baking soda. A confederate in a white lab coat posed as a pharmaceutical researcher from a fictitious drug company and was present for the entirety of the session. Subjects were informed that R273 had previously been shown in other drug trials to be safe and effective in 'enhancing mental alertness, attention and focus.' Additionally, they were told that a close cousin of R273 had been tested on military radar operating personnel and had made them, "better able to detect changes in their visual fields, and quickly and accurately distinguish enemy target signatures from simple environmental noise" (Clifasefi et al. 2007, p. 114). Subjects were weighed and measured ostensibly so that they could be administered the exact amount of R273 and subjects had their drug formula prepared in full view by the confederate. Subjects were informed that they were either getting R273 (Told R273) or the inactive version of the drug (Told placebo). After the drug administration phase, subjects took part in a misinformation effect study.

The results of the study showed two key findings. First, the subjects who were told that they had taken R273 rated themselves as feeling more effects of the sham drug than subjects who were told that they had taken the placebo. Told R273 subjects rated themselves as having: enhanced senses, better concentration, better memory and quicker responses. Second, when subjects were told that they were getting R273, they were resistant to misleading information. That is, Told R273 subjects were equally accurate for both control and misled items and rarely capitulated to the erroneous PEI. By contrast, Told Placebo subjects showed the classic misinformation effect.

The research reviewed in this chapter demonstrates that a placebo can reduce people's susceptibility to memory distortion. That is, people who were led to believe they had taken a cognitive enhancing drug were less susceptible to memory distortions and rated their cognitive abilities as higher, compared to people who were told they were receiving a matched placebo. This effect was observed even though both groups received the same substance: a mixture of lime flavored baking soda and water. Although the finding that a placebo can positively affect memory is a first in the psychological literature, memory drug manufacturers and their marketing departments have capitalized on this knowledge for years. Over the past decade, herbal remedies containing extracts of guarana, ginseng, and ginkgo biloba have been marketed and sold as memory aid supplements. Do these herbs really work? If they do, do they work because people believe that they do, or because of their physiological properties? The following experiment that we report here addresses this question.

Present Study

As Eastern medicine influences Western medicine, herbal supplements have experienced a surge of popularity among Western consumers. One herb believed by many to have memory enhancing qualities is *ginkgo biloba.* Some manufacturers of ginkgo claim that this nutrient, "helps maintain healthy memory function and mental alertness," (Nature's Resource®) others say it, "...improves memory, concentration and mental focus" (http://www.ginkoba.com). And one product manufacturer even insinuates that their Brainwash® Shampoo and Conditioner, which contains extract of the ginkgo leaf, gives you an extra edge with regards to mental performance (http://www.ermall.com/brain.html). Although the majority of these claims remain unsubstantiated and unsupported by the scientific literature, consumers still turn to pill popping and quick fix solutions to combat memory loss, as evidenced by the high sales in "smart" supplements.

Over the past five years, the efficacy of ginkgo on human cognitive functioning has been investigated in clinical drug trials (see for example, Hofferberth, 1994; Kennedy, Scholey, and Wesnes, 2000; LeBars, Katz, Berman, Itil, Freedman, and Schatzberg, 1997; McKenna, Jones, and Hughes, 2001; Moulton, Boyko, Fitzpatrick, and Petros, 2001; Rigney, Kimber, and Hindmarch, 1999; Soholm, 1998; Solomon, Adams, Silver, Zimmer, and DeVeaux, 2002; Stough et al., 2001). These studies suggest that ginkgo improves some aspects of cognitive functioning, but only in special populations. For example, Hofferberth (1994) showed that Alzheimer's and dementia patients improved on memory and attention tasks after taking an extract of ginkgo for one month compared to subjects who were taking a placebo. LeBars et al. (1997) found that ginkgo improved cognitive performance and social functioning in demented patients.

These results, coupled with clever marketing strategies, have contributed to a growing popular belief that ginkgo improves memory. Although the majority of research investigating ginkgo has focused on an elderly population with particular emphasis on Alzheimer's and dementia patients, only a handful of studies have investigated subjects from the general population (see for example, Kennedy et al., 2000; Stough et al., 2001). In general, however, results from ginkgo studies have been inconclusive and little is actually known about the effects of ginkgo on a healthy adult population (see Gold, Cahill, and Wenk, 2002 for a review). Thus, in the study we report here, we not only investigate the psychological effects associated with taking "a memory herb," we also investigate whether there are indeed pharmacological effects in relation to eyewitness memory performance in a population of normal adults.

The current study was set up so that it aligned closely with how a real world drug trial would be carried out. For example, most drug trials investigating the efficacy of a new drug are conducted over an extended period of time, to allow the pharmacological properties of the drug to take effect and to assess the long-term effects of the substance. These trials also take place outside of a laboratory setting, and are often double blind. In other words, neither the researcher nor the participant is aware of their condition until after the study is over. One of the key problems with the double blind procedure is that it does not align with the way drug administration is carried out in the real world. That is, when a doctor prescribes a medication for an ailment or an individual buys a product that they believe to work, the individual knows that what they are taking is an active substance. In a double blind trial, because subjects do not know the nature of the substance, the situation is analogous to a person reaching for an aspirin to relieve a headache while thinking that they only have a 50:50 chance of pulling out an active pill out of the bottle. Because the person does not know if they have taken an active drug or a placebo, they may try to introspect and guess about what they have received, thus altering their behavior. In fact, an extensive database search on ginkgo trials using human subjects yielded a 100% hit rate on double-blind administration procedures (National Library of Medicine (PubMed) database, 2003; Ovid Technologies, 2000-2003). Thus, our ginkgo study was unique in that we were essentially conducting a double blind trial for 30 days, but then attempted to remove the guessing variable and account for subject introspection by providing subjects with an instruction about their condition prior to giving them any memory tests.

We made several predictions about how the instructional manipulation coupled with the physiological properties of ginkgo may affect eyewitness memory. First, if ginkgo aids memory through both physiological and psychological mechanisms, then there should be an interaction between the actual drug and the instructional manipulation. That is, if ginkgo actually works to *prevent* memory decay and the instructional manipulation is successful, then Got Ginkgo/Told Ginkgo subjects should show superior performance over all other combinations. Similarly, Got Placebo/Told Placebo subjects should show the poorest performance on all dependent measures of memory.

However, if ginkgo does not have any pharmacological properties that work to enhance memory, then like the Clifasefi et al. (2007) study, the instruction should be the most important variable in determining whether ginkgo affects memory performance. In such a case, regardless of their actual drug condition, what subjects are told about their condition should predict their performance on eyewitness memory measures. A third outcome is also possible. If what subjects' thought about their condition during the DBT portion of the trial matters, then this thought variable may affect subjects' memory performance.

METHOD

Participants. Forty-one adults between the ages of 18-40 years volunteered for the study, with a mean age of 25.13 years (SD=4.44) and a median age of 25. Participants responded to radio and magazine advertisements, and posters placed around campus and on public notice boards.

Materials and Procedures. The study used a 2 (drug condition; Got Ginkgo or Got Placebo) x 2 (instruction; Told Ginkgo or Told placebo) between subjects design evaluating control performance and misled performance independently. Unlike the Clifasefi et al. (2007) study, subjects first received the supplement for 30 days, then the instructional manipulation (BPD), and then the memory test. The majority of drug trials investigating ginkgo's efficacy on cognitive functioning have concluded that the minimum treatment should be no less than 3 weeks, although some studies have shown positive results within 2 days (Kleijnen and Knipschild, 1992; Soholm, 1998; Stough et al., 2001). Based on this research, we decided upon a 30-day trial to increase the chances of detecting whether ginkgo had any physiological effects on eyewitness memory measures, as well as to lend credibility to the fact that we were testing the physiological properties of the herbal supplement.

Session 1. In the initial phase, participants viewed a television program describing a study that had shown positive cognitive effects of ginkgo biloba (The Holmes Show, 1999). In this video segment, subjects learned that people who took ginkgo improved their cognitive test scores by 10-15% after 30 days of taking the supplement, whereas the placebo group showed little change[3]. Additionally, subjects read some information about the intended trial. The experimenter explained the structure of the sessions and volunteers were given the opportunity to ask questions before deciding to participate. Once consent forms and questionnaires were collected, a research assistant assigned subjects to their drug condition in a double blind fashion. Half of the subjects were blindly assigned ginkgo tablets (extract 40mg equivalent to dry leave 2000mg; and standardized to contain ginkgo flavonglycosides 10.7mg and ginkgolides and bilobalide 2.7mg), which they took once a day for 30 days. The other half of the subjects was assigned placebo tablets, which were identical in appearance to the active ginkgo, for the same period of time[4]. Because telling subjects about which drug condition they were in before they returned for session 2 posed a threat to potential dropout rates, the trial operated blindly for the 30 days preceding this session. At the end of the 30-day trial, subjects returned for session 2 where the instructional manipulation was introduced.

Session 2. Thirty-nine of the original 41 participants returned for session 2. Prior to taking any memory tests, subjects were asked whether they thought they had been taking ginkgo or a placebo over the past 4 weeks. This measure was used as a manipulation check for the double blind portion of the trial, and the research assistant recorded participants' responses. Next, in an attempt to remove the guessing variable prevalent in double blind trials (DBTs) subjects were given an instruction about their drug condition—Told Ginkgo or Told Placebo—and what they were told was either true or false. Put another way, the research assistant told subjects either truthfully or falsely that they had been taking ginkgo or placebo. After receiving this instructional manipulation, subjects took part in the standard three-phase

[3] This program was based on a study conducted by Stough et al. (2001).

[4] I am grateful to Blackmores® pharmaceutical company for providing the ginkgo and placebo tablets for this experiment.

misinformation effect. Subjects first watched an event of a man stealing various items from a bookstore, then received some erroneous PEI about that event, and finally took a memory test. For the last experimental task subjects completed a questionnaire asking them to rate the extent to which they agreed with statements pertaining to ginkgo's effectiveness. After subjects filled out this questionnaire, they were debriefed.

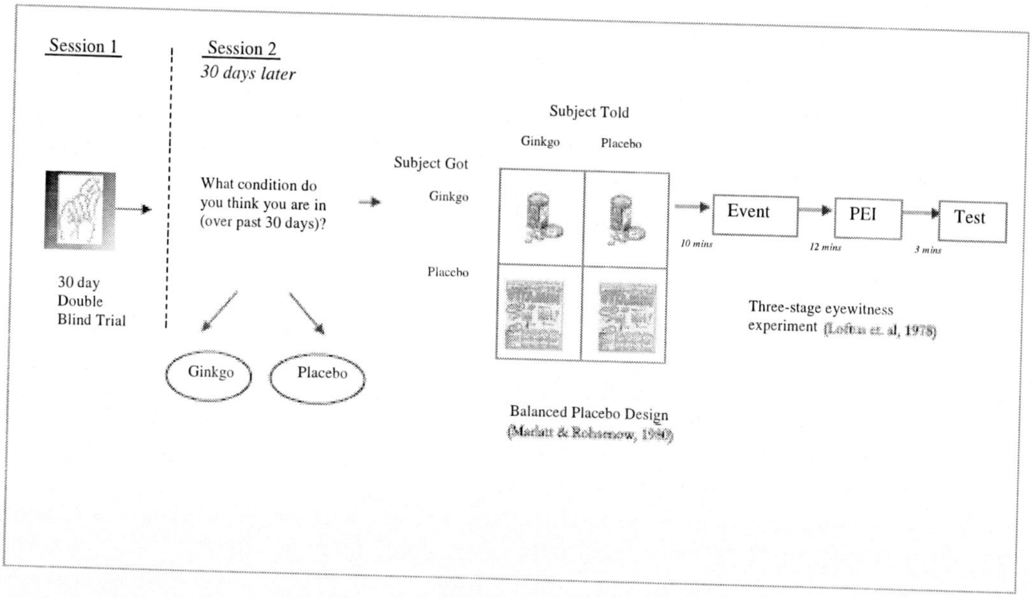

Figure 1. Overview of the method used in the Ginkgo experiment.

Results and Discussion

Overall, 38 students (21 females and 17 males) completed all phases of the study[5]. Before we examine whether ginkgo physiologically or psychologically affected eyewitness memory performance, we were first interested in whether our instructional manipulation was effective. That is, did subjects report self improved cognitive abilities based on what they were told about their substance? The simple answer is yes: Participants who were told that they had received Ginkgo rated their cognitive abilities higher overall than Told Placebo subjects $F(1, 36) = 5.43$, $p = .03$, $f = 1.50$. Specifically, Told Ginkgo subjects reported that their senses were enhanced, they had an easier time remembering, and their responses were quicker.

We next focus our attention on the effects on ginkgo on eyewitness memory performance. It is important to note that there were no interactions between what participants got and what they were told in relation to eyewitness memory performance, thus, we report the separate physiological and psychological effects of ginkgo on this memory measure.

Physiological Properties. Did ginkgo have any physiological effects on either control or misled test performance? The simple answer is no. Performance was identical on both memory measures. That is, two separate one way ANOVAs for drug condition on control and misled performance revealed that neither control nor misled performance was affected by

[5] Two subjects discontinued their participation during the trial, and one subject did not complete all the tests.

what subjects got, *Fs <1.* This finding suggests that ginkgo does not have any pharmacological properties that affect eyewitness memory performance.

Psychological Properties. We next direct our attention to the psychological properties of ginkgo. If what subjects are told is the primary factor affecting performance, then subjects who are told that they have received ginkgo should show better performance on misled items (i.e. be resistant to the misleading information) and equal performance on control items, regardless of what they actually got. Unlike the previous two studies reported, our results showed that being told that one was receiving ginkgo was not enough to affect test performance in the predicted direction. That is, both Told Ginkgo and Told Placebo subjects displayed equal performance on control items and equal performance on misled items as shown by the results of two, one-way ANOVASs, *Fs* <1.

Thought. We then decided to look at whether what subjects initially believed about their condition affected their results in the eyewitness task. Recall that we collected information about what subjects thought they were taking, prior to administering the instructional manipulation. Interestingly, if subjects thought that they had received ginkgo (Thought Ginkgo), regardless of what they were told about their condition, they were less susceptible to the misleading PEI compared to Thought Placebo subjects, F, (1, 36) = 6.88, p=. 01, f = .96. This pattern of results is similar to Clifasefi et al. (2007) where subjects who were told that they had received R273 were less susceptible to misleading information than their told placebo counterparts.

Overall, participants who were told that they had been taking ginkgo rated their perceived cognitive abilities as higher than those who were merely told they were getting a placebo, a finding that fits with our previous two reported studies on self reported measures. However, unlike the previous two studies, the instructional manipulation was not enough to affect susceptibility to misleading information. In other words, Told Ginkgo and Told Placebo subjects demonstrated equal performance on misleading test items. One possible account for why we were not entirely able to replicate Clifasefi et al. 2007's findings may have been due to the differences in design between the two studies, namely that in the ginkgo trials participants had 30 days to introspect about their condition. Interestingly, what subjects thought about their condition *did* predict whether they were susceptible to misleading information. That is, if participants initially reported that they believed they were taking Ginkgo, regardless of what they were told about their condition, they were less susceptible to the misinformation effect.

Taken together, these studies highlight some important findings. First, they offer evidence that a placebo can affect certain aspects of memory and, that belief plays a powerful role in memory performance, suggesting that at some level, people do have control over their memories. However, these studies also fit with the previous placebo literature showing that the cognitive part of memory remains unaffected by suggestion.

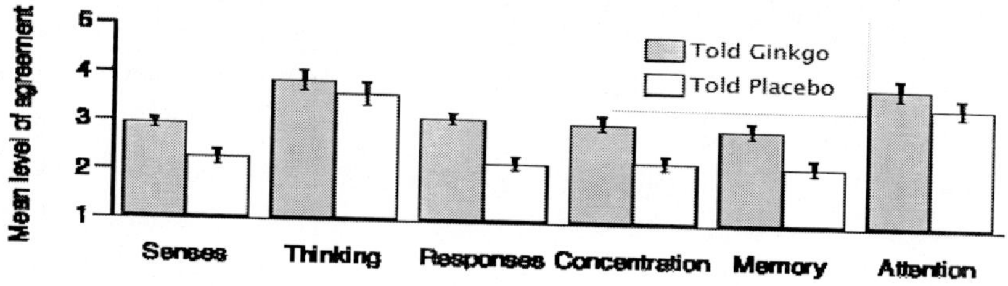

Figure 2. Subjects perceived cognitive abilities as as function of Told instruction. Error bars represent standard error for each individual mean.

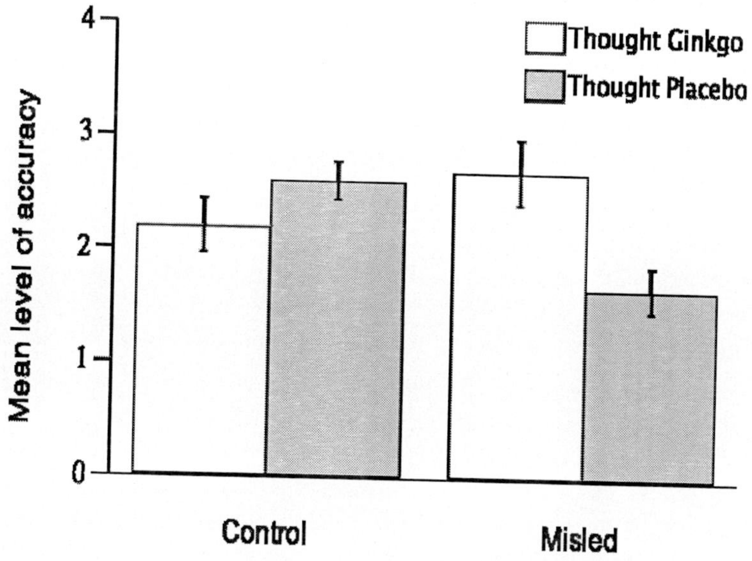

Figure 3. Performance on control and misled items by what subjects thought during the experiment. error bars represent the standard error for each individual mean.

Mechanisms of the R273 Effect

If the drug administered in the Clifasefi et al. (2007) study was nothing more than lime-flavoured baking soda and the alcohol administered in the Assefi and Garry (2003) study was nothing more than flat tonic water, and only subjects who believed that they were getting ginkgo, regardless of what they actually got, showed memory improvement, how is it that memory is made more or less susceptible to distortion through a placebo? One potential explanation comes from the *source monitoring (SM)* literature: the process by which we evaluate and attribute sources of information to a specific person, place or time (Johnson, Hashtroudi and Lindsay, 1993). According to the framework, the type of SM that people engage in can affect the likelihood that an individual will attribute the correct piece of information to the correct source. Since placebos can only affect behaviors that are under our control, they may cause people to either increase or decrease their SM behaviors depending on what substance they believe they have taken. That is, if people believe that they have been given a "smart drug", they may increase their SM behaviors accordingly by scrutinizing the information that they receive. By contrast, if people believe that they are taking a substance that decreases their cognitive abilities, they may decrease their SM behaviors in line with this expectation by paying less attention or exerting less cognitive effort to the information that they encounter.

How would we expect to see SM behaviors manifest themselves in the misinformation effect? SM may occur at any of the three phases of the misinformation effect. During the event, an individual who thinks they have taken a "smart drug" may pay closer attention to the information that they encounter. When they receive the PEI, they may scrutinize the information more closely and compare it to their memory of the original event. And finally, during the test, they may spend more time deliberating between the different sources of information. If a "smart drug" placebo causes people to pay closer attention to the event and take in more information than they normally would, then we may expect to see better performance in both control and misled performance. Recall that control performance is a straightforward measure of the cognitive component of memory, since there is no discrepant information to be considered and no social influence. That is, subjects view the event, receive generic information about it, and then are tested on what they remember. In fact, we find no differences in control item performance between groups in either the alcohol or the R273 studies (Assefi and Garry, 2003; Clifasefi et al., 2007; Parker, Garry, Engle, Harper and Clifasefi, 2008). This lack of difference in control performance indicates that at least during the event phase of the misinformation paradigm, placebos do not affect attentional mechanisms, and do not result in increased cognitive effort.

If a placebo is not contributing to increased cognitive effort during the encoding of the event, how else may this change in cognitive effort manifest itself? In stage two of the misinformation paradigm, subjects encounter verbal information in the form of a written narrative. One way of examining SM during this phase is to measure reading speed of the PEI. Studies have shown that when people increase the attention that they pay to the PEI this increased attention improves their ability to detect differences between what they have seen in the event and what they a reading in the PEI – this has become known as the *principle of discrepancy detection* (Tousignant et al., 1986). Thus, going back to our individual who believes that she has taken a "smart drug", we may expect to see her scrutinizing and paying closer attention to the PEI. This increased scrutiny may result in measurable differences in reading speed of the narrative depending on the type of substance the individual believes they have taken. In fact, Parker et al. (2008) recently showed that when participants were given a fictitious cognitive enhancing drug, their reading speed was equivalent to those individuals who were given what they were told was the "inactive version of the drug". Thus, there is no overt evidence that placebos are operating on SM behaviors during the second stage of this task.

Since Parker et al. (2008) showed no apparent difference in reading speed during the PEI, we now look to final phase of the misinformation design to assess whether increased SM is occurring here. Again, recall our participant who thinks she has taken a "smart drug". During the test phase of the misinformation task, increased SM behaviors may result in her taking longer to respond to test questions while she deliberates and evaluates the characteristics and quality of the information she has obtained and holds in her memory. Interestingly, Parker et al. examined how long subjects took to respond to the misleading test items and found that the subjects who had been told they were taking a "smart drug" exhibited longer reaction times on misled items compared to the subjects who were told they were taking the "inactive" version of the drug.

Taken together, these results indicate that placebos may affect memory in the misinformation paradigm by operating on SM behaviors that people engage in during the memory test. This finding is good news for law officials and legal investigators who strive to get the most accurate information from eyewitnesses. For instance, if individuals are given a "smart drug" placebo before they make an eyewitness identification, perhaps it could result in the individual exerting more cognitive effort into determining the correct source of information and help to reduce inaccurate testimony.

The findings that placebos can affect memory as well as subjects' self reports about memory, has both theoretical and practical implications for the study of memory as well as practical aspects of the legal and medical professions.

Theoretical Implications

From a theoretical perspective, the findings that placebos can affect certain components of memory that are subject to external suggestions fit with the notion that memory is multifaceted and serves more than just a cognitive function. Neisser, for example, has long argued that memory has a social function (Neisser, 1980, 1991; Neisser and Harsch, 1993; Neisser and Hyman, 2000). He argues that the importance of a memory does not lie with its accuracy, but in the fact that we can relate to other people by sharing our experiences about specific momentous events in history. In Neisser's view, then, the social function often outstrips the need for accuracy. Others have put forth compatible views (see for example, Conway, 1996; Gergen, 1994; Pillemer, Goldsmith, Panter and White, 1988, Ross and Buehler, 1994). For instance, Ross and Buehler (1994) describe how people recreate their pasts—through recollection—to fit in with their current schema of themselves. Viewed in this way, there is enough evidence to suggest that certain aspects of memory are not fixed, and can be influenced and manipulated by a variety of external social factors, including placebos.

Furthermore, the findings that memory distortions can be affected by placebos fit with the idea that memory distortions are also a function of social influence (see for example, Bless, Strack and Walther, 2001; Bruner, 1986; Middleton and Edwards, 1990; Wade, Garry, Read, and Lindsay, 2002). For example, Bless et al. (2001) suggest that just as individuals are likely to adopt other people's opinions when they are uncertain about their own (see Festinger, 1954 for a review on *social comparison theory*), those who are tentative about the nature of a memory tend to rely on information provided to them by others. The studies reported in this chapter show that simply the power of belief can be enough to give people the ability to place more trust and certainty in their own memory and rely less on an external suggestion.

Practical Implications

The finding that people's beliefs can dictate their susceptibility to memory distortions—as well as contribute to their self-perceptions—has wider implications for any person in the position of prescribing or recommending medication for memory related deficiencies. Physicians and treatment providers need to be aware that what they communicate about a medicine may play a substantial role in how subjects respond to that medicine. As noted earlier, law officials can use "smart drug" placebos to enhance the quality of eyewitness memory accounts.

The studies that we have described in this chapter highlight that placebos can influence some components of memory, but not others. In this vein, researchers may wish to continue using placebos as a tool to uncover the complexities of this multifaceted phenomenon. In the meantime, individuals need to know that the power of the mind may be the best and most effective memory enhancer currently available on the market today.

References

Assefi, S., and Garry, M. (2003). Absolut memory distortions: Alcohol placebos influence the misinformation effect. *Psychological Science, 14,* 77-80.

Bless, H., Strack, F., and Walther, E. (2001). Memory as a target of social influence: Memory distortions as a function of social influence and metacognitive knowledge. In J.P.F. and K.D. Williams (Eds.), *Social Influence: Direct and Indirect Processes. The Sydney Symposium of Social Psychology* (pp. 167-183).

Benedetti, F., Pollo, A., and Colloca, L. (2007). Opioid-mediated placebo responses boost pain endurance and physical performance: Is it doping in sport competitions? *The Journal of Neuroscience, 27,* 11934-11939.

Bruner, J. (1986). *Actual Minds, Possible Worlds*. Cambridge, MA: Harvard University Press.

Ceci, S., and Bruck, M. (1993). Suggestibility of the child witness: A historical review and synthesis. *Psychological Bulletin, 113*, 403-439.

Cherek, D. R., Steinberg, J. L., and Manno, B. R. (1985). Effects of alcohol on human aggressive behavior. *Journal of Studies on Alcohol, 46*(4), 321-328.

Clifasefi, S., Garry. M., Harper, D., Sharman, S. J., and Sutherland, R. (2007). Psychotropic placebos create resistance to the misinformation effect. *Psychonomic Bulletin and Review, 12,* 112-117.

Clifasefi, S. L., Takarangi, M. K. T., and Bergman, J. S. (2006). Blind drunk: The effects of alcohol on inattentional blindness. *Applied Cognitive Psychology, 20*, 697-704.

Collins, R. L., Gollnisch, G., and Izzo, C. V. (1996). Drinking restrain and alcohol-related outcomes: Exploring the contribution of beverage instructions, beverage content and self-monitoring. *Journal of Studies on Alcohol, 57*, 563-571.

Conway, M. A. (1996). Autobiographical knowledge and autobiographical memories. In D. C. Rubin (Ed.), *Remembering our Past: Studies in Autobiographical Memory* (pp.67-93). New York: Cambridge University Press.

Crum, A. J., and Langer, E. J. (2007). Mind-set matters: Exercise and the placebo effect. *Psychological Science, 18,* 165-171.

Dodd, D. H., and Bradshaw, J. M. (1980). Leading questions and memory: Pragmatic constraints. *Journal of Verbal Learning and Verbal Behavior, 19,* 695-704.

Festinger, L. (1954). A theory of social comparison processes. *Human relations, 7,* 117-140.

Fillmore, M., Mulvihill, L., and Vogel-Sprott, M. (1994). The expected drug and its expected effect interact to determine placebo responses to alcohol and caffeine. *Psychopharmacology, 115*, 383-388.

Fillmore, M., and Vogel-Sprott, M. (1992). Expected effect of caffeine on motor performance predicts the type of response to placebo. *Psychopharmacologia, 106*, 209-214.

French, L. Y., Garry, M., and Mori, K. (2008). You say tomato? Collaborative remembering leads to more false memories for intimate couples than strangers. *Memory, 16*, 262-273.

Gergen, K. J. (1994). Mind, test, and society: Self-memory in social context. In U. Neisser and R. Fivush (Eds.), *The Remembering Self: Construction and Accuracy in the Self-Narrative* (pp. 78-104). New York: Cambridge University Press.

George, W. H., and Marlatt, G. A. (1986). The effects of alcohol and anger on interest in violence, erotica, and deviance. *Journal of Abnormal Psychology, 95*, 150-158.

George, W. H., Stoner, S. A., Norris, J., Lopez, P. A., and Lehman, G. L. (2000). Alcohol expectancies and sexuality: A self-fulfilling prophecy analysis of dyadic perceptions and behavior . *Journal of Studies on Alcohol, 61*, 168-176.

Gold, P., Cahill, L., and Wenk, G. (2002). Ginkgo biloba: A cognitive enhancer? *Psychological Science in the Public Interest, 3*, 2-11.

Hofferberth, B. (1994). The efficacy of Egb 761 in patients with senile dementia of Alzheimer type, a double-blind, placebo-controlled study on different levels of investigation. *Human Psychopharmacology, 9*, 215-222.

Holmes, P. (1999). The Holmes Show [Television Broadcast]. New Zealand, TV1.

Hull, J. G., and Bond, C. F. (1986). Social and behavioral consequences of alcohol consumption and expectancy: a meta-analysis. *Psychological Bulletin, 99*(3), 347-360.

Johnson, M. K., Hashtroudi, S., and Lindsay, D. S. (1993). Source monitoring. *Psychological Bulletin, 114,* 3-28.

Kennedy, D.O., Scholey, A.B., and Wesnes, K.A. (2000). The dose dependent cognitive effects of acute administration of Ginkgo biloba to healthy young volunteers. *Psychopharmacologica, 151*, 416-423.

Kirsch, I. (1985). Response expectancy as a determinant of experience and behavior. *American Psychologist, 40*, 1189-1202.

Kirsch, I. (1997). Response expectancy theory and application: A decennial review. *Applied and Preventive Psychology, 6,* 69-79.

Kirsch, I., and Saperstein, G. (1999). Listening to prozac but hearing placebo: A meta-analysis of antidepressant medication. In Kirsch I. (Ed.), *How Expectancies Shape Behavior*. Washington, DC: American Psychological Association, 303-320.

Kvavilashvili, L., and Ellis, J. A. (1999). The effects of positive and negative placebos on human memory performances. *Memory*, 7(4), 421-437.

Lang, A. R., Goeckner, D. T., Adesso, V. J., and Marlatt, G. A. (1975). Effects of alcohol on aggression in male social drinkers. *Journal of Abnormal Psychology*, *84*, 508-518.

Lansky, D., and Wilson, G. T. (1981). Alcohol, expectations, and sexual arousal in males: An information processing analysis. *Journal of Abnormal Psychology, 90*(1), 35-45.

Lebars, P. L., Katz, M. M., Berman, N., Itil, T. M., Freedman, A. M., and Schatzberg, A. F. (1997). A placebo-controlled, double blind, randomized trial of an extract of Ginkgo biloba for dementia. *Journal of the American Medical Association, 276*, 1327-1332.

Lindsay, D. S. (1990). Misleading suggestions can impair eyewitness' ability to remember event details. *Journal of Experimental Psychology: Learning, Memory, and Cognition, 16*, 1077-1083.

Loftus, E. F. (1991). Made in memory: Distortions in recollection after misleading information. In G. H. Bower (Ed.), *The psychology of learning and motivation: Advances in research and theory* (pp. 187-215). San Diego, CA: Academic Press.

Loftus, E. F., Levidow, B., and Duensing, S. (1992). Who remembers best? Individual differences in memory for events that occurred in a science museum. *Applied Cognitive Psychology, 6*, 93-107.

Loftus, E. F., Miller, D. G., and Burns, H. J. (1978). Semantic integration of verbal information into a visual memory. *Journal of Experimental Psychology: Human Learning and Memory, 4,* 409-420.

Marlatt, G. A., and Rohsenow, D. J. (1980). Cognitive processes in alcohol use: Expectancy and the balanced placebo design. In N. K. Mello (Ed.), *Advances in Substance Abuse* (Vol. 1). Greenwich, CT: JAI Press.

Maylor, E. A., and Rabbitt, P. M. A. (1993). Alcohol, reaction time and memory: A meta analysis. *British Journal of Psychology, 84*, 301-317.

McDaniel, M. A., Maier, S. F., and Einstein, G. O. (2003). "Brain-specific" nutrients: A memory cure? *Nutrition, 19*, 957-975.

McKenna, D. J., Jones, K., and Hughes, K. (2001). Efficacy, safety, and use of Ginkgo biloba in clinical and preclinical applications. *Alternative Therapy, Health Medicine, 7*, 70-86; 88-90.

McMillan, D. L., Smith, S. M., and Wells-Parker, E. (1989). The effects of alcohol, expectancy and sensation seeking on driving risk taking. *Addictive Behaviors, 14*, 477–483.

Middleton, D. and Edwards, D. (1990). *Collective Remembering*. London: Sage.

Moulton, P. L., Boyko, L. N., Fitzpatrick, J. L., and Petros, T. V. (2001). The effect of Ginkgo biloba on memory in healthy male volunteers. *Physiology and Behavior, 73*, 659-665.

Neisser, U. (1980). On "social knowing." *Personality and Social Psychology Bulletin, 6,* 601-605.

Neisser, U. (1991). A case of misplaced nostalgia. *American Psychologist, 46,* 34-36.

Neisser, U., and Harsch, N. (1993). Phantom flashbulbs: False recollections of hearing the news about the Challenger. In E. Winograd (Ed.), *Affect and Accuracy in Recall: Studies of "Flashbulb" Memories* (pp. 9-31). New York: Worth.

Neisser, U., and Hyman, I. E. Jr. (Eds.). (2000). *Memory Observed* (2nd ed.) New York: Worth.

Nelson, T. O., McSpadden, M., Fromme, K., Marlatt, G. A. (1986). Effects of alcohol intoxication on metamemory and on retrieval from long-term memory. *Journal of Experimental Psychology: General, 115*(3), 247-254.

Parker, S., Garry, M., Engle, R. W., Harper, D., and Clifasefi, S. L. (2008). Psychotropic placebos reduce the misinformation effect by increasing monitoring at test. *Memory, 16,* 410-419.

Pillemer, D. B., Goldsmith, L. R., Panter, A. T., and White, S. H. (1988). Very long-term memories of the first year in college. *Journal of Experimental Psychology: Learning, Memory, and Cognition, 14*, 709-715.

Rigney, U., Kimber, S., and Hindmarch, I. (1999). The effects of acute doses of standardized Ginkgo biloba extract on memory and psychomotor performance in volunteers. *Phytotherapy research, 13*, 408-415.

Ross, R. M., and Buehler, R. (1994). Creative remembering. In U. Neisser and R. Fivush (Eds.), *The Remembering Self: Construction and Accuracy in the Self-Narrative. Emory Symposia in Cognition, 6*, (pp. 205-235).

Rowling, J. K. (2005). *Harry Potter and the Half-Blood Prince. Arthur A. Levine Books. 652p.*

Shaprio, A. K., and Morris, L. A. (1978). The placebo in medical and psychological theories. In S.L. and A.E. Bergin (Eds.), *Handbook of Psychotherapy and Behavior Change* (2nd ed.) (pp.369-410). NY: Wiley.

Shapiro, A. K., and Shapiro, E. (1997). The placebo: Is it much ado about nothing? In A.E. Harrington (Ed.). *The Placebo Effect: An Interdisciplinary Exploration* (pp. 12-34). Cambridge, MA: Harvard University Press.

Soholm, B. (1998). Clinical improvement of memory and other cognitive functions by Ginkgo biloba: A review of relevant literature. *Advanced Therapy, 15*, 54-65.

Solomon, P., Adams, F., Silver, A., Zimmer, J., and DeVeaux, R. (2002). Ginkgo for memory enhancement: A randomized controlled trial. *Journal of the American Medical Association, 288*, 835-840.

Stewart-Williams, S. (2004). The placebo puzzle: Putting together the pieces. *Health Psychology, 23,* 198-206.

Stough, C., Clarke, J., Lloyd, J., and Nathan, P.J. (2001). Neuropsychological changes after 30-day Ginkgo biloba administration in healthy participants. *International Journal of Neuropsychopharmacology, 4*, 131-134.

Sutherland, R., and Hayne, H. (2001). The effect of postevent information on adults' eyewitness reports. *Applied Cognitive Psycholoy, 15*, 249-263.

Takarangi, M. K. T., Parker, S., and Garry, M. (2006). Modernising the misinformation effect: The development of a new stimulus set. *Applied Cognitive Psychology, 20,* 583-590.

Tousignant, J. P., Hall, D., and Loftus, E. F. (1986). Discrepancy detection and vulnerability to misleading postevent information. *Memory and Cognition, 14,* 329-338.

Vornik, L. A., Sharman, S. J., and Garry, M. (2003). The power of the spoken word: Sociolinguistic cues influence the misinformation effect. *Memory, 11*, 101-109.

Vuchinich, R. E., Tucker, J. A., Sobell, M. B. (1979). Alcohol, expcectancy, cognitive labeling, and Mirth. *Journal of Abnormal Psychology, 88*(6), 641-651.

Wade, K. A., Garry, M., Read, J. D., and Lindsay, D. S. (2002). A picture is worth a thousand lies: Using false photographs to create false childhood memories. *Psychonomic Bulletin and Review, 9*, 597-603.

In: Applied Memory
Editor: Matthew R. Kelley

ISBN 978-1-60692-143-2

Chapter 8

FLASHBULB MEMORY FOR SEPTEMBER 11 AND THE COLUMBIA SPACE SHUTTLE DISASTER

***Trina C. Kershaw*[*1], *Joshua A. Hemmerich*[2], *and Sadia Ahmed*[3]**

[1] Department of Psychology, University of Massachusetts Dartmouth, North Dartmouth, MA, USA

[2] Department of Medicine, Section of Geriatrics),University of Chicago, Chicago, IL, USA

[3] Department of Psychology, University of Illinois at Chicago, Chicago, IL, USA

ABSTRACT

Flashbulb, or strong episodic, memories are no more consistent over time than other memories, but people are highly confident in these memories and report them as being salient and vivid. Consistency for flashbulb memories, as with other episodic memories, can be influenced by group membership or by personal assessment of an event's importance and consequentiality. An individual's emotional reaction to the event helps to determine assessment of importance and consequentiality, thus leading to rehearsal of the event. Incidence of flashbulb memory and emotional reaction were compared for two events, September 11th (n = 26) and the Columbia Space Shuttle Disaster (n = 30). We found that participants showed equivalent memory consistency when comparing the two events, and that memory consistency and emotional reaction were only marginally related. Participants in the September 11th group maintained their strong emotional reactions over time, but the emotional reaction of participants in the Columbia group decreased between T1 and T2. Analysis of free-recall responses revealed group differences in the kind of emotions that were experienced. The results are evaluated in light of current flashbulb memory theories, and suggestions are given for conducting rigorous flashbulb memory research.

---

* Corresponding author.

Introduction

Some memories seem to stick out more than others. They seem more vivid and easier to recall. Some of these memories are for personal events, like your first kiss or the death of a grandparent. Other memories are for shared public events, such as presidential elections, the deaths of public figures, and the events of September 11, 2001. In the following chapter, we will address what makes some events seem more memorable than others, even if our memories for these events are not better than our everyday memories. We will consider how these strong episodic memories, called *flashbulb memories*, are formed, and why some people are more likely than others to have a flashbulb memory of a particular event. Specifically, we will compare students' autobiographical memories for September 11th and the Columbia Space Shuttle disaster to illustrate the issues involved in the flashbulb memory phenomenon.

Cognitive psychologists define *flashbulb memory* as the memory of learning of a consequential, surprising, and emotionally arousing event (Brown and Kulik, 1977). Examples of flashbulb memory events that have been studied in recent history include the Columbia Space Shuttle Disaster (Coluccia, Bianco, and Brandimonte, 2006), the September 11th attacks (e.g., Budson et al., 2004; Curci and Luminet, 2006; Luminet et al., 2004 Pezdek, 2003; Shapiro, 2006; Smith, Bibi, and Sheard, 2003; Talarico and Rubin, 2003, 2007), the death of Princess Diana (Kvavilashvili, Mirani, Schlagman, and Kornbrot, 2003), the death of former French President Mitterand (Curci, Luminet, Finkenauer, and Gisle, 2001), and the verdict of the O.J. Simpson trial (Schmolk, Buffalo, and Squire, 2000).

Flashbulb Memory Characteristics

Brown and Kulik (1977) coined the term *flashbulb memory* and suggested that two main factors contribute to the development of flashbulb memories: that the event is very surprising and that it is consequential for the person who receives the news. They proposed that unexpected deaths constitute some of the most surprising events, and therefore centered their inquiries on the sudden deaths of nine public figures, most of whom were assassinated.

To determine whether the respondents experienced flashbulb memories of these events, Brown and Kulik (1977) administered questionnaires to 80 adult participants. Participants were asked if they could recall the circumstances surrounding each event, and to write a description of those circumstances if they could. From these descriptions, the authors were able to assess the intensity of the flashbulb memory, using number of words and amount of elaboration as indicators. To assess consequentiality, the authors asked participants to report, on a five-point scale, how consequential each event was for them.

Content analyses of the flashbulb descriptions indicated that participants recalled similar details across accounts. Based on these recalled details, Brown and Kulik (1977) established a set of canonical variables related to the features of flashbulb memory: the *time* at which one learned of an event, the *location* where one learned of an event, the *concomitant activity* that one was engaged in when he or she learned of the event, the *source* of the news of the event, and the *others present* when one learned of the event.

Brown and Kulik (1977) suggested that flashbulb memory is formed via a special, distinct memory mechanism that is triggered when an event exceeds critical levels of surprise and consequentiality. However, many researchers have challenged the conception of flashbulb memory as a different kind of memory (e.g., Weaver, 1993; Talarico and Rubin, 2007). Rather, many researchers have found that flashbulb memory is a product of the same formation processes as other autobiographical memories, and is subject to the same potential distortions as other episodic memories (e.g., McCloskey, Wible, and Cohen, 1988; Neisser and Harsch, 1992; Pillemer, 1990; Talarico and Rubin, 2003, 2007). In the literature as a whole, there is mixed evidence concerning the consistency of flashbulb memories; that is, the match between details in initial and later recollections. Neisser and Harsch (1992) found that participants' memories for the Challenger Space Shuttle explosion were not consistent (average consistency score of 2.95 out of a possible 7, with 50% of the sample scoring 2 or less), but that participants had high confidence for these memories (average 4.17 out of 5). In contrast to Neisser and Harsch, Schmolk et al. (2000) found 80% consistency among their participants for learning the news of the O.J. Simpson verdict up to two and a half years after the event.

As a further example, McCloskey et al. (1988) studied the Challenger space shuttle explosion, an event that was both surprising and consequential, and should therefore be likely to induce flashbulb memories. Unlike Brown and Kulik (1977), who tested participants one time up to several years after the events of interest, McCloskey et al. tested participants within one week of the explosion, and then again nine months later (repeated testing group), both times using questions that tapped Brown and Kulik's canonical variables. Additionally, 31 participants were tested only nine months after the explosion (nine-month only group).

Over 80% of the participants in both the repeated testing and nine-month only groups were able to provide detailed responses to the canonical variables questions, meeting Brown and Kulik's (1977) criteria for flashbulb memory. McCloskey et al. (1988) then compared the immediate and delayed responses of the participants in the repeated testing groups, and coded the responses as consistent between immediate and delayed tests, more specific, more general, or inconsistent. About 60% of the responses were consistent across immediate and delayed tests. Although the majority of the responses were consistent across the delay, 40% of the responses changed. About 20% of the responses became more general, which is in line with the memory phenomenon that the amount of accessible information decreases over time. Additionally, 15% of the participants claimed that they could not remember some of the information requested on the delayed test.

McCloskey et al. (1988) concluded that "...memories for the circumstances of learning about a surprising, consequential event are subject to reconstructive errors, and to a decline over time in the amount of information that can be retrieved from memory" (p. 177). Like regular memories, flashbulb memories can be inaccurate. The consistency of flashbulb memories was assumed in other studies, including Brown and Kulik (1977), because researchers only measured memory once long after the event of interest. Instead of supporting flashbulb memory as a special type of memory, McCloskey et al. suggested that flashbulb memories fall prey to the distortions that regular memories experience. Likewise, they concluded that normal memory mechanisms explain why flashbulb memories appear to be "special" – they are memories that are linked to personally distinctive, surprising, and vivid experiences that are likely to be rehearsed more often than everyday experiences (c.f. Conway, 1995; Weaver, 1993).

Individuals report very high levels of confidence in flashbulb memories. In fact, reported confidence is often at ceiling levels (e.g., Christianson and Engelberg, 1999; Neisser and

Harsch, 1992). Neisser and Harsch found a positive correlation between vividness of the memory and confidence in the memory, but neither vividness nor confidence predicted consistency. Recently, Talarico and Rubin (2003, 2007) compared students' memories for September 11th and an everyday memory that occurred on September 10, 2001. The details that students recalled for September 11th and the everyday event were equivalent in consistency. Belief in the accuracy of memory and vividness remained high and constant for the September 11th memories, but decreased over time for the everyday memories.

Group Differences in Flashbulb Memory

In general, flashbulb memories are no more accurate than other memories, but they seem stronger and more vivid (Conway, 1995; Talarico and Rubin, 2003, 2007). Group differences, however, can affect the level of consistency observed. For example, there are age effects on flashbulb memory consistency. Cohen, Conway, and Maylor (1994) found 90% consistency among younger participants for former British Prime Minister Margaret Thatcher's resignation, but only 42% consistency among older participants. Poorer memory in older adults may be due to the declining cognitive abilities of subgroups of older adults. Budson et al. (2004) found that adults with Alzheimer's disease showed lower recall for their memories of the September 11th attacks (45%) than adults with mild cognitive impairment (70%) and healthy older adults (74%), who did not differ.

Most group differences in flashbulb memory consistency are due to shared perceptions of the importance and consequentiality of an event. For example, Conway et al. (1994) found 86% consistency for Thatcher's resignation in a United Kingdom sample, but only 29% in a non-United Kingdom sample. Similar nationality differences have been found between British and Italian samples for the death of Princess Diana (Kvavilashvili et al., 2003) and between French and Belgian samples for the death of former French President Mitterand (Curci et al., 2001). Conway et al., Curci et al., and Kvavilashvili et al. postulated that the events they studied were more important to some national groups than others, thus leading to the difference.

Varying group perceptions of the importance and consequentiality of events have also been observed within nationalities. For example, Wright, Gaskell, and O'Muircheartaigh (1998) found that British men had stronger memories than British women of the Hillsborough football disaster because men found the event to be more important and had a stronger emotional reaction to it. Er (2003) found that victims of the Marmara earthquake in Turkey had stronger memories for the event than non-victims. Finally, Edery-Halpern and Nachson (2004) found that Israeli participants' memories for terrorist attacks were determined by their personal proximity to the attack and concern for a particular person who might have been involved in the attack.

Emotional Reaction and the Formation of Flashbulb Memories

Individual differences may also affect the consistency of flashbulb memories. One key individual difference is an individual's emotional reaction to an event. Talarico, LaBar, and Rubin (2004) suggest that the intensity of emotional reaction predicts the strength of memories. However, prior research has provided mixed evidence about the role of emotional reaction in flashbulb memory consistency. For example, Schmolk et al. (2000) found a positive correlation between emotional reaction and emotional consistency. In contrast, Pezdek (2003) and Smith, Bibi, and Sheard (2003) found a negative correlation between emotional reaction and consistency for autobiographical flashbulb memory, but a positive correlation of emotional reaction and event memory. Finally, Neisser and Harsch (1992) and Talarico and Rubin (2003) found no correlation between emotional reaction and consistency.

Just as the consistency of flashbulb memories is measured by comparing remembered details at two or more time points, flashbulb memory researchers have also studied the consistency of emotional reactions to the events by comparing emotional ratings across two or more time points. Here, however, most evidence supports the consistency of emotional reactions across time. For example, Bohannon and Symons (1992) found that their participants showed consistent emotional reactions over three years for the Challenger explosion. Likewise, Curci et al. (2001) found consistent emotional reactions one year after the death of French President Mitterand. However, Curci and Luminet (2006) found large decreases in emotional reaction for September 11th in a multinational sample approximately one and a half years after the event. Curci and Luminet followed up on the multinational sample used by Luminet et al. (2004) with subgroups from the United States, Belgium, Italy, the Netherlands, Romania, and Japan. Although all participants showed a significant drop in their emotional reaction, the largest effects were seen in the US, Romanian, and Dutch participants.

Emotional reaction is considered to be one of the important factors in the formation of flashbulb memories, with different researchers postulating different ways in which an individual's emotional reaction influences the saliency and longevity of his or her flashbulb memories. Brown and Kulik (1977) stated that the event must be novel, therefore leading to surprise. If the event is surprising enough, it is then evaluated in terms of its importance/ consequentiality and emotional reaction. The level of emotional reaction, as well as perceived consequentiality, leads to overt rehearsal. Surprise, consequentiality, emotional reaction, and rehearsal all contribute directly to flashbulb memory formation.

In contrast to Brown and Kulik's (1977) model, Conway et al. (1994) postulate that prior knowledge (in this case prior knowledge of Margaret Thatcher's government and level of interest in politics) directly influences assessment of consequentiality, emotional reaction (includes surprise), and overt rehearsal. Emotional reaction and overt rehearsal are also affected by assessment of consequentiality. Unlike in Brown and Kulik's model, emotional reaction and overt rehearsal make the only direct contributions to flashbulb memory formation.

The most detailed model of how emotional reaction affects flashbulb memory formation was proposed by Finkenauer et al. (1998; c.f. Er, 2003). In Finkenauer et al.'s emotional-integrative model, the original event is appraised for novelty and consequentiality. Novelty leads to surprise and consequentiality, which, along with level of surprise, determine the emotional feeling state. Consequentiality and emotional feeling state are determined by personal characteristics, in this case, attitude toward King Baudouin of Belgium and the royal family. Surprise directly affects flashbulb memory formation. In contrast to the models of Brown and Kulik (1977) and Conway et al. (1994), emotional feeling state indirectly affects flashbulb memory formation by influencing the amount of overt rehearsal, which in turn forms the memory for the original event, which then directly influences flashbulb memory formation (along with surprise). Finkenauer et al. compared their model to the models of Brown and Kulik and Conway et al. using structural equation modeling and found that their emotional-integrative model provided the best fit for the data, as shown by the highest GFI and CFI scores (.926 and .967, respectively) and the lowest RMSEA score (.043). According to Finkenauer et al.'s model, emotional reaction has no direct influence on the formation of flashbulb memories.

The mixed results concerning the connection between emotional reaction and flashbulb memory accuracy may be due to experimenter differences in measuring emotional state and accuracy. Another explanation is that the connection between emotional reaction and flashbulb memory consistency may depend upon the nature of the event (c.f. Er, 2003). Due to the inconsistent nature of the evidence concerning the link between emotional reaction and flashbulb memory formation, additional research is needed before any conclusions can be drawn.

Summary and Introduction to the Study

In sum, flashbulb memories are no more consistent over time than other memories (e.g. McCloskey et al., 1988), but people are highly confident in these memories (e.g. Neisser and Harsch, 1992) and report them as being salient and vivid (e.g. Talarico and Rubin, 2003, 2007). Consistency for flashbulb memories, as with other episodic memories, can be influenced by group membership (e.g. Conway et al., 1994; Curci et al., 2001; and Kvavilashvili et al., 2003) or by personal assessment of an event's importance and consequentiality (e.g. Edery-Halpern and Nachson, 2004; Er, 2003; Wright et al., 1998). An individual's emotional reaction to the event helps to determine assessment of importance and consequentiality (Finkenauer et al., 1998), thus leading to rehearsal of the event. Neisser (1982) suggests that individuals' ability to provide vivid detailed recollections may be a product of rehearsal of the reception event associated with learning the flashbulb memory event.

In the current study, we compared flashbulb memory among college students for two events: the terrorist attacks of September 11, 2001, and the Columbia Space Shuttle disaster on February 1, 2003. We sought to answer the following questions:

1) *Do participants show equivalent consistency of flashbulb memory for each event?* The flashbulb memory literature has mixed results as to the consistency of recall for events. Some events show high consistency (e.g., the O.J. Simpson trial verdict, Schmolk et al., 2000) while other events show low consistency (e.g., Margaret Thatcher's resignation, Wright et al., 1998). There are even cases where different

participants have different consistency outcomes for the same event. For example, for the Challenger explosion, McCloskey et al. (1988) found that 60% of their participants provided consistent memories across two time points, but Neisser and Harsch (1992) reported an average consistency score of 2.95 (out of a maximum of seven). We compared students' memories of two events, September 11th and the Columbia Space Shuttle disaster. Other studies, such as Kvavilashvili et al. (2003) and Brown and Kulik (1977), have compared two or more events within the same sample, but in our study both events were sampled within days of their occurrence.

2) *Is emotional reaction related to consistency?* Several models of flashbulb memory formation suggest that emotional reaction only plays an indirect role in determining the strength of the memory trace (Er, 2003; Finkenauer et al., 1998). On the other hand, there is mixed evidence about the connection between emotional reaction and consistency of flashbulb memory. Schmolk et al. (2000) found a positive correlation between emotional reaction and consistency, Pezdek (2003) and Smith et al. (2003) found a negative correlation, and Neisser and Harsch (1992) and Talarico and Rubin (2003) found no correlation between emotional reaction and consistency. We conducted correlational analyses of the connection between memory consistency and emotional reaction to further explore this issue.
3) *Do participants report equivalent emotional reactions to each event?* Kvavilashvili et al. (2003) found that British participants had equivalent emotional reactions to September 11th and the death of Princess Diana, but that Italian participants had greater emotional reactions to September 11th. Because emotional reaction is predicted by personal assessment of the importance and consequentiality of the event (Finkenauer et al., 1998), it is possible that participants in our study would differ in their emotional reactions to September 11th and the Columbia Space Shuttle disaster because they might perceive the importance and consequentiality of September 11th and Columbia differently.
4) *Do emotional reactions change over time?* The flashbulb memory literature suggests that emotional reaction is stable (e.g., Bohannon and Symons, 1992; Curci et al., 2001). However, Curci and Luminet (2006) found large decreases in emotional reaction for September 11th in a multinational sample approximately one and a half years after the event. By comparing two events, we explored if emotional reactions to flashbulb memory events change.

METHOD

Participants and Procedure. The participants in the September 11th group included 68 students in an undergraduate cognition and memory course taught by the second author, with the first author serving as the teaching assistant, at the University of Illinois at Chicago (UIC). Students filled out a survey two days after the event (T1). Eleven weeks later, on November 29, 2001, surveys were again distributed (T2). Because some students who filled out the T1 survey were not in class for the administration of the T2 survey, only 26 students completed this second survey, leaving 26 participants in the sample. No demographic data were collected about the participants.

The participants in the Columbia group included students in two undergraduate cognition and memory courses: one taught at UIC by the first author, and the other one taught at Governor's State University (GSU) by the second author. Twenty students at UIC completed the first survey on February 4, 2003, three days after the event, and 38 students at GSU completed the first survey on February 5, 2003, four days after the event (T1). Seven weeks later, on April 16, 2003 (GSU) or April 17, 2003 (UIC), students again completed the surveys (T2). Because some students who filled out the T1 survey were not in class for the administration of the T2 survey, only 17 UIC students and 13 GSU students completed the second survey, leaving 30 participants in the sample. No demographic data were collected about the participants.

Survey Characteristics. For both the September 11th and Columbia events, participants completed 15-question surveys that were modeled after those used by Neisser and Harsch (1992; see Appendix A). The survey first asked for a free recall of their learning of the event. Participants reported their personal reactions and were asked to include as much information as they could remember. They then answered a series of short-answer questions based on Brown and Kulik's five canonical categories: time, location, concomitant activity, source, and others present. Participants also rated their emotional reaction to the event on 1 to 5 scale, with 1 = indifferent to 5 = extremely upset/devastated.

Coding. We transcribed and coded answers to the free response question. The first and third authors calculated the number of words and propositions (idea units) in each response. Then we developed a coding scheme in a bottom-up fashion from themes present in participants' responses. The first and third authors coded the entire set of data. Interrater reliability was high (kappa = .75) and differences were resolved via discussion.

ANALYSIS

We compared the content of participants' responses to the short-answer questions at both time points to estimate the consistency of their memories. Classification of consistency for each variable proceeded in a similar fashion because we required same or very similar content in responses at T1 and T2 (c.f. Talarico and Rubin, 2003). The only exception was the time variable, for which we allowed a 15-minute window in the report of time learned. For example, if a participant listed at T1 that her concomitant activity was "getting up" and then listed at T2 that her concomitant activity was "just awakening," this was considered to be consistent. However, if a participant wrote that he was at work on the T1 survey but then wrote that he was at home on the T2 survey, this would not be considered consistent. If a participant provided more information at T2, the answer was considered consistent as long as the T1 information was included. For example, it would be considered consistent if at T1 a participant stated that her mother was present when she heard news of the event, but at T2 stated that her mother and sister were present when she found out the news. The converse of this rule was not considered as a consistent answer; that is, if a T2 answer left out information that was part of the T1 answer, the T1 and T2 answers were not considered to be consistent.

RESULTS

Flashbulb Memory Consistency. Participants exhibited flashbulb memories if they remained consistent on at least four of the five canonical categories (c.f. Conway et al., 1994; Schmolk et al., 2000). Eighty-one percent (21/26) of the participants in the September 11 group, and 67% (20/30) of the participants in the Columbia group showed flashbulb memory. This was not a significant difference between the events, χ^2 (1, 56) = 1.41, ns.

Relationship between Consistency and Emotional Reaction. Only participants who exhibited flashbulb memories were considered in this analysis. These participants had change scores of zero or one because they were consistent on at least four out of five variables. Therefore consistency was measured through a change score of zero or one. Mean emotional reactions for the events at T1 and T2 were as follows: September 11 T1, 4.24 (SD = .83); September 11 T2, 4.14 (SD = .66); Columbia T1, 3.40 (SD = .94), Columbia T2, 2.80 (SD = 1.20). There was only a marginally significant positive correlation between emotional reaction at T1 and consistency in the September 11th group, r (21) = .40, p = .07. No other relationship between emotional reaction and consistency reached significance: September 11th T2, r (21) = .06, ns; Columbia T1, r (20) = -.11, ns; or Columbia T2, r (20) = -.34, ns.

Change in Emotional Reaction over Time. A mixed design analysis of variance (ANOVA) was conducted, with event (September 11th or Columbia) as the between-subjects factor, time as the within-subjects factor, and participants' ratings of emotional reaction as the dependent variable only using the participants who exhibited flashbulb memory, as determined as being consistent on at least four of the five canonical variables. Emotion ratings were significantly higher for T1 than T2, F (1, 39) = 7.85, $p < .05$, $\eta^2 = .17$, and were higher for September 11th than Columbia, F (1, 39) = 17.57, $p < .05$, $\eta^2 = .31$. There was also an interaction between time and event, F (1, 39) = 4.14, p = .05, $\eta^2 = .10$. Emotion ratings were consistent for September 11th between T1 and T2, F (1, 39) < 1, ns, but emotion ratings decreased for Columbia between T1 and T2, F (1, 39) = 9.24, $p < .05$, $\eta^2 = .33$.

ANALYSIS OF FREE-RECALL RESPONSES

Words and Propositions. Open-ended responses were first analyzed for both events in terms of the number of words participants used and the number of propositions, or idea units, present in the responses. The flashbulb memory literature suggests that more detailed responses are associated with stronger memories (Brown and Kulik, 1977; Er, 2003; Kvavilashvili et al., 2003; Pezdek, 2003). Participants in the September 11th group used more words in their free recalls at T1 (M = 93.19, SD = 43.03) than participants in the Columbia group (M = 62.40, SD = 34.58), *t* (54) = 2.97, $p < .05$. There was no difference between the groups in number of words used in the free recalls at T2 (September 11th, M = 59.96, SD = 36.62; Columbia, M = 46.07, SD = 25.16, *t* (54) = 1.67, ns). More propositions were used by participants in the September 11th group than the Columbia group at T1 (September 11th [M = 3.52, SD = 1.02] > Columbia [M = 2.87, SD = 1.26], *t* [54] = 2.23, $p < .05$) and T2 (September 11th [M = 3.43, SD = 1.33] > Columbia [M = 2.76, SD = 1.15], *t* (54) = 2.01, *p* = .05).

Event Differences in Coding Categories. Coding categories emerged through a bottom-up examination of themes that were present in the free-recall responses. Table 1 presents a complete list of the coding categories and examples from the free-recall responses that fit in each category, while Table 2 displays the frequency of coding categories present for each event.

A series of chi-square tests revealed no differences between the events for the mention of the following coding categories: sadness, anger, relief, prayer, need for information, and terrorism. There was a marginally significant difference between the September 11th and Columbia groups for mention of disbelief at T1, χ^2 (1, 56) = 3.37, p = .07, λ = .12, and at T2, χ^2 (1, 56) = 4.69, p < .05, λ = .15, with participants in the September 11th group mentioning they felt more disbelief than participants in the Columbia group.

Table 1. Examples of Coding Categories from Free Recall Responses

Coding Category	September 11th Example	Columbia Example
Disbelief/unreality	It seemed like it was a movie. I couldn't believe it.	It didn't seem real.
Sadness/grief	Later when I began to see the images on television, I was so saddened and awestruck that I don't think words can describe it.	I felt really sad when we saw photos of all the astronauts.
Anger/revenge	I actually feel really angry at the terrorists and pretty much their community especially when I saw how happy they were after the terror. I feel that they should pay "BIG TIME!"	I felt sick, upset, angry, and outraged at the same time.
No reaction/neutrality	N/A	I didn't really feel anything.
Sympathy/concern for victims/families	I felt sorry for all the people who were in the airplanes and for the people working in the WTC towers.	I felt deep sorrow for the people that lost their lives and also for their families.
Fear/could happen to me	When I heard about it, I was at first shocked and then became scared and frightened. I thought to myself that what would happen if a plane came towards us.	N/A
Relief	N/A	I was kind of relieved to see that we were not being attacked.

Coding Category	September 11th Example	Columbia Example
Religious/praying/God reference	And I immediately began to pray for the children who may have lost parents and just everyone involved directly.	Also, I prayed for the victims families on their loss of their loved one.
Surprise/shock/alarm	I was horrified and shocked all at once.	I was shocked. I couldn't believe it.
Need for information	I was kind of curious to find out all the details.	I felt like talking to everyone on the train on the way to school about the event and find out what else they knew that I didn't.
Talked to others	First thing I did was to call my family.	My coworker had discussions about it for a while.
Mention of terrorism/war	All I could think about was that this would start World War III.	At first I thought there was another terrorist attack.
Confusion/not understanding what was happening	I didn't understand what was happening at the moment.	I just plopped myself on the couch and stared at the TV screen very dumbfounded.
Mention of change to normal day	So I turned around after hearing that everyone from downtown was racing back to their hometowns!	N/A
Knew someone involved in event/lived there	Then I talked to my best friend in Brooklyn.	My fiance was worried because his mom lives in Houston and is actually good friends with many astronauts.

Participants in the September 11th group reported being more fearful than the Columbia group, both at T1, χ^2 (1, 56) = 9.23, $p < .05$, $\lambda = .21$, and at T2, χ^2 (1, 56) = 12.37, $p = .07$, $\lambda = .28$. At T1 only, participants in the September 11th group mentioned the following categories marginally more often than participants in the Columbia group: the need to talk to others, χ^2 (1, 56) = 3.37, $p = .07$, $\lambda = .12$, a change to their day, χ^2 (1, 56) = 3.66, $p = .06$, $\lambda = .10$, and knowing people involved in the event, χ^2 (1, 56) = 3.66, $p = .06$, $\lambda = .10$. At T2 only, participants in the September 11th group mentioned being confused more often than participants in the Columbia group, χ^2 (1, 56) = 4.97, $p < .05$, $\lambda = .13$.

Table 2. Frequency and Percentage of Each Coding Category per Event

	September 11th		Columbia	
Coding Category	T1	T2	T1	T2
Disbelief/unreality	10 (38.5%)	10 (38.5%)	5 (16.7%)	4 (13.3%)
Sadness/grief	9 (34.6%)	5 (19.2%)	11 (36.7%)	11 (36.7%)
Anger/revenge	3 (11.5%)	3 (11.5%)	1 (3.3%)	2 (6.7%)
No reaction/neutrality	1 (3.8%)	1 (3.8%)	6 (20%)	7 (23.3%)
Sympathy/concern for victims/families	4 (15.4%)	2 (7.7%)	14 (46.7%)	7 (23.3%)
Fear/could happen to me	7 (26.9%)	9 (34.6%)	0	0
Relief	0	0	2 (6.7%)	2 (6.7%)
Religious/praying/God reference	2 (7.7%)	2 (7.7%)	1 (3.3%)	1 (3.3%)
Surprise/shock/alarm	6 (23.1%)	10 (38.5%)	6 (20%)	12 (40%)
Need for information	5 (19.2%)	3 (11.5%)	10 (33.3%)	7 (23.3%)
Talked to others	10 (38.5%)	7 (26.9%)	5 (16.7%)	4 (13.3%)
Mention of terrorism/war	5 (19.2%)	2 (7.7%)	3 (10%)	3 (10%)
Confusion/not understanding what was happening	4 (15.4%)	4 (15.4%)	3 (10%)	0
Mention of change to normal day	3 (11.5%)	1 (3.8%)	0	0
Knew someone involved in event/lived there	3 (11.5%)	2 (7.7%)	0	1 (3.3%)

More participants in the Columbia group were neutral than participants in the September 11th group at both T1, χ^2 (1, 56) = 3.32, p = .07, λ = .03, and T2, χ^2 (1, 56) = 4.32, $p < .05$, λ = .06. At T1 only, participants in the Columbia group mentioned sympathy for those involved in the event (and their families) more often than participants in the September 11th group, χ^2 (1, 56) = 6.25, $p < .05$, $\lambda = .14$.

Differences Across Time in Frequency of Coding Categories. In addition to examining group differences (by event) in the types of codes mentioned by participants, we also examined the changes to codes mentioned between the two surveys (T1 and T2).

There were no changes from T1 to T2 in the coding categories that the September 11th participants mentioned. However, the Columbia participants showed a variety of marginally significant changes. The mention of sympathy for those involved in the events and their families changed in the Columbia group, with the number of participants reporting sympathy decreasing, χ^2 (1, 56) = 3.59, $p = .06$, $\lambda = .14$. There was also a decrease in mention of confusion, with fewer participants in the Columbia group mentioning they were confused at T2 than at T1, χ^2 (1, 56) = 3.18, $p = .08$, $\lambda = .09$. Finally, there was a change in mention of surprise in the Columbia group, with more participants mentioning surprise at T2 than T1, χ^2 (1, 56) = 2.86, $p = .09$, $\lambda = .13$.

CONCLUSION

Our aim in this paper was to answer four questions concerning flashbulb memory differences between two recent events, the terrorist attacks of September 11th and the Space Shuttle Columbia disaster. These questions concerned memory consistency for both events, whether emotional reaction predicted consistency, if participants showed the same emotional reactions for both events, and if their emotional reactions changed over time.

Memory Consistency. We found that participants showed equivalent consistency in flashbulb memory when comparing the two events. Participants in the September 11th group were no more consistent than participants in the Columbia group. Our finding of a medium to high level of memory consistency (74% averaged across the two events) falls in the middle of the spectrum of the prior research on the consistency of flashbulb memories. In contrast to our results, Schmolk et al. (2000) found 80% consistency, and Wright et al. (1998) found 12% consistency.

Emotional Reaction for Each Event and its Relation to Consistency. Participants showed stronger emotional reactions to September 11th than Columbia. Several prior studies suggest that differences in emotional reactions to flashbulb memory events are due to nationality differences in the assessment of importance and consequentiality (e.g. Conway et al., 1994; Curci et al., 2001; Kvavilashvili et al., 2003).

Even though participants in the September 11th group showed stronger emotional reactions, these emotional reactions were only marginally related to their consistency, and only at T1. This marginal correlation was positive, supporting the results of Schmolk et al. (2000). However, the general lack of relationship between emotional reaction and consistency supports the findings of Neisser and Harsch (1992) and Talarico and Rubin (2003). The lack of direct relationships between emotional reaction and consistency lends support to flashbulb memory models that posit an indirect influence of emotional reaction on the strength of the memory trace (Er, 2003; Finkenauer et al., 1998).

Change in Emotional Reaction over Time. Participants in the September 11th group maintained their strong emotional reactions over time, but the emotional reaction of participants in the Columbia group decreased between T1 and T2. This observation of decreased emotional reaction to memories of Columbia is comparable to Curci and Luminet's (2006) findings about September 11th, but it stands in contrast to many other studies (e.g., Bohannon and Symons, 1992; Curci et al., 2001)..

Why did the emotional reaction of Columbia participants decrease between T1 and T2? This is not a common finding in the flashbulb memory literature (e.g. Bohannon and Symons, 1992; Curci et al., 2001, but see Curci and Luminet, 2006). The examination of the free recall responses may provide a reason for the decrease in emotion ratings between T1 and T2. Participants in the Columbia group expressed less sympathy for those involved in the event and less confusion about the event at T2. Unexpectedly, they expressed more surprise about the event at T2. These changes in free recall responses may explain why participants in the Columbia group rated their emotional reaction to the event lower at T2.

Differences in the perceived consequentiality of each event might also explain our findings. Prior works by Brown and Kulik (1977), Conway et al. (1994), Finkenauer et al. (1998), and Er (2003) have all stressed how flashbulb memories only form in reaction to consequential events. It is possible, therefore, that although both events were surprising[6], the events may not be equally consequential. In an informal survey of the consequentiality of each event, students from an undergraduate psychology course were asked on April 12, 2004 to provide free recalls of how they learned the news of September 11th and Columbia. All of the students had substantive memories for September 11th (31 months after the event), but 42% could not recall how they learned the news of Columbia (14 months after the event). Similar results were obtained in undergraduate psychology courses during the Fall 2006, Spring 2007, and Fall 2007 semesters. Students' recall for the reception event of September 11th was 100%. For Columbia, however, 57%, 67%, and 58% of the students had no recall of the event in the Fall 2006, Spring 2007, and Fall 2007 semesters, respectively.

The reasons that September 11th may have been perceived as more consequential than Columbia are varied. For example, September 11th had more media coverage, and changes to everyday life (tightened security in airports and public areas) followed, as well as a war. Although the Columbia disaster halted shuttle missions for over two years, it did not affect the daily lives of many people. When an event's effects are as pervasive as those of September 11th, individuals have increased chances for rehearsal of both their experiences in learning of the event and their emotional reactions of the event. As noted by Finkenauer et al. (1998) concerning the death of Belgian King Badouin, "...it seems that Belgian citizens could hardly avoid participating in the rehearsal process. It is possible that less intense national events give people the possibility to deliberately choose whether they want to engage in rehearsal or not" (p. 525, c.f. Er, 2003). When comparing September 11th to Columbia, it is possible we have exemplified Finkenauer et al.'s statement: Americans could not avoid rehearsing their reactions to September 11th, but could avoid engaging in rehearsal about Columbia. Using Finkenauer et al.'s model, it is likely that a reassessment of the importance and consequentiality of the Columbia Space Shuttle disaster led to a decreased emotional reaction, and thereby less rehearsal of the reception event. In turn, according to Finkenauer et al.'s model, this should affect memory for the original reception event, and therefore the

[6] Although the Columbia Space Shuttle disaster can be compared to the Challenger Space Shuttle disaster, most of the participants in the Columbia group were too young to recall the Challenger. For example, a college junior who was 20 or 21 years old in 2003 would have been three or four years old in 1986, when the Challenger exploded.

flashbulb memory consistency. In our sample, the T2 survey occurred seven weeks after the original survey. That may have been enough time to affect emotional reaction, but not enough to affect memory consistency. However, at the later dates that the informal surveys were held, the importance of the event had likely paled to such a degree that it degraded memory for the Columbia event.

In conclusion, although individuals may show equal accuracy in flashbulb memories to two very different events, their initial emotional reactions, as well as how these emotional reactions may change over time, may differ greatly. Comparing the events of September 11, 2001 to the Columbia Space Shuttle disaster helps us to understand the complex emotional reactions that are associated with national events, and the role of these emotional reactions in the formation of memory. In addition, the comparison of these two events provides support for theories of flashbulb memory formation that emphasize the role of perceived consequentiality.

Despite the contributions of the current study to our understanding of the nature of flashbulb memory, research in this area is far from complete. For example, although differences in emotional reaction to an event can be explained by personal or group consequentiality, these are ad hoc explanations. Comparisons of different events either have to be accomplished by comparing different samples to catch initial reactions to an event soon after it occurs (as in the current study), or by querying one sample about multiple events that have happened at different times (e.g. Brown and Kulik, 1977, Kvavilashvili et al., 2003; Wright et al., 1998). Although Weaver (1993) compared two recently occurring events in one sample, only one event (the bombing of Iraq) would qualify as an event typically expected to lead to flashbulb memory (the second event was the personal meeting of a roommate or friend).

The nature of research on flashbulb memory is largely opportunistic. Because researchers cannot fully predict when a nationally (or internationally) shared surprising and consequential event will occur, convenience samples are often used, and questionnaires are not consistent across studies. In order to conduct the most rigorous research on flashbulb memory, several steps should be taken. First, researchers must pick a common survey instrument. At minimum, the survey should assess surprise, consequentiality, rehearsal, and emotional reaction as well as Brown and Kulik's (1977) canonical variables. In addition, much of the current flashbulb memory research compares autobiographical memory to event memory (e.g. Coluccia et al., 2006; Er, 2003; Pezdek, 2003), so measures of both of these areas should be included. Second, memory should be assessed as soon as possible after the event of interest (within a few days), and should be then assessed again after a period of time (see Coluccia et al., 2006; Shapiro, 2006; and Talarico and Rubin, 2003 for discussions of when this second testing should occur).

In this way, flashbulb memory can be measured using consistency across responses instead of the amount of detail provided in a single response. Although there will likely be some dropout of participants between T1 and subsequent assessment, researchers should make an effort to keep participant retention high. Third, an ideal situation for research would be if multiple flashbulb memory events could be initially assessed soon after their occurrence within the same sample. This situation would allow for the best evaluation of the ways in which emotional reaction and personal consequentiality differ among events. Although no one would wish for the disasters and deaths that characterize most events studied in flashbulb memory research to occur in quick succession, being able to study two or more events within the same sample would allow for the best evaluation of flashbulb memory theories.

Author Notes

Trina C. Kershaw, Department of Psychology, University of Massachusetts Dartmouth; Joshua A. Hemmerich, Department of Medicine, Section of Geriatrics, University of Chicago; Sadia Ahmed, Department of Psychology, University of Illinois at Chicago. This research was conducted with students in undergraduate cognitive psychology courses at the University of Illinois at Chicago (Fall 2001, Spring 2003) and Governor's State University (Spring 2003). The authors thank these students for their participation. The authors also thank Susan Goldman and Jason Braasch for their explanations of proposition coding for the free recall responses, and Jordan Lippman and Maria Hines for comments on a draft of this chapter.

Appendix: Flashbulb Memory Questionnaire

1) Please describe how you heard the news about the disasters on September 11/Space Shuttle Columbia Space explosion on Saturday, February 1, 2003. Where were you when you found out about the news? How did you feel? Please describe your personal reaction; do not write as if you were reporting the news. Please include as much information as you can remember.
2) Please answer the following questions as briefly as possible.

1. What time was it when you found out about the news/Space Shuttle explosion?

__:__

2. Where were you when you found out about the news/Space Shuttle explosion?

____

3. What were you doing when you found out about the news/Space Shuttle explosion? __________________

4. Who told you the news/about the Space Shuttle explosion? _______________

5.Who else was there when you found out the news?______________________

6. Please rate your overall feelings about the news on the following scale (place x next to number):

1 = indifferent
2 = slightly upset
3 = moderately upset
4 = very upset
5 = extremely upset/devastated

7. Please rate how you think the person who told you felt about the news (place x next to number):
   1 = indifferent
   2 = slightly upset
   3 = moderately upset
   4 = very upset
   5 = extremely upset/devastated

8. What did you do after you found out about the news/Space Shuttle explosion?

REFERENCES

Bohannon, J.N., and Symons, L.V. (1992). Flashbulb memories: Confidence, consistency, and quantity. In E. Wingograd and U. Neisser (Eds.), *Affect and accuracy in recall: Studies of "flashbulb" memories* (pp. 65-91). Cambridge, England: Cambridge University Press.

Brown, R., and Kulik, J. (1977). Flashbulb memories. *Cognition, 5*, 73-99.

Budson, A.E., Simons, J.S., Sullivan, A.L., Beier, J.S., Solomon, P.R., Scinto, L.F., Daffner, K.R., and Schacter, D.L. (2004). Memory and emotions for the September 11, 2001, terrorist attacks in patients with Alzheimer's disease, patients with mild cognitive impairment, and healthy older adults. *Neuropsychology, 18*(2), 315-327.

Christianson, S.-A., and Engelberg, E. (1999). Memory and emotional consistency: The MS Estonia ferry disaster. *Memory, 7*, 471–482.

Cohen, G., Conway, M.A., and Maylor, E.A. (1994). Flashbulb memories in older adults. *Psychology and Aging, 9*, 454–463.

Coluccia, E., Bianco, C., and Brandimonte, M.A. (2006). Dissociating veridicality, consistency, and confidence in autobiographical and event memories for the *Columbia* shuttle disaster. *Memory, 14*(4), 452-470.

Conway, M.A. (1995). *Flashbulb memories*. Hillsdale, NJ: Lawrence Erlbaum Associates.

Conway, M.A., Anderson, S.J., Larsen, S.F., Donnelly, C.M., McDaniel, M.A., McClelland, A.G.R., Rawles, R.E., and Logie, R.H. (1994). The formation of flashbulb memories. *Memory and Cognition, 22* (3), 326-343.

Curci, A., and Luminet, O. (2006). Follow-up of a cross-national comparison of flashbulb and event memory for the September 11th attacks. *Memory, 14*(3), 329-344.

Curci, A., Luminet, O., Finkenauer, C. and Gisle, L. (2001). Flashbulb memories in social groups: A comparative study of the memory of French president Mitterand's death in a French and a Belgian Group. *Memory, 9*, 81-101.

Edery-Halpern, G., and Nachson, I. (2004). Distinctiveness in flashbulb memory: Comparative analysis of five terrorist attacks. *Memory, 12*(2), 147-157.

Er, N. (2003). A new flashbulb memory model applied to the Marmara earthquake. *Applied Cognitive Psychology, 17*, 503-517.

Finkenauer, C., Luminet, O., Gisle, L., El-Ahmadi, A., van der Linden, M., and Philippot, P. (1998). Flashbulb memories and the underlying mechanisms of their formation: Toward an emotional-integrative model. *Memory and Cognition, 26*(3), 516-531.

Kvavilashvili, L., Mirani, J., Schlagman, S., and Kornbrot, D. (2003). Comparing flashbulb memories of September 11 and the death of Princess Diana: Effects of time delays and nationality. *Applied Cognitive Psychology, 17*, 1017-1031.

Luminet, O., Curci, A., Marsh, E.J., Wessel, I., Constantin, T., Gencoz, F., and Yogo, M. (2004). The cognitive, emotional, and social impacts of the September 11 attacks: Group differences in memory for the reception context and the determinants of flashbulb memory. *The Journal of General Psychology, 131*(3), 197-224.

McCloskey, M., Wible, C.G., and Cohen, N.J. (1988). Is there a special flashbulb-memory mechanism? *Journal of Experimental Psychology: General, 117*(2), 171-181.

Neisser, U. (1982). Snapshots or benchmarks? In U. Neisser (Ed.), *Memory observed:Remembering in natural contexts* (pp. 43-48). San Francisco: Freeman.

Neisser, U., and Harsch, N. (1992). Phantom flashbulbs: False recollections of hearing the news about Challenger. In E. Winograd and U. Neisser (Eds.), *Affect and accuracy in recall:Studies of "flashbulb" memories*. Cambridge, UK: Cambridge University Press.

Pezdek, K. (2003). Event memory and autobiographical memory for the events of September 11, 2001. *Applied Cognitive Psychology, 17*, 1033-1045.

Pillemer, D.B. (1990). Clarifying the Flashbulb Memory concept: Comment on McCloskey, Wible, and Cohen (1988). *Journal of Experimental Psychology: General, 119*, 92-96.

Schmolck, H., Buffalo, E.A., and Squire, L.R. (2000). Memory distortions develop over time: Recollections of the O.J. Simpson trial verdict after 15 and 32 months. *Psychological Science, 11*(1), 39-45.

Shapiro, L.R. (2006). Remembering September 11th: The role of retention interval and rehearsal on flashbulb and event memory. *Memory, 14*(2), 129-147.

Smith, M., Bibi, U., and Sheard, E. (2003). Evidence for the differential impact of time and emotion on personal and event memories for September 11, 2001. *Applied Cognitive Psychology, 17*, 1047-1055.

Talarico, J.M., LaBar, K.S., and Rubin, D.C. (2004). Emotional intensity predicts autobiographical memory experience. *Memory and Cognition, 32*(7), 1118-1132.

Talarico, J.M., and Rubin, D.C. (2003). Confidence, not consistency characterizes flashbulb memories. *Psychological Science, 14*(5), 455-461.

Talarico, J.M., and Rubin, D.C. (2007). Flashbulb memories are special after all; in phenomenology, not accuracy. *Applied Cognitive Psychology, 21*, 557-578.

Weaver, C.A. III. (1993). Do you need a "flash" to form a flashbulb memory? *Journal of Experimental Psychology, 122*(1), 39-46.

Wright, D.B., Gaskell, G.D., and O'Muircheartaigh, C.A. (1998). Flashbulb memory assumptions: Using national surveys to explore cognitive phenomena. *British Journal of Psychology, 89*(1), 103-121.

In: Applied Memory
Editor: Matthew R. Kelley

ISBN 978-1-60692-143-2

Chapter 9

The Magnitude Gap: Revealing Differences in Recall Between Victims and Perpetrators

Robert N. Kraft
Department of Psychology,
Otterbein College, Westerville, OH, USA

Abstract

The magnitude gap refers to the consistent differences in recall between victims and perpetrators (Baumeister, Stillwell, and Wotman, 1990). Victims recall a series of provocations leading up to an incident as well as the consequences afterwards, whereas perpetrators recall an incident as bracketed in time, omitting previous provocations and later consequences. Victims omit situational influences and recall more emotion, whereas perpetrators recall incidents as resulting from situational factors, often with the victim overreacting. This chapter introduces new research on the magnitude gap in free recall, with a focus on *metamemory*. In free recall, victim accounts were almost 20% longer than perpetrator accounts, showing significantly more description of the aftermath, more remembered conversation, and more quantitative detail, whereas perpetrators' accounts included more justification for their behavior. The metamemory analysis revealed that time was experienced as slowing down in a majority of victim incidents but that there was no reported change in experienced time with a majority of perpetrator incidents, though nearly one-third of the perpetrator incidents led to the experience of time moving more quickly. In addition, with victim incidents the most frequently reported reason for retrieval was that these incidents still generated emotion. This chapter applies the experimental findings on the magnitude gap to *truth commissions*, where victims and perpetrators confront each other with discrepant accounts of the same events. The chapter focuses on South Africa's Truth and Reconciliation Commission (TRC) as an exemplar for the twenty-eight national truth commissions conducted to date. During the TRC, victims of apartheid recalled events to document the crimes committed against them and to seek reparations, whereas perpetrators recalled events to detail the crimes they committed during apartheid and to obtain amnesty. Consistent with the experimental literature, the TRC hearings revealed dramatic and predictable discrepancies between the memories of perpetrators and victims. Perpetrators bracketed their criminal incidents within narrow time frames and in the context of doing their jobs; victims recalled the incidents as an extended series of events that continued to generate emotion. Moreover, many victims did not believe the discrepancies between their own personal memories and those of the perpetrators, and they went on record stating that the perpetrators failed to disclose fully, potentially denying them amnesty. Research on the magnitude gap can help explain the profound differences in recall between victims and perpetrators during truth commissions, ultimately contributing to the overall effectiveness of these commissions.

INTRODUCTION

In July of 1997, Captain Jeffrey Benzien of the South African Police (SAP) sat before the amnesty committee of South Africa's Truth and Reconciliation Commission and gave testimony about his illegal activities during apartheid. In the course of this testimony, Benzien provided extended free recall of his duties with the "terrorist tracking unit" of the SAP, finding and detaining anti-apartheid activists and locating their ammunition and weapons. He then recalled in detail his most notorious expertise: the "wet bag" method of torture interrogation. He recounted how he would force a wet canvas bag over the head of a bound prisoner and then alternately tighten and release the bag, repeatedly bringing the prisoner to the brink of asphyxiation while conducting his interrogation.

During these hearings, as Benzien's former victims listened to his sworn testimony and asked questions, they became increasingly distressed about his memory for the events. At one point, for example, Benzien described his relationship with one of his torture victims in the following way: "Apart from those two occasions where I questioned him in an unconventional way, we built up an excellent rapport" (Benzien, 14 July 1997). The former victim did not agree, and he said so. But even more distressing to his former victims was what Benzien could *not* remember. In three days of testimony – in free recall and in answering questions – Benzien cited his inability to remember more than sixty times (Benzien, 14-16 July 1997). He could not remember who helped him during his interrogations, the length of time he interrogated prisoners, or the particular methods (beatings, repeated suffocation, or suspending prisoners in handcuffs so their feet could not touch the ground). Each of his former victims expressed deep suspicion at Benzien's failure to recall events that they considered central to their mistreatment.

In fact, serious discrepancies between the memories of perpetrators and the memories of victims occurred throughout the amnesty hearings of the Truth and Reconciliation Commission. As the hearings proceeded, in one instance after another, the memories of the perpetrators came into direct conflict with the memories of the victims. There was, in short, an unbridgeable gap in memory.

The memory effect elaborated and applied in this chapter is this gap: the consistent pattern of differences in personal event memory between victims and perpetrators, known as the *magnitude gap* (Baumeister, Stillwell, and Wotman, 1990; Baumeister and Newman, 1994; Baumeister, 1997; Stillwell and Baumeister, 1997). The primary application of this memory effect is to *truth commissions*, which are mandated to investigate widespread abuses of human rights and to reconcile the profound differences between the victims of violence and the perpetrators. This chapter reviews the literature on the magnitude gap, introduces new experimental work on memory differences between victims and perpetrators, and applies the overall findings on the magnitude gap to the difficult problem of resolving long-standing national conflicts through truth commissions.

The Magnitude Gap

In the seminal study of Baumeister, Stillwell, and Wotman (1990), participants freely recalled incidents of angering someone else (a perpetrator memory) and of being angered by someone else (a victim memory).[7] The memory descriptions were then analyzed in terms of dichotomous codings that specified the presence or absence of particular contents. Comparison of victim accounts and perpetrator accounts revealed several categories of difference with respect to the time frame of the memory description, the aftermath of the actions, the intentions of the perpetrator, the responses of the victim, and the emotions experienced. Victim accounts placed the incident in an extended time frame that included a series of provocations, whereas perpetrator accounts bracketed the incident in a narrower time frame. Victim accounts described the incidents as having lasting consequences, whereas perpetrator accounts described the events as isolated and closed. Victim accounts blamed the perpetrator, whereas perpetrator accounts were more situational, describing the incident as something that could not be helped, often with the victim overreacting. Finally, victim accounts related more emotion.

Critiquing the original study, Stillwell and Baumeister (1997) noted that deviations from factual accuracy could not be assessed because victim memories and perpetrator memories involved different sets of incidents. To ensure that victim accounts and perpetrator accounts were based on the same incident, Stillwell and Baumeister provided all the participants with identical detailed descriptions of an interpersonal transgression involving two main characters: a victim and an offender. While reading the descriptions, one group assumed the perspective of the victim, another the perspective of the offender, and a third served as a control, simply reading the information without taking the perspective of either character. All participants were then required to recall the detailed description. The experimenters assessed systematic differences in the accuracy of victim memories and perpetrator memories by comparing the recalled information to the original description of the incident. This assessment showed that offender accounts and victim accounts did not differ in the total number of errors but did differ significantly in the *type* of information selectively omitted. Victim accounts were as accurate as control accounts in including details that exacerbated the transgression, but they omitted information that mitigated the offense or that emphasized its positive aspects. Offender accounts were as accurate as control accounts in including details that mitigated or emphasized the positive aspects of the transgressions, but they omitted information that exacerbated the transgressions. That is, victims and offenders remembered identical transgressions differently, with victims omitting details that justified the offenders' actions and perpetrators omitting details that emphasized the unpleasantness of the acts. These results suggest that a readily accessible schema for victim or offender guided the initial

[7] With most research on the magnitude gap, the words "victim" and "perpetrator" are used in the published discussions of the results, but they are not used with the participants. In some of these discussions, an alternative word for perpetrator is "offender." The incidents themselves are usually referred to as "transgressions" or "offenses."

selection of information to be remembered and that inconsistent information was not encoded as part of the instantiated schema (Rumelhart, 1980).

The concept of "magnitude gap" was first labeled and summarized by Baumeister (1997). In general, when asked to remember an incident, victims recall a series of provocations leading up to the incident and the long-term consequences afterwards, whereas perpetrators recall the incident as bracketed in time, omitting the provocations leading up to the incident and the consequences afterwards. Victims recall the incident as arbitrary; perpetrators recall the incident as comprehensible. Victims omit situational factors, whereas perpetrators emphasize these factors. A common example of the magnitude gap in popular culture is the acceptance of disproportionate revenge in narratives that take the perspective of those who are initially victimized. In the typical revenge narrative, the ultimate punishment of the perpetrators far exceeds the original crime. Such punishment appears justified when the narrative is encoded from the perspective of the victims because it is based not on a dispassionate assessment of the perpetrators' actions but on the victims' representation of their own experience.

Later studies of the magnitude gap focused on variables that could potentially affect the gap and account for the differences in memory. Schütz and Baumeister (1999) focused on linguistic features in the recall of transgressions versus the recall of incidents of making someone happy. Compared to memory descriptions of having made a person happy, descriptions of transgressions had fewer concrete details and longer introductions that explained background and mitigating circumstances. Kearns and Fincham (2005) elaborated Baumeister et al. (1990) by distinguishing between romantic and non-romantic transgressions, replicating the magnitude gap between victim and perpetrator accounts with both types of offenses. With both offenses, most of the variability was accounted for by perpetrators remembering the transgressions as less severe than the victims.

As in Baumeister et al. (1990), Zechmeister and Romero (2002) required participants to describe memories of events in which they were either victims or perpetrators, but with an additional distinction: events were divided into those in which the perpetrators were either forgiven later or not forgiven later. This distinction then provided an indirect method for separating encoding effects from later memory effects. That is, after an offense occurs, it is then represented in the form of a personal event memory, and memory descriptions will reveal the standard magnitude gap between victims and perpetrators. If the offense is subsequently forgiven, any changes in the magnitude gap would then be due to memory activities that occurred *after* the original encoding of the event. In general, Zechmeister and Romero (2002) replicated the memory patterns of Baumeister, et al. (1990): victim accounts elaborated the time frame of the incident as a set of multiple offenses and portrayed events as arising from arbitrary and unjustified actions by the perpetrator; perpetrator accounts bracketed the incident in time and portrayed events as arising from external or mitigating circumstances. Later forgiveness, however, altered the victims' remembered time frame of the incident: victim accounts of *forgiven* offenses were more likely to recall the offenses as closed and less likely to report multiple provocations leading to the incident. Nonetheless, victims who forgave still recalled their emotions resulting from the offenses and the unpleasant consequences of the offenses that justified these emotions. In this study, forgiveness affected the *bracketing* of the incident but not the encoding and representation of the central actions and emotions.

In terms of Schacter's (1999) "seven sins of memory," three basic memory processes contribute to the magnitude gap after the initial encoding of the incident: misattribution, bias, and persistence. *Misattribution* contributes to the magnitude gap when people mistakenly draw from an elaborated, general schema that characterizes other, similar instances and then report information from this schema as being part of a different specific memory (Kraft, 2000). *Bias* results from the distorting influences of present knowledge. In particular, a bias for consistency alters memories of past events so that they are more congruent with present behavior and attitudes. Similarly, a bias for *in*consistency alters memories of past events so that they are more discordant with previous behavior – if people believe they have changed considerably over time. This inconsistency bias would be especially pertinent in the case of perpetrators who conceive of themselves as different people years after their transgressions. *Persistence* refers to the tendency for victims to remember events that they would rather forget, ruminating on past injustices and increasing the frequency of rehearsal.

Reexamining the Magnitude Gap

The experimental research introduced in this chapter analyzed the magnitude gap in freely recalled incidents, with a focus on *metamemory* for the incidents.[8] That is, after freely recalling incidents of being treated unfairly and of treating others unfairly, what do participants report about their own memory processes and how do their metamemory analyses inform the magnitude gap? More broadly, to what extent are people *aware* of the magnitude gap and the processes underlying this gap in their own memory system? An assessment of this awareness would be integral in applying the basic research on the magnitude gap to the profound discrepancies that exist between the accounts of victims and perpetrators during truth commissions.

Method

There were 70 participants in this study, with an age range of 18 to 38 and a mean age of 23. The procedure involved two separate steps. First, all participants freely described four personal event memories: two perpetrator memories and two victim memories. For a perpetrator memory, participants were instructed as follows: "Describe an incident in which *you* treated *another person* unfairly or unjustly. Tell as much as you can about the incident. Be thorough and provide the full story." For a victim memory, the first sentence of the instructions was, "Describe an incident in which *you* were treated unfairly or unjustly *by someone else*." Order was balanced.

The second step occurred approximately one week later when participants returned to analyze their own memory descriptions. They read their accounts and then answered the five questions shown in Table 1.

[8] This study began as part of an Advanced Research class at Otterbein College, with the following students: Emily Bennett, Shannon Fox, Seth Greene, Kara Kelly, Eric Miller, Elizabeth Moore, Cathrine Pace, Theresa Pryor, Matthew Williams, and Jonathan Wright. A preliminary report of the results was presented at the Experimental Psychological Society in Edinburgh, Scotland in July of 2007.

Table 1. Memory analysis questions

1) Why did you select this particular memory?
2) What parts of your description might be exaggerated or inaccurate? Why?
3) During the incident, how did you experience the passage of time? Describe your experience freely and then choose one of the following statements below.

a. My perception of time did not change.
b. Time seemed to move more slowly.
c. Time seemed to move more quickly.

4) Did you learn any long-term lessons from this incident? If so, what were they?
5) Describe what the other person was thinking and feeling.

Question 1 focused on the reasons that particular memories were retrieved and the retrieval cues used for accessing these memories. Question 2 focused on the participants' knowledge of their own inaccuracies, encouraging them to reexamine their memories and their beliefs about what transpired (Mazzoni and Kirsch, 2002; Scoboria, Mazzoni, Kirsch, and Relyea, 2004). What kinds of inaccuracies would participants identify in their own memory descriptions and what differences would occur between victim accounts and perpetrator accounts? Question 3 focused on time perception during the incidents. The rationale for this question was based on analysis of direct reports from victims about their encoding of extended trauma (Kraft, 2002, 2006a) and testimony from perpetrators about their transgressions (Kraft, 2006b). Question 4 was designed to elicit knowledge about the lessons of memory, termed "memory directives" by Pillemer (1998). Question 5 attempted to elicit more information about one's memory for others involved in the incident, in particular the reasons of the perpetrator (for a victim memory) and the reactions of the victim (for a perpetrator memory).

RESULTS

Almost all the remembered incidents were unexceptional injustices involving friends, school, relationships, family, athletics, work, or authority figures, such as police. The three most frequent categories of victim memories were misunderstandings at school and work, betrayal by friends and lovers, and injustices in the classroom – most notably being falsely accused by a teacher. The three most frequent categories of perpetrator memories were betraying friends, being deceptive or unfaithful in relationships, and being rude to a family member. While the injustices were in familiar categories, most were considered serious by the participants (e.g., being roughed up by a group of students and having the teacher do nothing or suffering an asthma attack in gym class and being yelled at for slacking off or being inconsiderate to a brother who was dying of leukemia).

In free recall of the incidents, victim accounts were almost 20% longer than perpetrator accounts: a mean of 205 words to recall being treated unfairly by others and a mean of 171 words to recall treating someone else unfairly ($t(69) = 4.20$, $p < .001$). The free recall accounts were then analyzed for general categories of content, as shown in Table 2.

Table 2. Categories of content in victim accounts and perpetrator accounts

	Victim Accounts	Perpetrator Accounts
Conversation	4.3	1.4
Numbers and quantities	1.9	1.2
Emotion	1.5	1.2
Perceptual experience	1.1	.78
Justification	5.9	22.16
Aftermath	11.7	7.2

Sample justifications in perpetrator accounts and descriptions of aftermath in victim accounts

Justifications

"I was doing him a favor by pointing out his behavior was reckless and would lead to misfortune."

"I remember having a very bad day at work and then came home and took it out big time on my housemate."

"I must have been daydreaming because I didn't really know what was going on."

"Unfortunately, I had to drive to Akron the previous night and I was exhausted."

Descriptions of aftermath

"That experience just increased my hatred for her as a teacher, making me dread going into her classroom. And from then on, I disliked math."

"We eventually stopped talking and it took a long time before we reconciled our differences and became friends again."

"To this day, I still have some built up hatred for this person."

"I don't think I've seen those friends since this incident: partly because we went our separate ways and partly because they refused to keep in touch with me."

Victim accounts showed significantly more words for remembered conversations ($t(69) = 3.99$, $p < .01$)[9] and more detail about numbers and quantities ($t(69) = 4.63$, $p < .01$). Victim accounts also showed more emotion words ($t(69) = 1.90$, $p > .05$) and more description of perceptual experience – sights, sounds, and physiological states ($t(69) = 1.94$, $p > .05$), but the use of these words was infrequent and the differences were not significant with a two-tailed test.

Perpetrator accounts included significantly more justification for their behavior as part of the memory description ($t(69) = 7.40$, $p < .01$), with almost four times as much justification than in victim accounts. Victim accounts included significantly more description of the aftermath ($t(69) = 2.85$, $p < .01$), with recall of the aftermath 60% longer in victim accounts than in perpetrator accounts. Table 2 presents specific examples of justifications in perpetrator accounts and descriptions of aftermath in victim accounts. Overall, the perpetrator accounts suggest that transgressions arise from the situation and that justification is necessary to describe the transgression accurately. The elaborated description of the aftermath in victim accounts suggests that the remembered incident can extend well beyond the specific transgression.

With regard to the second step of the study, participants showed appreciable awareness of their own memory processes. Consider a verbatim response from one participant, with the freely recalled incident involving victimization in school.

> I was rather a large child and I used to be teased for my weight. And my unique name. The teasing was so bad at one point that a group of older boys ganged up on me, ripped my shirt off, and made me sing to them as they pushed me around in a circle. When I got back to class, covered in mud, and shirtless, the teacher refused to punish the boys and yelled at me for being inappropriate and a liar.

---

[9] To assess remembered conversation, two kinds of statements were counted: those within quotation marks and implied quotations. The one exception to counting words within quotation marks was for phrases or words that were marked with quotations for emphasis. In the following two sentences, for example, "cool" and "spare time" were not counted. "One of the 'cool' kids asked me for a ride." "I guess she must have thought I was selling houses in my 'spare time.'" All other quoted entries were counted as remembered conversation. Phrases that were not enclosed in quotation marks had to meet several requirements in order to be counted as remembered conversation. To begin, the recalled statements had to be immediately preceded by words such as "said," "told," "called" or "asked." In the following four sentences, the italicized words were counted as remembered conversation. "Our teacher asked *would it be okay if Andi joined our group*." "I very politely asked *why wasn't I able to work on my project and the others were*." "She said *he has a family and doesn't need to talk to anyone else*." "He called me *Kike* under his breath." Several rules excluded the counting of unquoted statements as remembered conversation. If "that" was used as a conjunction to introduce the statement, it was not counted (e.g., "He told us that we should not throw the ball in the store any more."). Only the simple past tense was permitted; the past perfect simple ("he had said"), the progressive past ("he was asking"), and the past perfect progressive ("he had been telling us") were not. In general, if the introductory statement included an auxiliary verb, the phrase was not counted, as in the following two sentences from the memory descriptions. "I had been told not to cut across the neighbor's yard." "The other members were asked to be there around 6 o'clock to do this." When an implied statement was merely informational or a summary, it was not counted. For example, the following informational statement did not qualify as remembered conversation. "My dad asked about my hourly wage, which they told him would be $8.50 per hour." The following summary statements were also not counted. "He started to tell me what to do and how to do it." "He still continued to call and tell me he loved me." In short, all quoted passages were counted as remembered conversation, except those words that were in quotation marks for emphasis. Phrases not in quotations were counted as remembered conversation only when they were 1) preceded by statement words ("said," "told," "called" or "asked"), 2) in the past tense without auxiliary verbs, and 3) not strictly factual or summary statements.

One week later, this participant analyzed his memory description with respect to the five questions (Table 1). He selected the particular memory because, "It was a very painful experience that had no real cause, and it has stayed with me until the present." About inaccuracies or exaggerations, he said, "I may be exaggerating the teacher's reaction or the boys' cruelty because I was/am so upset by the incident." Concerning time perception, he said, "Time slowed down drastically. It seemed to last forever." The lesson of memory was, "Bad things happen for no reason, and sometimes people just like to be cruel." When asked to describe what the others were thinking or feeling, he said, "Empowered and superior, I don't really know."

With regard to the metamemory analysis, Table 3 shows the five most frequent reasons for selecting a particular memory, ordered in descending frequency of the responses for victim accounts. For victims, the most frequent reason was that the remembered incident still generated emotion, with twice as many victim accounts citing this reason: 35% of the victim accounts and 17% of the perpetrator accounts (χ^2 (1, N = 73) = 8.56, p < .01). For victims, the primary emotion was anger; for perpetrators, the emotions were guilt or regret.

Table 3. Most frequent reasons for selecting a particular memory as a function of type of memory

Reason for Retrieval	Percentages (and number of responses out of 140) Type of Memory: Victim	Perpetrator
1. Still generates emotion	35% (49)	17% (24)
2. Recency or vividness	15% (21)	14% (20)
3. Violation of expectations	14% (20)	18% (25)
Violation of assumptions about others	12% (17)	1% (2)
Violation of one's self concept	2% (3)	16% (23)
4. Most extreme example	11% (15)	9% (13)
5. First time for this type of event	6% (8)	8% (11)

Note. Percentages are rounded to the nearest whole number.

These differences in emotional memory can be accounted for by extrapolating the results of the metamemory analysis. According to the schema-theoretic approach of Harber and Pennebaker (1992), emotions arise when there is a discrepancy between our schema-based expectations and our direct encounters with events in the world. Emotions then function to direct our attention to the unprepared schemas so they can be restructured to accommodate the discordant events. If expectations are realigned to account for the specific events, emotions dissipate. If schema-based expectations are not aligned with specific memory of the events, then emotions persist. Moreover, the larger the discrepancy between general expectations and specific memory, the stronger the emotion.

In terms of the schema-theoretic explanation for emotional memory, victims experience anger when recalling a particular incident because of the discrepancy between the schema for what the offenders should have done and what they actually did. If the discrepancy is not resolved, the anger persists (Kraft, 2004). Perpetrators experience guilt from a particular memory because of the discrepancy between their *self*-concept and the representation of the specific incident. If this discrepancy is not resolved, then guilt persists.

The participants' answers to Question 5 suggest that some unresolved discrepancies remain between general schema and specific memories, and more so with victims. In answering Question 5, more victims than perpetrators stated that they could not explain the behavior of the other person, indicating that the discrepancy between their representation of the incident itself and their general schema for what ought to have happened remained, which in turn could lead to persisting emotion. With 31 victim accounts, participants said they did not know what the perpetrator was thinking or feeling, whereas only eight of the perpetrator accounts generated an "I don't know" response (χ^2 (1, N = 39) = 13.56, p < .01). This pattern also showed up in free recall, with many of the victim accounts stating that the perpetrators were arbitrary and without justification.

Almost all the participants listed only one reason for retrieving a memory, so the processes underlying the most frequent reason (still generates emotion) could not be directly assessed. An indirect approach, however, is to examine the distribution of answers in the third category of Table 3 (violation of expectations), which is further subdivided into subcategories of assumptions about the behavior of others and about one's self concept. In fact, violation of one's *self* concept accounted for 16% of the reasons for retrieving perpetrator memories and only 2% for victim memories. Violating an assumption about the behavior of *others* accounted for 12% of the reasons for retrieving victim memories and only 1% for perpetrator memories. One participant, for example, gave the following reason for selecting a *perpetrator* memory about being rude and not apologizing: "I chose this memory because I am a person who is nice to everyone no matter what, and this is the one time I remember not following through with being nice to everyone." Another participant gave the following reason for selecting a *victim* memory about being swindled by a customer at her cash register: "It shocked me to think there are people in the world that are so deceptive and take advantage of innocent people." The responses in the category of violated expectations were significantly different (χ^2 (1, N = 45) = 27.01, p < .01), with a large degree of association between the type of memory and the type of violated expectation (Cramer's ϕ = .774) (Cohen, 1988, 1992).

Both perpetrators and victims recognized the existence of mistakes, with no difference between the two (χ^2 (1, N = 153) = .16, p > .5). As shown in Table 4, just over half the accounts were judged to be inaccurate or exaggerated in some way, and of those, almost half were judged to arise from misremembering the *extent* of an emotion or a response. For example, in the metamemory analysis, one participant critiquing a victim account said of the perpetrator, "Maybe his temper wasn't as bad, but that's how I remember it." Another participant said, "The person wasn't as rude as I said, but that's how it seemed to me." One participant analyzing a perpetrator account said, "I didn't 'yell.' I over-annunciated." Another said, "I wasn't drunk – I just had a couple of beers."

Table 4. Inaccuracies and exaggerations

Percentage (and number) of accounts judged to be inaccurate or exaggerated	
Victim accounts	Perpetrator accounts
53% (74/140)	56% (79/140)

Percentage (and number) of the most frequent reasons cited for inaccuracies or exaggerations		
	Victim accounts	Perpetrator accounts
Extent of response	49% (36/74)	47% (37/79)
Details	17% (13/74)	18% (14/79)
Duration of incident	12% (9/74)	10% (8/79)
Number of responses	10% (8/74)	9% (7/79)
Sequence and timing	4% (3/74)	12% (9/79)

Note. Percentages are rounded to the nearest whole number.

One consistent set of differences between victims and perpetrators was how they remembered their experience of time during the recalled incidents (χ^2 (2, N = 285) = 38.9, p < .01). As shown in Table 5, the most frequent response in the analysis of victim accounts was that time *slowed down*, with participants reporting that 51% of these victim incidents resulted in a slowing of time. In contrast, only 16% of the perpetrator incidents led to an experienced slowing of time. In one victim account, for example, a participant described moving to a new state and starting in a new school: "Listening to people question me and call me names, it felt like time froze." Another participant said, "It felt like the longest hour of my life," when describing how a teacher singled her out at the beginning of class and announced to everyone how poorly she was doing in history. Several victim accounts said, "Time seemed to move on forever" or "I felt like time stopped."

In the analysis of perpetrator accounts, the most frequent response was that time perception did not change (52%), but 32% said that time went by *more quickly*. In contrast, only 20% of victim incidents led to a remembered experience of accelerated time. In referring to a perpetrator incident, one participant said, "I felt very confused, and time seemed to get away from me before I could organize my thoughts." Another said, "Time seemed to move more quickly for me because one incident seemed to lead to another." When analyzing perpetrator incidents, some participants reported that time moved too quickly even to think. With regard to memory, the experience of time slowing down during the initial encoding of a victim incident may lead to a memory representation that is more vivid and detailed, with a focus on one's thoughts at the time. The experience of time speeding up may lead to a memory representation that is less detailed and more about the overall situation, with less information about one's thoughts at the time.

Table 5. Memory for the passage of time

Percentage (and number) of accounts					
Victim accounts			Perpetrator accounts		
Slow	Quick	No change	Slow	Quick	No change
51% (73)	20% (28)	29% (42)	16% (23)	32% (45)	52% (74)

Note. Percentages are rounded to the nearest whole number. Due to several participants indicating two responses, the percentages are based on the following totals: 143 victim accounts and 142 perpetrator accounts.

Lessons or memory directives were prevalent, not just in the memory analysis but in free recall as well, before the participants were informed that they would be asked about lessons of memory. In the metamemory analysis, almost all the recalled events generated some type of lesson, although there was a significant difference in the number of accounts that did not generate one. Of the 140 victim accounts, 29 did not generate a lesson; of the 140 perpetrator accounts, only seven did not yield a lesson (χ^2 (1, N = 36) = 13.44, p < .01). One reason for this difference could be that perpetrators were more likely to use memory directives to resolve the discrepancy between their *self* schemas and what they remembered actually doing than victims were to use memory directives to adjust violated assumptions about others.

In summary, the accounts of being victimized were significantly longer than the perpetrator accounts, with more details, more remembered conversation, and more description of the aftermath – as part of the incident itself. The focus on details and on specific conversations could be due, in part, to the victims' experience of time slowing down during the incidents, which was identified in just over half the victim accounts. Victims were less likely to draw lessons from the incidents than perpetrators and less likely to understand the actions of the perpetrators than perpetrators were to understand the reactions of victims. With both types of incidents, participants identified inaccuracies and exaggerations, with the *extent* of the responses being the most frequently identified type of mistake. That is, both victims and perpetrators were equally aware of inaccuracies and exaggerations in their original memory descriptions. In terms of application, these findings can be integrated with earlier research on the magnitude gap to provide a framework for interpreting the critical differences in memory between victims and perpetrators in more extreme situations, such as those addressed by truth commissions.

TRUTH COMMISSIONS

For the past twenty-five years, the use of truth commissions to resolve long-standing national conflicts has continued to grow. Since the development of the modern truth commission in Latin America in the early 1980s, twenty-eight countries have conducted some form of truth commission, with another eleven calling for commissions before the end of this decade (Posel and Simpson, 2002; Hayner, 1994; United States Institute of Peace, 2005).[10] Currently, Iraq is a truth commission waiting to happen – along with Chechnya, Somalia, the Democratic Republic of Congo, Sudan, and North Korea.[11] Ideally, truth commissions function to disclose past abuses of human rights and to encourage reconciliation among former enemies. They perform their truth-gathering function by collecting material evidence and by documenting the memories of those who were directly involved in the human rights abuses.

The South African Truth and Reconciliation Commission

To date, the most extensive and well documented of the truth commissions has been South Africa's Truth and Reconciliation Commission (TRC), mandated by an act of the South African parliament in 1995 and conducted over a period of six years, from 1996 through 2001. The stated purpose of the TRC was to gather information about human rights violations during apartheid and to promote reconciliation in a country devastated by decades of violent struggle. To help accomplish its eponymous goals of truth and reconciliation, the TRC obtained testimony from the victims and from the perpetrators of apartheid. The victims gave testimony to document the crimes committed against them and their families and to apply for reparations. The perpetrators gave testimony to inform the nation of the specific crimes they carried out during apartheid and to obtain amnesty for these crimes. If the perpetrators' crimes were judged to be politically motivated, and if they made *full disclosure*, they were granted amnesty. If the perpetrators were in prison – and more than 70% of them were – the granting of amnesty meant immediate release from prison and permanent immunity from any legal or civil action (Boraine, 2000; Pigou, 2002; Truth and Reconciliation Commission [TRC], 2003). In the words of the TRC chairperson, Archbishop Desmond Tutu, "Freedom was granted in exchange for truth" (Tutu, 1999, 7). The very lives of the perpetrators depended on the perceived accuracy and comprehensiveness of their personal memories.

The profound consequences of personal memory and the reverberating discrepancies between victim accounts and perpetrator accounts argue persuasively for the application of memory research to the operation of truth commissions. Moreover, widespread destruction of documents by authoritarian central governments only amplifies the urgency for understanding personal memory in this context. In South Africa, for example, three years before the TRC began its work, the National Intelligence Services of the South African Government destroyed almost fifty *tons* of paper and microfilm records of their illegal activities during apartheid, an assault on evidence so massive that furnaces had to be used, with the result that

---

[10] There were eighteen truth commissions before the Truth and Reconciliation Commission in South Africa, and since then, there have been different forms of truth commissions implemented in nine countries: East Timor, Ghana, Panama, Peru, Serbia and Montenegro, Rwanda, Sierra Leone, South Korea, and Uruguay. By the end of this decade, countries calling for their own truth commissions include Afghanistan, Angola, Bosnia-Herzegovina, Cambodia, Colombia, Indonesia, Jamaica, Kenya, Mexico, Morocco, and Venezuela. For more documentation, refer to the United States Institute of Peace (2005) and Hayner (1994).

[11] After an extended conflict comes to an end, not with total victory for any side but through a negotiated peace, the truth commission is the most likely resolution. In the aftermath of widespread atrocities that each side inflicted on the other, coexistence among the hundreds of thousands of people directly involved in the conflict will require truth gathering and reconciliation – and probably conditional amnesty.

much historical truth about apartheid now resides only in the personal memories of the victims and the state perpetrators (Bundy, 2000; TRC, 1999a).

The TRC eventually collected 22,000 victim testimonies and received more than 7,000 applications for amnesty, with more than 1,600 perpetrators qualifying for the amnesty process (Posel and Simpson, 2002; Foster, Haupt, and de Beer, 2005). During the hearings of the amnesty committee the former victims were able to testify and to confront the perpetrators, which made available two different sets of memories for the same events. In fact, the hearings proceeded as a real-life suspense story: perpetrators testified before the TRC and then waited – sometimes more than a year – to hear whether or not they were granted amnesty. The members of the amnesty committee made their decisions case by case, balancing the accounts of the perpetrators and the accounts of the victims.

Consistent with the experimental literature on the magnitude gap, the testimonies collected by the TRC revealed dramatic and predictable discrepancies between the memories of the perpetrators and the memories of the victims (TRC, 1999b). Perpetrators bracketed the criminal incidents within the context of doing their jobs; victims encoded the incidents as part of a series of events, with abuses before and after remembered as parts of the incidents. From the perpetrator's perspective, the violence was justified – even if it was recognized later as morally wrong. From the victim's perspective, the violence was often incomprehensible and senseless. Moreover, many victims did not believe the discrepancies between their own personal memories and the memories of the perpetrators, and they went on record stating that the perpetrators had failed to disclose fully their involvement in the crimes committed during apartheid. Given that perpetrators were required to provide honest and comprehensive disclosure in order to receive amnesty, the discrepancy in recall between the perpetrators and the victims had life-changing implications.

The magnitude gap dominated the hearings of Paul van Vuuren, a member of the Security Forces known as "apartheid's electrician" because of his favored form of torture interrogation (Pauw, 1998; van Vuuren, 25 February 1997). One of the prisoners van Vuuren interrogated was Scheepers Morudu, who eventually testified against van Vuuren at his amnesty hearings. Van Vuuren described the interrogation and beating of Scheepers Morudu and admitted to administering electric shocks during questioning, but he failed to disclose that Morudu was detained after the interrogation (van Vuuren, 25 February 1997). Morudu said he was beaten and tortured by van Vuuren, and then detained for two months (Morudu, 26 February 1997). Factual evidence and other testimony revealed that Morudu had been detained for at least one week after the torture (Wilson, 26 February 1997). Consistent with the findings on the magnitude gap, van Vuuren's perpetrator account bracketed the incident to exclude the aftermath, whereas the victim, Morudu, recalled the series of provocations that led up to his capture and torture and emphasized the consequences afterwards – possibly exaggerating the extent of time he was detained.

With serious transgressions, such as those investigated during truth commissions, the magnitude gap may begin as an encoding phenomenon explained in part by *action identification theory* (Vallacher and Wegner, 1987; Wegner and Vallacher, 1986). That is, people encode and represent their own actions in terms of different levels of identification. For example, the act of calling an acquaintance who has just had minor surgery could be encoded as movements of one's fingers on a phone pad or as the gathering of medical information or as caring about a friend who has just undergone a stressful experience. Moving one's fingers and pushing numbers on a phone pad involves a low level identity as physical technician, with no moral meaning. Gathering medical information involves a cognitive understanding of surgery and outpatient procedures, with faithfulness to factual accuracy. Caring about the health of a friend entails the moral responsibilities of close relationships and empathy. Depending upon the level of action identification, the encoding and representation of the actions will differ.

As indicated by the testimony provided to the TRC, the perpetrators often maintained a low-level identity, focusing on specific actions and techniques (getting the job done, doing it well, not leaving marks on the detainees), whereas the victims maintained a high-level identity, experiencing the actions against them in terms of moral considerations of good and evil – or less extreme dimensions such as honest-dishonest or fair-unfair. Encoding of the events differed accordingly, with perpetrators more likely to encode specific situational factors and victims more likely to encode higher level meanings. Consistent with the predictions of action identification theory, the perpetrator's low-level identity led to representations primarily of contextual factors, whereas the victim's high-level identity led to representations of more personal considerations (Vallacher and Wegner, 1987; Wegner and Vallacher, 1986).

During the TRC hearings, when perpetrators consistently recalled events at the level of specific actions and not at a level where motive and morality could be considered, it proved unsatisfying for the victims and their families. Consider Robert McBride, an activist in the armed wing of the African National Congress (ANC), the largest of the liberation groups fighting against apartheid. McBride applied for amnesty for a number of violent attacks, including setting off a car bomb outside a crowded nightclub that killed three young women and seriously injured 60 others. During his lengthy hearing, McBride recalled the act of placing explosives that would eventually kill innocent people. "When you do an operation, you are trained, go and lay your charge, initiate it, and retreat. That's your frame of mind. I had been doing that on more than ten occasions: going, gaining entry and laying charges, and retreating. That's what it is. That's what your mind is on" (McBride, 5 October 1999). As McBride recalled the process of selecting a location for his car bomb, the juxtaposition of low-level and high-level encoding was especially jarring: when setting a car bomb, the main focus is on finding a good parking spot.

When McBride and his associates were confronted by the victims and their families, a dramatic magnitude gap appeared. The perpetrators recalled the justifications for their acts and the specifics of the operations, bracketing the incidents, whereas the victims recalled the suffering caused by the acts, the meaning of the events, and the aftermath. During these hearings, consensus was not reached – far from it. There was no meeting of minds and no healing. Both sides recalled the events, sometimes with considerable insult. The hearings went on for two weeks, and near the end, the daughter of one of the slain women said that Robert McBride's testimony had changed her position from supporting amnesty to opposing it (van der Linde, 13 October 1999).

Dawid Ackerman and his family were worshipping in the St. James Church in Kenilworth when three members of the armed wing of the Pan African Congress attacked the congregation, killing eleven people and seriously wounding another 58. After the attack, Ackerman found his mortally wounded wife and rushed her to the hospital, where she died soon afterwards. Four years later, during the amnesty hearings of the TRC, Ackerman confronted the leader of the armed attack and asked if he remembered seeing his wife sitting in the front of the church. The perpetrator answered by saying that all he could remember was entering the church and firing his weapon. Ackerman then told all three perpetrators, “I want you to know that I forgive you unconditionally.” Yet even with this sincere forgiveness, when Ackerman was asked if he was satisfied that he had heard all the relevant facts, he replied, “My subjective answer is *no*, I don’t think that I’ve heard everything. I think there might yet be something more” (Ackerman, 10 July 1997). For the perpetrators, memory of the incident was bracketed in time, with the focus on the technical aspects of the operation. For Ackerman, the incident was recalled as a detailed sensory experience, evaluated as moral act, and placed within a longer series of events that extended into the present.

The confrontation of discrepant memories during the TRC hearings can be interpreted through an analogy to the principles of physical *parallax* (Žižek, 2006). In physics, parallax is the apparent displacement of a distant object against its background, caused by a change in the position of the observer. A star, for example, appears to be in a different position depending on the location of the astronomer. Moreover, by observing parallax and performing the appropriate calculations, one can precisely specify the position of the distant object. In other words, parallax creates two different perceptions of the same distant object *and* it can be used to locate the object in question. In fact, only by considering the different perceptions can we know the nature of the elusive object.

The physical principles of parallax can be transposed to the problem of the magnitude gap. When recalling an incident, victims and perpetrators create parallax in memory: discrepant accounts of the same incident. By characterizing this discrepancy and by applying what has been learned from basic research on the magnitude gap, we can more accurately specify the incident in question. In particular, research on the magnitude gap tells us the following: perpetrators bracket the incidents in time, emphasize situational influence and mitigating events, shorten the time span of the events, and deemphasize consequences; victims remember antecedents and consequences as part of the incidents, emphasize active, personal choice on the part of the perpetrator, recall the incidents as unjustified and often inexplicable, lengthen time span, and recall details of their own experience caused by the perpetrator’s actions.

Regarding the difference between the memories of victims and of perpetrators, Baumeister (1997) asked, “Who is telling the truth?” (46). The answer is that *both* the victims and the perpetrators can describe their memories honestly and still construct appreciably discrepant accounts. Did Jeffrey Benzien plan to kill the anti-apartheid activist, Ashley Kriel, as his sisters testified, or was the killing the result of reflexive judgments during a physical struggle, as Benzien testified? The facts and the remembered accounts suggested both. In truth commissions, events often remained unreconciled, and the commission must agree on a satisfactory version of the events, often within the gap between the discrepant accounts. In fact, we cannot rely solely on the narratives of victims *or* perpetrators; we need both, which only occurs during the confrontation between the victims and the perpetrators. By applying the research on the magnitude gap, we can understand more about the elusive incidents of the past from the memory lapses of the perpetrators and the memory elaboration of the victims.

In his controversial minority report, TRC Commissioner Wynand Malan criticized the bias in favor of the victim’s point of view, writing that, “Exaggeration is a natural consequence of human suffering” (Malan, 1999, 441). Malan’s statement was oddly insensitive and was rebuked by the majority report, but it also revealed an intuitive awareness of the magnitude gap. But what exactly is exaggerated? Research on the magnitude gap reveals an answer relevant to the testimonies in the TRC hearings: factual information regarding *number* or *extent* – the duration of an incident, the number of shots fired, the number of people involved. Victims widen the event, include earlier events, emphasize the aftermath, and do not recall mitigating factors that might lessen the severity of their evaluation of the transgression. In contrast, perpetrators bracket the transgression within a narrow time frame, deemphasize or forget provocations before the central transgression, emphasize mitigating factors, and exclude the aftermath. In fact, the official report of the TRC referenced the magnitude gap of Baumeister (1997) but did not specifically apply Baumeister's findings (TRC, 1999b). The point here is that truth commissions are open to the application of such research, but they do not have the findings in an accessible, applicable form.

Future research should codify the findings on the magnitude gap and apply them in more naturalistic settings. The focus in this chapter is on truth commissions, but there are other relevant settings with different particulars, such as conflict resolution and divorce mediation (Petersen, 2005). Research on the magnitude gap should also focus on a fundamental question of applied metacognition: What criteria do we use to judge the comprehensiveness and honesty of memory descriptions? (Bond and DePaulo, 2006; Ekman and O'Sullivan, 1991; Ekman, O'Sullivan, and Frank, 1999). With regard to this question, Judge Bernard Ngoepe of the TRC amnesty committee made a particularly discerning observation during the final day of hearings for Captain Jeffrey Benzien:

> How do you reconcile the ability not to remember certain things with the ability to remember not having done certain things? In other words the person says he has forgotten about certain things, he has blocked them out of his mind, but when other things are put to him he says, "No, I remember very well, it did *not* happen." I think that's what the problem is: he's able to remember that such and such a thing did *not* happen, but at the end of the same breath, he's saying, "I am not able to remember that, I've lost my memory or part of it, I am not able to can say whether certain things did or did not happen" (Ngoepe, 21 October 1997).

A final implication from the research on the magnitude gap is the role of the truth commission in specifying what is *not* accurate. One stated goal of the TRC was to elicit, "as much truth as possible about past atrocities" (TRC, 1999a, 120), but also important is the documentation of what is *un*true: the truth commission as national lie detector – a polygraph, using multiple measures to identify falsehoods in public discourse. By applying the specific findings on the magnitude gap, we can validate the differences that honestly occur between victims and perpetrators and characterize the contours of the gap between the different accounts. But if an account lies *outside* the contours of the memory gap, we can state with confidence that it is *not* accurate. After the TRC, for example, the National Party could no longer claim that police hit squads did not exist, that torture was carried out by only a few delinquent members of the security forces, that only violent activists were targeted by the apartheid government (Mamdani, 2000; Posel, 2002). Detecting what is not accurate may be as essential to the function of truth commissions as finding truth (Mamdani, 2000, 58-61).

In the context of truth commissions, the opportunities for applied research on the magnitude gap will continue to grow. When a country decides to promote reconciliation after widespread, long-term conflict, the honest memories of victims and perpetrators will necessarily come into conflict. Applied research on the magnitude gap will contribute to the effectiveness of these truth commissions and help interpret the profound differences in memory between the perpetrators and the victimized.

REFERENCES

Ackerman, D. J. (1997, July 10). Comments provided to the Amnesty Committee of the Truth and Reconciliation Commission, Cape Town.

Baumeister, R. F. (1997). *Evil: Inside human violence and cruelty*. New York: Holt.

Baumeister, R.F., and Newman, L.S. (1994). How stories make sense of personal experiences: Motives that shape autobiographical narratives. *Personality and Social Psychology Bulletin, 20,* 676-690.

Baumeister, R. F., Stillwell, A. M., and Wotman, S. R. (1990). Victim and perpetrator accounts of interpersonal conflict: Autobiographical narratives about anger. *Journal of Personality and Social Psychology, 90*, 994-1005.

Benzien, J. T. (1997, July 14-16). Testimony provided to the Amnesty Committee of the Truth and Reconciliation Commission, Cape Town.

Bond, C. F., and DePaulo, B. M. (2006). Accuracy of deception judgments. *Personality and Social Psychology Review*, *10*(3), 214–234.

Boraine, A. (2000). *A country unmasked: Inside South Africa's Truth and Reconciliation Commission*. Cape Town: Oxford.

Bundy, C. (2000). The beast of the past: History and the TRC. In W. James and L. van de Vijver (Eds.), *After the TRC: Reflections on truth and reconciliation in South Africa.* (pp. 9-20). Cape Town, South Africa: David Philip Publishers.

Cohen, J. (1988). *Statistical power analysis for the behavioral sciences*. Hillsdale, NJ: Erlbaum.

Cohen, J. (1992). A power primer. *Psychological Bulletin, 112*, 155-159.

Ekman, P., and O'Sullivan, M. (1991). Who can catch a liar? *American Psychologist*, *46*(9), 913–920.

Ekman, P., O'Sullivan, M., and Frank, M. (1999). A few can catch a liar. *Psychological Science*, *10*(3), 263–265.

Foster, D., Haupt, P., and de Beer, M. (2005). *The theatre of violence: Narratives of protagonists in the South African conflict*. Cape Town: HSRC Press.

Harber, K. D. and Pennebaker, J. W. (1992). Overcoming traumatic memories In S.-Å. Christianson (Ed.), *The handbook of emotion and memory: Research and theory* (pp. 359-387). Hillsdale, NJ: Erlbaum.

Hayner, P. B. (1994). Fifteen truth commissions – 1977 to 1991: A comparative study. *Human Rights Quarterly, 16*, 597-655.

Kearns, J. N., and Fincham, F. D. (2005). Victim and perpetrator accounts of interpersonal transgressions: Self-serving or relationship-serving biases? *Personality and Social Psychology Bulletin*, *31*, 321-333.

Kraft, R. N. (2000, November). *Revealing mistakes in personal memory*. Paper presented at the 41st annual meeting of the Psychonomic Society, New Orleans.

Kraft, R. N. (2002). *Memory perceived: Recalling the Holocaust*. Westport, CT: Praeger.

Kraft, R. N. (2004). Emotional memory in survivors of the Holocaust: A qualitative study of oral testimony. In D. Reisberg and P. Hertel (Eds.), *Memory and emotion* (pp. 347-389). New York: Oxford University Press.

Kraft, R. N. (2006a). Archival memory: Representations of the Holocaust in oral testimony. *Poetics Today*, *27*, 311-330.

Kraft, R. N. (2006b, May). *Crimes of allegiance: An analysis of perpetrator testimony.* Invited paper presented at the annual meeting of the Midwestern Psychological Association, Chicago.

van der Linde, C. (1999, October 13). Testimony provided to the Amnesty Committee of the Truth and Reconciliation Commission, Durban.

Malan, W. (1999). Minority report. Truth and Reconciliation Final Report, Vol. 5, 441.

Mamdani, M. (2000). A diminished truth. In W. James and L. van de Vijver (Eds.), *After the TRC:Reflections on truth and reconciliation in South Africa* (pp. 58-61). Cape Town, South Africa: David Philip Publishers.

Mazzoni, G., and Kirsch, I. (2002). Autobiographical memories and beliefs: A preliminary metacognitive model. In T. L. Perfect and B. L. Schwartz (Eds.), *Applied metacognition* (121-145). Cambridge, UK: Cambridge University Press.

McBride, R. (1999, October 5). Testimony provided to the Amnesty Committee of the Truth and Reconciliation Commission, Durban.

Morudu, S. (1997, February 26). Testimony Provided to the Amnesty Committee of the Truth and Reconciliation Commission, Pretoria.

Ngoepe, B. (1997, October 21). Comments made to the Amnesty Committee of the Truth and Reconciliation Commission, Cape Town.

Pauw, J. (1998). Inside the mind of torture: The story of apartheid's electrician. *Covert Action Quarterly*, 63, 17- 25.

Petersen, V. (2005). Therapeutic child-focused mediation. In S. M. Harris, D. C. Ivey, and R. A. Bean (Eds.), *A practice that works: Strategies to complement your stand alone therapy practice* (pp. 115-125). New York: Routledge.

Pigou, P. (2002). False promises and wasted opportunities? Inside South Africa's Truth and Reconciliation Commission. In D. Posel and G. Simpson (Eds.), *Commissioning the past: Understanding South Africa's Truth and Reconciliation Commission* (pp. 37-65). Johannesburg: Witwatersrand University Press.

Pillemer, D. B. (1998). *Momentous events, vivid memories*. Cambridge MA: Harvard.

Posel, D. (2002). The TRC Report: What kind of history? What kind of truth? In D. Posel and G. Simpson (Eds.), *Commissioning the past*: *Understanding South Africa's Truth and Reconciliation Commission* (pp. 147-172). Johannesburg: Witwatersrand University Press.

Posel, D., and Simpson, G. (2002). The power of truth: South Africa's Truth and Reconciliation Commission in context. In D. Posel and G. Simpson (Eds.), *Commissioning the past*: *Understanding South Africa's Truth and Reconciliation Commission* (pp. 1-13). Johannesburg: Witwatersrand University Press.

Rumelhart, D. E. (1980). Schemata: The building blocks of cognition. In R.J. Spiro, B.C. Bruce, and W.F. Brewer (Eds.), *Theoretical issues in reading comprehension* (pp. 33-58). Hillsdale, NJ: Erlbaum.

Schacter, D. L. (1999). The seven sins of memory: Insights from psychology and cognitive neuroscience. *American Psychologist*, *54*, 182-203.

Schütz, A., and Baumeister, R. F. (1999). The language of defense: Linguistic patterns in narratives of transgressions. *Journal of Language and Social Psychology*, 18, 269-286.

Scoboria, A., Mazzoni, G., Kirsch, I., and Relyea, M. (2004). Plausibility and belief in autobiographical memory. *Applied Cognitive Psychology*, *18*, 791-807.

Stillwell, A. M., and Baumeister, R. F. (1997). The construction of victim and perpetrator memories: Accuracy and distortion in role-based accounts. *Personality and Social Psychology Bulletin*, *23*, 1157-1172.

Truth and Reconciliation Commission of South Africa. (1999a). *Truth and Reconciliation Commission of South Africa Report*. (Vol. 1). London: Macmillan.

Truth and Reconciliation Commission of South Africa. (1999b). *Truth and Reconciliation Commission of South Africa Report*. (Vol. 5). London: Macmillan.

Truth and Reconciliation Commission of South Africa. (2003). *Truth and Reconciliation Commission of South Africa Report*. (Vols. 6-7). Cape Town: Truth and Reconciliation Commission.

Tutu, D. (1999). Foreword. *Truth and Reconciliation Commission of South Africa Report*. (Vol. 1). (pp. 1-23). London: Macmillan.

United States Institute of Peace (2005). Truth commissions digital collection. Retrieved from *http://www.usip.org/library/truth.html*

Vallacher, R. R., and Wegner, D. M. (1987). What do people think they're doing? Action identification and human behavior. *Psychological Review*, *94*, 3-15.

van Vuuren, P. (1997, February 25). Testimony provided to the Amnesty Committee of the Truth and Reconciliation Commission, Pretoria.

Wegner, D. M., and Vallacher, R. R. (1986). Action identification. In R. M. Sorrentino and E. T. Higgins (Eds.), *Handbook of motivation and cognition: Foundations of social behavior* (pp. 550-582). New York: Guilford.

Wilson, A. (1997, February 26). Examination conducted with the Amnesty Committee of the Truth and Reconciliation Commission, Pretoria.

Zechmeister, J. S., and Romero, C. (2002). Victim and offender accounts of interpersonal conflict: Autobiographical narratives of forgiveness and unforgiveness. *Journal of Personality and Social Psychology*, *82*, 675-686.

Žižek, S. (2006). *The parallax view*. Cambridge, MA: MIT Press.

In: Applied Memory
Editor: Matthew R. Kelley

ISBN 978-1-60692-143-2

Chapter 10

PROSPECTIVE PERSON MEMORY

***James Michael Lampinen*[*1], *Jack D. Arnal*[1], *and Jason L. Hicks*[2]**

[1] Department of Psychology, University of Arkansas, Fayetteville, AR, USA

[2] Department of Psychology Louisiana State University, Baton Rouge, LA, USA

ABSTRACT

We explore a new application of prospective memory, namely, *prospective person memory*. Prospective person memory refers to situations in which one is asked to "be on the lookout" for a particular person who may be encountered during one's day to day activities. Specific examples include being on the lookout for a missing child, a wanted fugitive, or a terrorist. Three lines of ongoing research are described. First, in the laboratory studies, participants engaged in simulated tasks on a computer (e.g., grocery shopping). While engaged in these tasks, participants were asked to "be on the lookout" for a group of "wanted" individuals. If they spotted these individuals, they were asked to press a key (i.e., 'alt' button) thereby alerting authorities. Second, in the field experiments, participants viewed a mock news broadcast describing two "wanted" individuals. Participants were told that if they spotted the individuals and alerted the experimenter they would receive a portion of a $100 prize. Seemingly unrelated to this experiment, participants had an opportunity to identify the wanted individuals at a departmental cookie sale. We then examined the probability that the experimenter was contacted. Prospective person memory in the laboratory studies was relatively poor and in the field studies it was even worse. Third, field research was designed to determine how much attention customers pay to posters of missing children. In the project, posters of missing children were placed at the exits of participating supermarkets. As patrons left the stores, they were asked to complete a survey. The survey asked them to indicate the degree to which they looked at the posters and to complete a recognition memory test for the children's pictures. We also describe research on the utility of forensic age progression in the recovery of missing children. The research reported in this chapter represents the first program of research specifically aimed at using basic research and theory on prospective memory in order to help better understand these important applied memory issues.

* Corresponding author.

INTRODUCTION

The general public serves as an important resource in helping law enforcement track down individuals (Witkin, 1995). When investigators are attempting to apprehend a suspect or fugitive in an investigation, they sometimes release his/her picture to the general public, with the hope that someone will see the suspect and contact authorities (e.g., Lafayette, 1998). Military, intelligence, and anti-terrorist applications of person identification also exist. When intelligence agencies or the F.B.I. learn that particular terrorist suspects may be present in the United States or abroad, they may provide the news media with pictures of the suspected terrorists and ask them to alert the general public (USA Today, 2004). Law enforcement also relies on the news media in cases in which a missing child is sought (Office of Juvenile Justice and Delinquency Prevention, 2004). Particular approaches include "Amber Alerts" (Zgoba, 2004) and placing pictures of missing children on products such as milk cartons (Brown, 1997) or at the exits of stores such as Walmart (Walmart Foundation, 2001).

The purpose of the research described in this chapter is to better understand the mechanisms by which persons are identified in these forensic contexts, in the hopes of developing approaches that will increase the probability of a "hit" when an individual is being sought by law enforcement, military, or anti-terrorism personnel. The examples described above all involve *prospective person memory*. Prospective memory refers to a set of processes that allows one to remember to engage in a future activity such as mailing a bill the next time one is near a post office (Ellis and Kvavilashvili, 2000; Guynn, McDaniel, and Einstein, 1998; Marsh, Hicks, Cook, Hansen, and Pallos, 2003). In the case of prospective person memory, successful completion of the task requires members of the general public to contact authorities (delayed intention) when they encounter a particular person (PM cue) as they go about other attention demanding tasks during their daily lives (ongoing activities).

The program of research described in the present chapter follows analogous research on eyewitness identification, and seeks to identify both system and estimator variables that influence prospective person memory (Wells, 1978). We have examined these questions in the context of both laboratory analog experiments and in field experiments. The research is important for a number of reasons. First, it is the first systematic program of research aimed at understanding prospective person memory. Second, the research has made use of well-established paradigms within the field of event based prospective memory. Third, the research has been informed by a theoretical understanding of prospective memory, as well as being heuristically guided by the system variable / estimator variable distinction that has been useful in studies of retrospective eyewitness memory. Fourth, the research has combined tightly controlled laboratory based experiments with ecologically valid field experiments, providing an opportunity to answer important scientific questions at the intersection between behavioral science and the law.

TRACKING DOWN FUGITIVES AND RESCUING MISSING CHILDREN

Law enforcement has been seeking the help of the general public for years in tracking down wanted fugitives. For instance, pictures of wanted fugitives may be publicized in local and national news media, sometimes receiving extensive coverage (Lafayette, 1998). Since

1949, the Federal Bureau of Investigation has maintained a most wanted list (Witkin, 1995) by which it publicizes the identities of criminal suspects and fugitives. Since its inception, 479 fugitives have been placed on the F.B.I.'s most wanted list. Overall, 147 fugitives have been caught because of tips from the public (Johnson, 2005). More recently, the syndicated television program, *America's Most Wanted,* has publicized the identities of wanted fugitives (Russell, 1997). The show features weekly sequences on fugitives being sought by law enforcement. Eight-hundred and fifty-one of these fugitives have been apprehended (America's Most Wanted, 2005). Law enforcement also uses a number of additional venues to seek help from the public in tracking down fugitives (e.g., press releases, news conferences, Internet). Prospective person memory is thus important in tracking down fugitives wanted by U.S. law enforcement agencies.

Anti-terrorist and military personnel also rely on prospective person memory. U.S. military personnel in Iraq were given playing cards with faces of 55 wanted individuals (Stone, 2003). The global war against terrorism has also made use of publicity in order to track down terrorist suspects (USA Today, 2004). The F.B.I. has released a most wanted terrorist list, in addition to their most wanted fugitive list (Levitt, 2001). In the second wave of terror bombings in London, during the summer of 2005, British police publicized pictures of four suspects and sought the aid of the public in finding them (Cable News Network, 2005a). Improving prospective person memory has the potential to aid U.S. military operations and the global war against terrorism.

Another important law enforcement function involves finding and recovering missing children (Blomquist, 1990). Estimates of the number of missing and exploited children in the United States are staggering (Tedisco and Paludi, 1996). According to the second *National Incidence Study of Missing, Abducted, Runaway, and Thrownaway Children* (NISMART2), 797,500 children were reported missing in the year 1999 (Sedlak, Finkelhor, Hammer, and Shultz, 2002). Approximately 9% of all cases involve abductions either by family members or strangers. Law enforcement in many states put out "Amber Alerts" when children go missing, resulting in the child's photograph being made available to media outlets, to be shown to the general public (Office of Juvenile Justice and Delinquency Prevention, 2004; Zgoba, 2004). Some missing children cases receive a great deal of media attention, whereas other cases receive far less attention (Office of Juvenile Justice and Delinquency Prevention, 2004). The National Center for Missing and Exploited Children (NCMEC) maintains a national database of missing children (Girouard, 1990). The NCMEC also sends out direct mail advertisements featuring the pictures of missing children to about 75 million homes every week (Office of Juvenile Justice and Delinquency Prevention, 2004). Missing children have also been publicized by corporations. One early strategy was to place the pictures of missing children on products such as milk cartons (Brown, 1997). Since 1996, Walmart Corporation has been posting photographs of missing children at the exits of its stores leading to many recovered children (Walmart Foundation, 2001). In addition to these efforts, parents of missing children often institute their own grass-roots efforts to publicize details about their child's disappearance (Office of Juvenile Justice and Delinquency Prevention, 2004).

A recent example of the successful use of these strategies occurred with the case of Shasta Groene (Cable News Network, 2005b). Shasta was abducted in the course of a triple homicide and later recovered. After extensive national media coverage, a waitress at a Denny's restaurant recognized Shasta and contacted authorities. Although this case ended with a successful recovery, it is noteworthy that news reports indicate that just hours earlier,

Shasta had been in the plain view of a number of people at a local convenience store, none of whom identified her. Unfortunately, many missing children cases do not end with the child being safely recovered (Blomquist, 1990).

Note that the prospective person memory problem has two components. The first problem concerns missed opportunities for identification by members of the general public. When Shasta Groene was taken by her abductor to a local convenience store, she was not disguised in any way. If the customers and employees at the store had seen the extensive news reports, then they had an opportunity to contact authorities. For whatever reasons, they did not. A second problem with prospective person memory concerns false identifications. When a fugitive from justice or a missing child receives a great deal of media attention, authorities receive a large number of leads that end up being false alarms. Although law enforcement prefers to receive information, even if it uncertain, false leads necessarily consume investigative resources that might be better utilized elsewhere in the investigation. Because of these dual problems, the research in the present proposal measures both the correct identification rate in prospective person memory tasks, as well as the false identification rate.

THEORETICAL ACCOUNTS OF PROSPECTIVE MEMORY

There has been growing interest among basic memory researchers on the topic of prospective memory (e.g., Einstein and McDaniel, 1990; Marsh et al., 2003; Marsh, Hicks, and Landau, 1998; McDaniel, Robinson-Riegler, and Einstein, 1998). Prospective memory concerns the ability of people to remember to engage in some action in the future. The present chapter focuses on a particular type of prospective memory called *event based prospective memory*. Event based prospective memory refers to situations in which a person has to remember to engage in an action when they encounter a particular cue in the environment (e.g., remembering to mail the letter the next time one is by a mailbox). Research on event based prospective memory has been dominated by a series of clever laboratory based paradigms (e.g., McDaniel and Einstein, 1993; McDaniel et al., 1998).

In a typical study, participants are presented with one or more *prospective memory cues* (i.e., *PM cue*) that they are to be on the lookout for during the course of the experiment. For instance, a participant might be told to be on the lookout for the words *chair, monkey,* and *toothbrush.* Participants are told to make a specific response, such as pressing the 'alt' key on the computer keyboard, when they encounter these items (i.e., *PM response*). Because prospective memory involves remembering to engage in a behavior during the course of one's normal day to day activities, laboratory based prospective memory tasks embed the target items in an attention demanding *ongoing activity*. For instance, participants may be presented with several hundred words and might be asked to make pleasantness ratings for each of these words. During the course of this ongoing activity, participants encounter the PM cues and the main dependent measure is whether or not they remember to make the PM response (e.g., pressing the 'alt' key). It is also important to note that in order to discourage active item-by-item monitoring, participants often engage in filler activities during which the prospective memory targets are never presented.

Theoretical accounts suggest that prospective memory tasks involve both a prospective and retrospective component, and that performance of the tasks engage both automatic and controlled processing (Cohen, Dixon, Lindsay, and Masson, 2003; Einstein and McDaniel, 1990; Ellis, 1996). To successfully perform a prospective memory task, participants need to remind themselves when encountering the PM target that it is significant in some way (e.g., "I was supposed to do something when I saw the word *monkey.*")—this has typically been considered the prospective component of the task. Once the target has been identified as significant, participants have to successfully remember the delayed intention associated with the target (e.g., "*Monkey* is associated with pressing the 'alt' key")—this has typically been considered the retrospective component of the task. This distinction is important, because it would hardly be surprising if participants failed at a PM task, if they are unable to remember what targets they were supposed to be on the lookout for or the relationship between the PM target and the delayed intention. Many studies of event based prospective memory, therefore, include standard measures of retrospective memory subsequent to the performance of the PM task.

Theoretical accounts of prospective memory also make a distinction between automatic processes leading to the recognition of PM cues and controlled processes that lead to the recognition of PM cues (McDaniel and Einstein, 2000). Note that in the course of an experiment, it is possible that participants could actively prompt themselves, during each item's presentation, whether or not it is one of the PM cues. This process has been referred to in the literature as *conscious monitoring,* or *strategic checking* (Guynn, 2003). Conscious monitoring involves comparing each item as it is presented with a mental representation of the PM targets. With regard to this view, Smith and Bayen (2004) have proposed a model that suggests that successful prospective memory always requires monitoring. Smith (2003; Experiment 3) found that working memory capacity was positively correlated with performance on prospective memory tasks (see also Reese and Cherry, 2002; West and Craik, 2001). Researchers have also found that prospective memory tasks often interfere with performance on the ongoing task, suggesting that a monitoring process was using some of the capacity available for working memory (Marsh et al., 2003). Other theorists, however, argue that there are some situations where recognition of the prospective memory targets occurs automatically (Einstein and McDaniel, 2005; McDaniel and Einstein, 2000). According to these multi-process views, whether the PM task is performed automatically or strategically depends on the importance of the task, how distinctive the PM cue is, how stereotypical the PM cue is, planning strategies and characteristics of the participant engaged in the task.

System Variables and Estimator Variables

Some time ago, Wells (1978) argued that the variables that influence eyewitness accuracy can be divided into two categories, estimator and system variables. Estimator variables are factors that are likely to influence eyewitness accuracy but that are not under control of the legal system. For instance, some research suggests that witnesses are more accurate when identifying members of their own race than members of a different race (Anthony, Copper, and Mullen, 1992; Bothwell, Brigham, and Malpass, 1989; Chance and Goldstein, 1996; Platz and Hosch, 1988). Eyewitness accuracy can also be influenced by the amount of stress the witness experienced at the time of the event (Deffenbacher, 1983; Kramer, Buckhout, Fox, Widman, and Tusche, 1991; Loftus and Burns, 1982) and the amount of time the witness had to view the event (Memon, Hope, and Bull, 2003). Estimator variables are useful because they provide investigators with information that can help them assess the reliability of the witness's recollection. For instance, a police investigator may put more stock in an eyewitness identification when the witnessing conditions are good than when they are poor.

System variables, on the other hand, are factors that are under the direct control of the police investigator. For instance, simply informing witnesses that the perpetrator may or may not be present in the lineup can considerably reduce false identifications without reducing correct identification (Malpass and Devine, 1981). Lindsay and Wells (1985) proposed that the photographs in a photo-array should be presented sequentially rather than simultaneously. Recently, it has also been suggested that the lineup administrator should be blind as to the identity of the suspect so as not to inadvertently influence the witness's choice or level of confidence (Garrioch and Brimacombe, 2001; Phillips, McAuliff, Kovera, and Cutler, 1999). The system variable approach is useful in that it provides practical guidance as to how police can limit false identifications rather than merely diagnosing the problems after the fact. The program of research described in the present chapter has been informed by a theoretical understanding of the nature of prospective memory and empirically derived factors known to influence success at event based prospective memory tasks. The research is also informed by the system variable / estimator variable distinction, which provides a heuristic for generating forensically useful research questions concerning prospective person memory.

To Catch a Thief

One important application of research on prospective person memory concerns law enforcement efforts to catch missing fugitives or wanted terrorists. We have examined this issue with laboratory analog experiments, as well as with field experiments in which participants have had an opportunity to win a reward if they identify a particular individual during the course of their day to day lives. In one laboratory study, we presented participants with pictures of 4 individuals and asked them to imagine that these individuals were wanted by police. In one condition, participants were asked to imagine that the fugitives were wanted for a serious felony (armed robbery). In another condition, participants were asked to imagine that the fugitives were wanted for a relatively trivial misdemeanor (unpaid parking tickets). In both conditions, participants were told that if they saw the fugitives at any point during the experiment that they should immediately press the space bar to inform authorities. A control condition was also used in which participants were not asked to be on the lookout for anyone.

Participants also performed two ongoing tasks. The prospective memory targets were embedded in the second ongoing task. In the first ongoing task, participants viewed a slide presentation on a computer screen of a trip through a grocery store. Participants were given a shopping list and were asked to press a response key every time they saw one of the items on their grocery list indicating whether the item was on the left or right side of the screen. In the second ongoing task, participants viewed a slide presentation depicting a walk through the campus. As students watched the presentation they had a series of goals to accomplish (e.g., mail a letter, recycle a soda bottle). The ongoing task involved pressing a response key every time an opportunity to accomplish one of the goals occurred (e.g., a mailbox was shown, a recycling bin was shown). Students pressed the 'z' key if the opportunity to accomplish the goal occurred on the left side of the screen and the '/' key if the opportunity to accomplish the goal occurred on the right side of the screen. A number of people, including the four missing fugitives, appeared in the slides making up this second ongoing task. In the felony condition, only 26.61% of the "fugitives" were correctly identified during the prospective person memory task. In the misdemeanor condition, 36.76% of the "fugitives" were correctly identified. This difference was not statistically reliable and was in the opposite direction of what we had predicted. Consistent with the view that prospective memory engages strategic processing, participants in the control condition responded about 200 msec faster on ongoing task than did participants in either of the prospective person memory conditions.

We have also conducted field research aimed at understanding prospective person memory. In one study, students in five introductory psychology classes were shown pictures of two male suspects with one of the suspects being the critical suspect who the students would have an opportunity to identify later. Students were asked to imagine that these individuals were wanted by authorities. The participants were told that if they spotted these individuals and contacted the experimenter that they would win a portion of a $100 prize. For half of the subjects, the picture of the critical suspect was shown with facial hair and, for the other half of the subjects, the picture of the critical suspect was shown clean shaven. Participants were allowed to study the pictures for four minutes. Two days later, the critical suspect came to the classroom and delivered some papers to the class instructors. The suspect turned and faced the class, said "Good morning", paused for a few seconds, and then left the classroom. In his appearance, the critical suspect was clean shaven. Only 5% of the students present at during both class sessions contacted the experimenter and correctly identified the suspect. Of those who identified the suspect, 75% had seen a picture of the suspect without facial hair, although it is important to note that the number of identifications was too low to provide a reliable comparison between the facial hair and no facial hair conditions.

In another study, participants from four different introductory psychology classes watched a mock news broadcast showing pictures of two individuals. The news broadcast was meant to simulate a search for two wanted bank robbers. Participants were told that the individuals shown in the news broadcast were not actually wanted by authorities, but that if they spotted the individuals on campus and contacted their instructor, they would win a portion of a $100 prize. Two days later, the wanted individuals held a cookie sale for the psychology club on the second floor of the psychology building. The classrooms for general psychology were all on the third floor, and the only way students could get to their class or leave their class required that the students walk past the cookie sale. Overall, less than 4% of the students who were present in class both on the day of the cookie sale and on the day of the mock news broadcast made a correct identification. To examine focus of attention, students for half of the classes were sent an email, prior to the cookie sale, telling them about the cookie sale and providing them with a coupon promising two cookies for the price of one. This additional manipulation increased identifications, but only slightly. Students who had been told of the cookie sale correctly identified the "fugitives" 6.67% of the time compared to 2.47% of the time for the control condition.

The studies described above suggest that the ability of members of the general public to correctly identify wanted fugitives in realistic real world conditions is quite limited. In no study that we have conducted has the identification rate exceeded 7%. This is in spite of the fact that the wanted suspects have appeared either in the very same classroom where the initial encoding of the suspects occurred, or immediately outside the classroom. Indeed, initially we were concerned that we were making the task too easy for subjects. Apparently we were mistaken.

FINDING MISSING CHILDREN

Since the 1980s there has been an increased awareness in the United States of the problem of missing children (Asdigian, Finkelhor, and Hotaling, 1995). To obtain data on the nature and extent of the problem, the Department of Justice funded the National Incidence Studies of Missing, Abducted, Runaway, and Thrownaway Children (Finkelhor, Hotaling, and Sedlak, 1990). These studies found that 797,500 children were reported missing in 1999 (Sedlak et al., 2002). Forty-three percent of these cases involve a benign explanation such as: the parent is temporarily unaware of where the child is, contacts police, and later determines that the child is safe after all (e.g., the child went to a friend's house without telling the parent). Forty-six percent of cases involve children who have either runaway or have been "thrownaway" (i.e., have been expelled from their domicile by their legal guardians). Eight percent of cases are children who are lost, injured, or otherwise missing. Family abductions, such as when a non-custodial parent takes a child from the parent with legal guardianship, represent 7 percent of cases. Non-family abductions occur for 2 percent of cases.[12] "Stereotypical abductions", in which a child is taken by a stranger, transported more than 50 miles, held for ransom, kept permanently or killed are rare, representing a little more than 100 cases per year (Finkelhor, Hammer, and Sedlak, 2002).

Missing children represent an important problem and society has been aggressively responding to the problem in a number of different ways including direct mail advertising campaigns, supermarket posters, television coverage, and Amber Alerts. We believe that these efforts are laudable and important. A central goal of our program of research thus far has been to examine these approaches from the perspective of our theoretical understanding of prospective person memory with an eye towards making these approaches more effective.

In one early study we examined the effectiveness of campaigns which place posters of missing children at the exits of supermarkets (Lampinen, Arnal, and Hicks, in press). With the help of a local grocery store that does not currently have a missing children campaign, we placed posters of eight missing children at the exit of the store. The posters were closely modeled after those used by major national campaigns and the children depicted in the posters were active cases from the website of the National Center for Missing and Exploited Children. One week after we first placed the posters in the supermarket we surveyed customers as they left the store. Customers were asked how important they thought the problem of missing children was, the degree to which they looked at the posters in the supermarket, as well as a number of other questions. Participants were also shown pictures of 16 missing children and were asked to circle the 8 pictures that were depicted in the grocery store.

[12] The authors of the NISMART studies point out that these totals sum to more than 100% because some children are involved in more than one incident.

Results of the survey are shown in Figures 1, 2 and 3. About 90% of people indicated that the problem of missing children is either a very important problem or an extremely important problem. Despite this concern, most customers did not look at the posters. More than 90% of customers either did not look or looked only briefly. The memory data were equally discouraging. Memory for the photographs shown in the store did not reliably differ from chance. Note that the results indicated that participants could not distinguish between presented and non-presented pictures within minutes of their visit to the store, even when the pictures on the test were identical with the pictures in the store.

In a follow up survey, we asked participants to indicate why they did not spend more time looking at the posters that were in the grocery store. The reasons given by customers were coded and are depicted in Figure 4. About 40% of customers indicated that they simply walked by the posters without taking note of them. About a third of customers indicated that they were simply too busy to look. A little over 10% indicated that they simply did not think to look. The results of these initial surveys are discouraging, although not especially surprising. Customers at grocery stores are typically busy people, eager to get home or to continue on to other errands. Placing posters at the exits of grocery stores requires that customers will interrupt their important ongoing activities long enough to look at the posters and attempt to commit them to memory. This may not be a realistic expectation.

However, there is reason for hope. Customers are concerned about the problem of missing children and many of our respondents were downright apologetic about the fact that they did not stop to look at the posters. Moreover, the contributions of large corporations in publicizing the problem of missing children are both laudable and promising. We believe that it should be possible to take advantage of work in marketing psychology to develop more effective campaigns for publicizing missing children. In particular, we are currently working on making use of point of purchase advertising approaches to help find missing children. Point of purchase campaigns place advertisements at and around cash registers. Marketing psychologists have shown that point of purchase advertising can dramatically increase sales and product memory (Bennett, 1998; Woodside and Waddle, 1975). We believe that these same techniques can be used to better publicize missing children cases.

Another problem that arises with regards to missing children has to do with obtaining pictures of the children that match their current appearance. Sometimes children go missing and remain missing over extended time periods. The longer a child is missing, the more likely they are to suffer physical and psychological harm (Plass, Finkelhor, and Hotaling, 1996). These problems are complicated by the fact that children change dramatically as they age, hampering attempts to find them (McQueen, 1989).

The dominant strategy for dealing with this problem has been to make use of forensic age progression (McQueen, 1989). In forensic age progression, a child's picture at one age is digitally altered by a forensic artist to project what the child would look like at another age. For instance, if a child goes missing at age 5 and is still missing 5 years later, a forensic artist might be asked to make use of the picture from age five to project what the child likely looks like at age 10. The forensic use of age progression is a relatively recent technique. In 1985, medical illustrators Barrows and Stadler conducted the first forensic age progressions for law enforcement (McQueen, 1989; Sadler, 1986). They based their technique on a large database of children's faces that provided them with statistical information about the craniofacial growth patterns of typical children as they age. In their technique, a computer program projects changes in the relative location of 40 anatomical landmarks on the child's face.

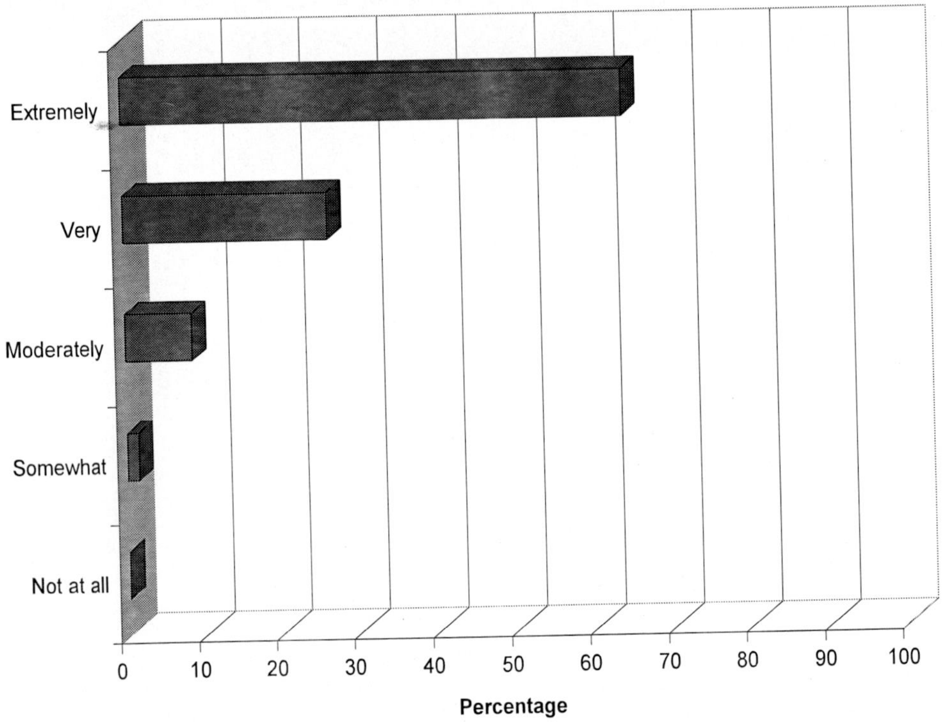

Figure 1. How important is the problem of finding missing children?

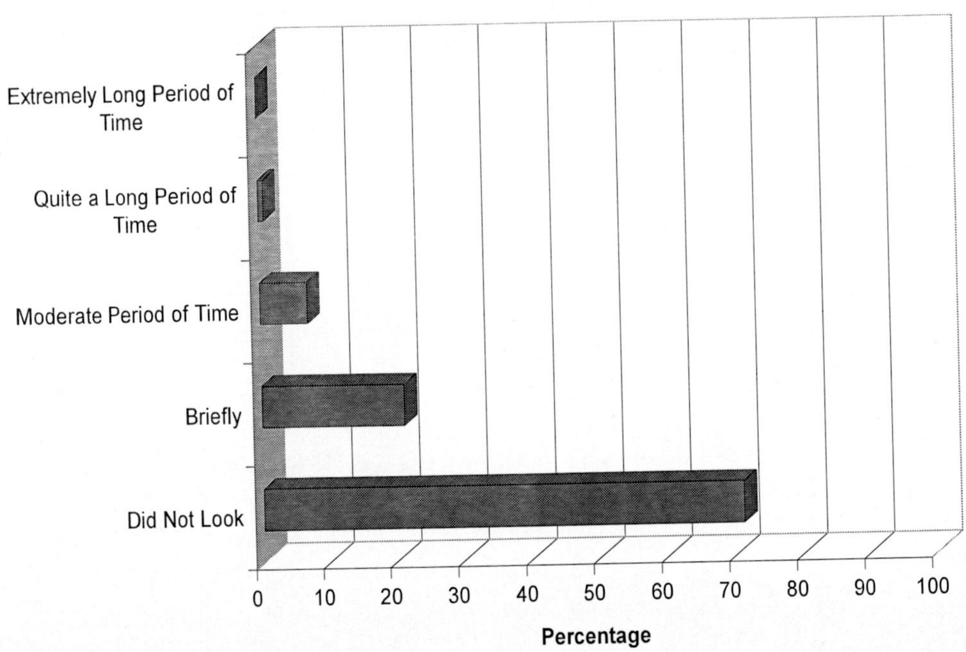

Figure 2. How long did you look at the posters of the missing children?

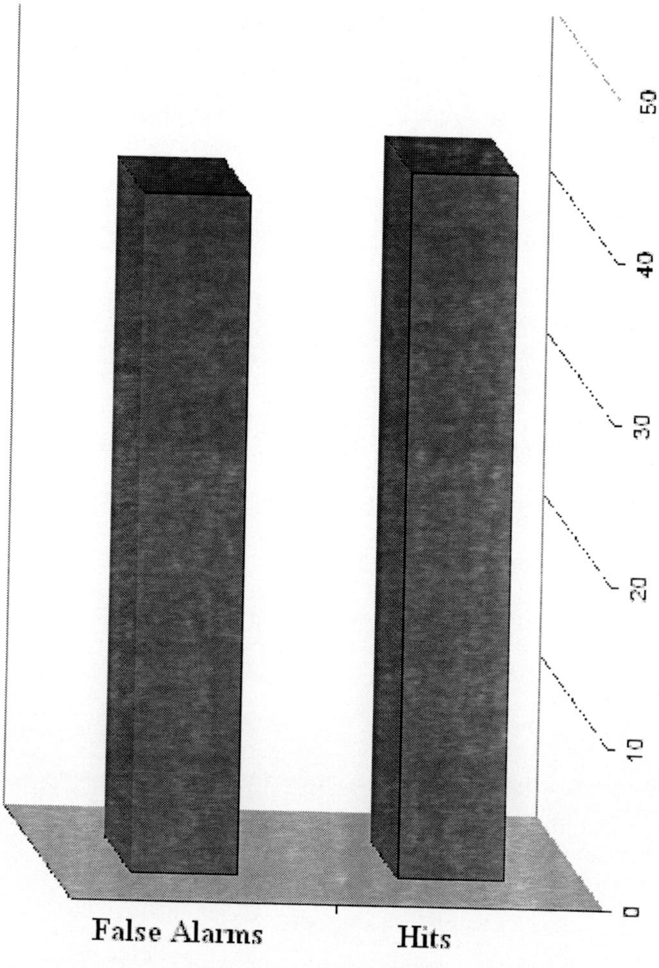

Figure 3. Memory accuracy in recognizing children that were depicted in the supermarket posters.

In addition to these techniques, some forensic artists make use of pictures of the child's biological relatives at the target age to help guide the projection. For instance, a picture of the missing child's father at age 10 might be used to help guide the projection of what the child looks like at age ten.

Forensic age projection is a very common technique in missing children cases. Recently, we randomly sampled 100 cases from the website of the National Center for Missing and Exploited Children. Thirty-nine percent of the cases we sampled involved a child that has been missing for more than 5 years, meaning there is no recent picture of the missing child. Forty-one percent of the cases we sampled made use of forensic age progression. Many of the cases involve a substantial amount of age progression. The median number of years a case has been age progressed is 11 years. Clearly, then, the effectiveness of forensic age progression is an important issue.

We recently undertook a study to examine the effectiveness of age progressed pictures in allowing participants to identify children. Undergraduate volunteers provided us with pictures of themselves at age 7, pictures of their parents at age 12, and pictures of siblings at age 12. The volunteers also provided us with pictures of themselves at age 12.

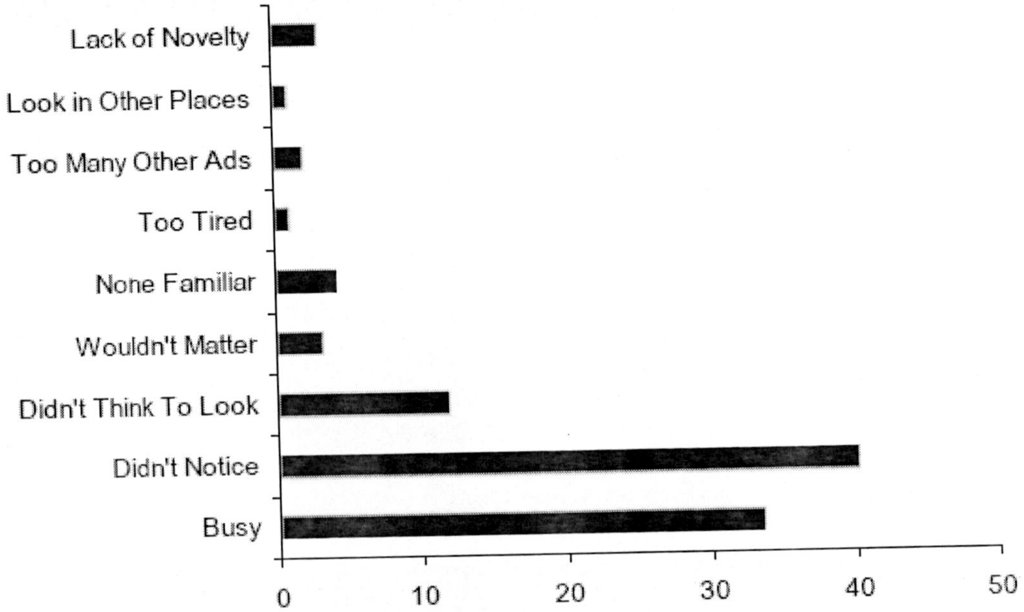

Figure 4. Reasons given by customers for not looking at posters of missing children.

Forensic artists who are experienced at conducting age progression for law enforcement were provided with pictures of the students at age 6-7, as well as the pictures of their siblings and parents. The artists were asked to provide us with age progressed pictures of the students with a target age of 12.

To examine the effectiveness of these age progressed photographs, participants engaged in a laboratory based prospective person memory task. Participants were asked to imagine that 4 children went missing, and that they went missing several years ago. In the *age matched condition*, participants studied 4 pictures of children at age 12, and they were later tested with different pictures of those same children at age 12. In the *age mismatched condition*, participants studied 4 pictures of children at age 7, and they were later tested with pictures of those same children at age 12. In the *age progressed condition*, participants studied pictures of 4 children that had been age progressed to age 12, and they were later tested with actual pictures of those same children at age 12. In all three conditions, participants were shown the pictures four times, at a presentation rate of 3 seconds per presentation.

After this study session, participants engaged in a prospective person memory task, followed by a retrospective person memory task. During the prospective person memory task, participants viewed 44 pictures of children who were approximately 11-12 years old. Four of the pictures were of the "missing children" and 40 of the pictures were new foils. Participants were told that they were to imagine they were placing children into two teams: the P team and the Q team. To place a child on the P team, they were to press the 'P' key on their keyboard. To place a child on the Q team, they were to press the 'Q' key on their keyboard. Participants were instructed to create teams that had an equal number of boys and girls. This ongoing task was moderately difficult because the pictures were randomly presented, requiring minimally that the participant keep track of which team they placed the last girl on and which team they placed the last boy on. In addition to this ongoing task, participants were told that if at any point they saw one of the "missing children," that they were to press the 'H' key on their keyboard.

Immediately following the prospective memory task, participants engaged in a retrospective memory task. In the retrospective memory task, participants were shown four lineups. Each lineup contained a picture of one of the "missing" children at age 12 and seven foils. All pictures were of children who had previously been in the prospective memory task. Participants were to select the picture of the "missing" child or to indicate that none of the pictures were of one of the "missing" children.

Results of the prospective and retrospective memory task are shown in Figure 5. Prospective memory was corrected by subtracting the proportion of false identifications of foils made. As can be seen, forensic age progression did not appear to be especially effective. With regard both to prospective memory and retrospective memory, age progressed photographs did not lead to better identifications than simply studying the picture of the child at age 7. Studying the picture of the child at age 12 led to significantly better prospective and retrospective memory than either of the other conditions. Regression analyses indicated that performance on the prospective memory task was predicted by performance on the retrospective memory task. This suggests that the type of picture shown is primarily influencing the retrospective component of the prospective memory task.

Forensic age progression is an extremely common technique in cases involving missing children. We had a forensic artist age progress childhood pictures given to us by adult volunteers. Age progressed pictures did not appear to improve prospective person memory for missing children relative to a condition where participants simply studied to pictures of the children at the younger age. Age progressed pictures also did not appear to improve lineup identification. These findings are troubling, because in a large proportion of cases a current photograph of the missing child is simply not available.

It is important to note, however, that this study represents simply an initial look at age progression and is part of a larger ongoing program of research. The results are based on one company that does age progression for law enforcement. Moreover, we looked only at age progressions from age 7 to age 12, and it is plausible that the success of age progression techniques may depend crucially on how much the pictures are age progressed, as well as the starting points and end points of the age progression. We also only looked only at age progression with Caucasian children, and it's important to note that there are a large number of missing children who are African American or Hispanic. All of these issues are currently being addressed in our ongoing work.

The problem of missing children is extremely important and the general public evinces great concern over the issue. Additionally, considerable societal resources are being devoted to the problem of helping to find missing children. We have argued that these efforts can best be characterized as an instance of prospective person memory. While efforts by law enforcement, the media and corporations is laudable, we believe that research on prospective person memory can be utilized to help improve the effectiveness of these programs. A major focus of our current research is on finding ways of accomplishing these objectives in hopes of helping secure the return of missing children.

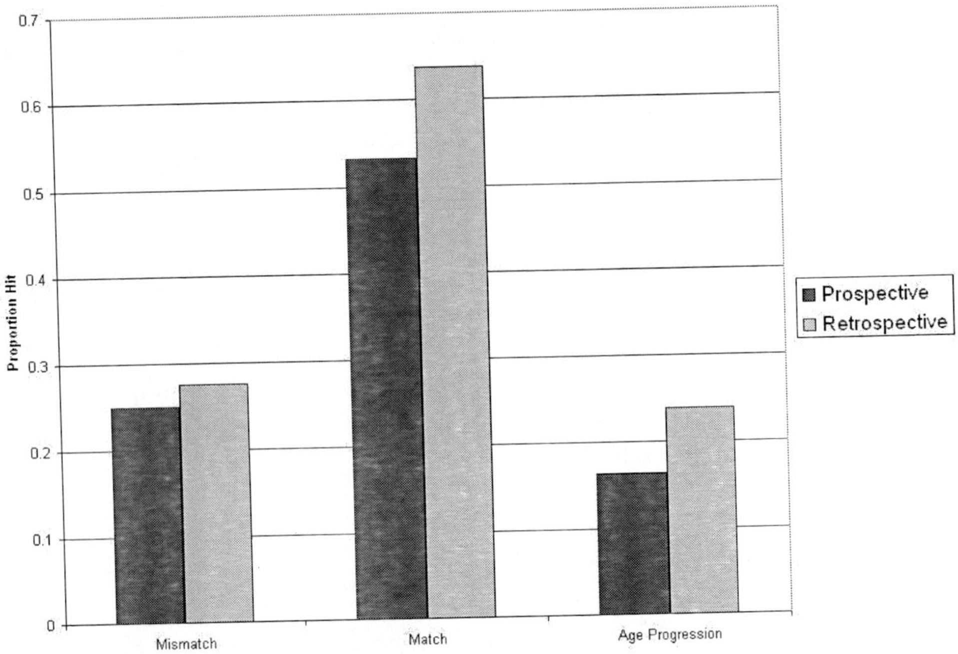

Figure 5. Mean proportion correctly recognized in the prospective and retrospective tasks in the forensic age progression study.

CONCLUSION

The contemporary, experimental study of prospective memory is now a couple of decades old, and the naturalistic study of prospective memory is even older. The research reviewed in this chapter represents a novel combination of both methods to address an important application of prospective memory in the real world, namely, identifying missing children and fugitives from the law. The study of person prospective memory holds promise for continued application and theoretical innovation in the prospective memory literature. What follows are some conclusions and thoughts regarding future directions in this area.

A notable feature of the research described in this chapter is that we are getting an idea of how often people naturally form intentions on their own. This can be contrasted with experimental work in which participants in studies are uniformly given the intention to respond to a cue in the future and are often asked to repeat those instructions for an experimenter to confirm the encoding. The supermarket survey study is an exemplar case for the study of naturally-formed intentions (Lampinen, Arnal, and Hicks, in press). Very few customers spent time even looking at photographs of missing children, which essentially limits the number of people that could have formed the intention to be on the lookout for those children, and only about 10% of customers reported forming a meaningful intention. Thus, more research needs to be done exploring how to get people to take the time needed for forming intentions about such photographs.

A promising area for further development in this regard may lie with implementation intentions (Gollwitzer, 1999). Implementation intentions are those that take the form "When situation x arises, I will perform response y" (Gollwitzer, p. 494). These are contrasted with goal intentions, which are more generally formed as "I will perform y." As applied to the routine aspects of life, people often form very general goal intentions (e.g., "I need to pick up the dry cleaning") without specifying the critical conditions under which the intentions are to be fulfilled (e.g., "I need to pick up the dry cleaning on my way to work just as I pass the local supermarket"). A number of recent papers have explored the utility of implementation intentions in both naturalistic and experimental prospective memory paradigms (e.g., Cohen and Gollwitzer, 2007; Liu and Park, 2004). Implementation intentions can be quite effective and take very little time and effort to encode. The potential combination of implementation intentions with imagery and pictorial encoding of faces holds great promise for the study of person prospective memory.

As a word of caution, we are careful not to assume that the study of *person* prospective memory is necessarily unique as compared with the traditional methods of investigating prospective memory. But what is unique about this research is the way in which both experimental and naturalistic (i.e., field) research is being done in tandem to uncover the theoretical principles of identifying people in service of carrying out intentions and the degree to which people develop such intentions on their own. Thus, our research program lies at the intersection of a budding theoretical interest in prospective memory and one of the more compelling everyday aspects of memory performance—remembering to carry out intentions.

References

America's Most Wanted (2005, July, 27). America's Most Wanted Fugitives. Retrieved July 27, 2005, from the World Wide Web: *http://www.amw.com/fugitives/*

Anthony, T., Copper, C. and Mullen, B. (1992). Cross-racial facial identification: A social cognitive integration. *Personality and Social Psychology Bulletin, 18,* 296-301.

Asdigian, N. L., Finkelhor, D., and Hotaling, G. (1995). Varieties of nonfamily abductions of children and adolescents. *Criminal Justice and Behavior, 22,* 215-232.

Bennett, R. (1998). Customer recall of promotional displays at supermarket checkouts: Arousal, memory and waiting in queues. *International Review of Retail, Distribution and Consumer Research, 8,* 383-398

Blomquist, M. E. (1990). Missing children: A legal framework. In M. L. Frost (Ed.), *Missing Children: The Law Enforcement Response.* (pp. 23-50). Charles C. Thomas Publishers: Springfield IL.

Bothwell, R. K., Brigham, J. C. and Malpass, R. S. (1989). Cross-racial identification. *Personality and Social Psychology Bulletin, 15,* 19-25.

Brown, J. (November 13, 1997). Groups take missing person search to the web. *Wired News.* Retrieved July 22, 2005, from the World Wide Web: *http://wired-vig.wired.com/news/culture/0,1284,8513,00.html.*

Cable News Network (2005a, July, 22). London police kill man in Underground. Retrieved July 22, 2005, from the World Wide Web: *http://www.cnn.com/2005/WORLD/europe/07/22/london.tube/index.html*

Cable News Network (2005b, July, 3). Missing Idaho girl reunited with her father. Retrieved July 22, 2005, from the World Wide Web: *http://www.cnn.com/2005 /US/07/02/ idaho.children/*

Chance, J. E. and Goldstein, A. G. (1996). The other-race effect and eyewitness identification. In S. L. Sporer, R. S. Malpass, and G. Koehnken (Eds.), *Psychological issues in eyewitness identification* (pp. 153-176). Mahwah, NJ: Erlbaum.

Cohen, A. L., and Gollwitzer, P. M. (2007). The cost of remembering to remember: Cognitive load and implementation intentions influence ongoing task performance. In M. Kliegel, M. A. McDaniel, and G. O. Einstein (Eds.), *Prospective Memory: Cognitive, Neuroscience, Developmental, and Applied Perspectives* (pp. 367-390). Mahwah, NJ: Erlbaum.

Cohen, A. L., Dixon, R. A., Lindsay, D. S., and Masson, M. E. J. (2003). The effect of perceptual distinctiveness on the prospective and retrospective components of prospective memory in young and old adults. *Canadian Journal of Experimental Psychology*, *57*, 274-289.

Deffenbacher, K. A. (1983). The influence of arousal on reliability of testimony. In S. M. A. Lloyd-Bostock and B. R. Clifford (Eds.), *Evaluating witness evidence* (pp. 235–251). Chichester, England: Wiley.

Einstein, G. O., and McDaniel, M. A. (1990). Normal aging and prospective memory. *Journal of Experimental Psychology: Learning, Memory, and Cognition, 16*, 717-726.

Einstein, G. O., and McDaniel, M. A. (2005). Prospective memory: Multiple retrieval processes. *Current Directions in Psychological Science, 14*, 286-290.

Ellis, J. and Kvavilashvili, L. (2000). Prospective memory in 2000: Past, present, and future directions. *Applied Cognitive Psychology, 14*, S1-S9.

Ellis, J. (1996). Prospective memory or the realization of delayed intentions: A conceptual framework for research. In M. Brandimonte, G. O. Einstein and M. A. McDaniel (Eds.), *Prospective memory: Theory and applications* (pp. 1-22). New Jersey: Lawrence Erlbaum Associates.

Finkelhor, D., Hammer, H., and Sedlak, A.J. (2002, October). Nonfamily abducted children: National estimates and characteristics. *National Incidence Studies of Missing, Abducted, Runaway and Thrownaway Children.* Office of Juvenile Justice and Deliquiency Prevention, United States Department of Justice. Washtington D.C.

Finkelhor, D., Hotaling, G., and Sedlak, A. (1990, May). *Missing, Abducted, Runaway, and Thrownaway Children in the United States.* Office of Juvenile Justice and Delinquency Prevenstion: Washington D.C.

Garrioch, L. and Brimacombe, C. A. E. (2001). Lineup administrators' expectations: Their impact on eyewitness confidence. *Law and Human Behavior, 25*, 299-314.

Girouard, C. (1990). *The National Center for Missing and Exploited Children.* Washington, DC: U.S. Dept. of Justice, Office of Justice Programs, Office of Juvenile Justice and Delinquency Prevention.

Gollwitzer, P. M. (1999). Implementation intentions: Strong effects of simple plans. *American Psychologist, 54*, 493-503.

Guynn, M. J. (2003). A two-process model of strategic monitoring in event-based prospective memory: Activation/retrieval mode and checking. *International Journal of Psychology, 38*, 245-256.

Guynn, M. J., McDaniel, M. A., and Einstein, G. O. (1998). Prospective memory: When reminders fail. *Memory and Cognition, 26,* 287-298.

Johnson, D. (2005). The ten most wanted list: A history. Infoplease Database. Retrieved July 22, 2005, from the World Wide Web: *http://www.infoplease.com/spot /tenmostwanted.html*

Kramer, T. H., Buckhout, R., Fox, P., Widman, E. and Tusche, B. (1991). Effects of stress on recall. *Applied Cognitive Psychology, 5,* 483-488.

Lafayette, J. (1998, July, 27). Manhunt coverage taxes station's resources. *Electronic Media, 17(31),* 35.

Lampinen, J. M., Arnal, J. D., Hicks, J. L. (in press). The effectiveness of supermarket posters in helping to find missing children. *Journal of Interpersonal Violence.*

Levitt, M. A. (2001, Summer). War on terrorism scorecard. *Middle East Quarterly,* 39-52.

Lindsay, R. C. L. and Wells, G. L. (1985). Improving eyewitness identifications from lineups: Simultaneous versus sequential lineup presentation. *Journal of Applied Psychology, 70,* 556-564.

Liu, L. L., and Park, D. C. (2004). Aging and medical adherence: The use of automatic processes to achieve effortful things. *Psychology and Aging, 19,* 318-325.

Loftus, E. F., and Burns, T. E. (1982). Mental shock can produce retrograde amnesia. *Memory and Cognition, 10,* 318–323.

Malpass, R. S. and Devine, P. G. (1981). Eyewitness identification: Lineup instructions and the absence of the offender. *Journal of Applied Psychology, 66,* 482-489.

Marsh, R. L., Hicks, J. L., and Landau, J. D. (1998). An investigation of everyday prospective memory. *Memory and Cognition, 26,* 633-643.

Marsh, R. L., Hicks, J. L., Cook, G. I., Hansen, J. S., and Pallos, A. L. (2003). Interference to ongoing activities covaries with the characteristics of an event-based intention. *Journal of Experimental Psychology: Learning, Memory and Cognition, 29,* 861-870.

McDaniel, M. A., and Einstein, G. O. (1993). The importance of cue familiarity and cue distinctiveness in prospective memory. *Memory, 1,* 23-41.

McDaniel, M. A., and Einstein, G. O. (2000). Strategic and automatic processes in prospective memory retrieval. *Applied Cognitive Psychology, 14,* S127-S144.

McDaniel, M. A., Robinson-Riegler, B., and Einstein, G. O. (1998). Prospective remembering: Perceptually-driven or conceptually driven processes? *Memory and Cognition, 26,* 121-134.

McQueen, I. (1989, June). Computer age. *Police,* 33-34, 42-43.

Memon, A., Hope, L., and Bull, R. (2003). Exposure duration: Effects on eyewitness accuracy and confidence. *British Journal of Psychology, 94,* 339-354.

Office of Juvenile Justice and Delinquency Prevention (May, 2004). *When Your Child is Missing: A Family Survival Guide.* NCJ 204958. Washington D.C.: U.S. Department of Justice.

Phillips, M. R., McAuliff, B. D., Kovera, M. B. and Cutler, B. L. (1999). Double-blind photoarray administration as a safeguard against investigator bias. *Journal of Applied Psychology, 84,* 940-951.

Plass, P. S., Finkelhor, D., and Hotaling, G. T. (1996). Family abduction outcomes: Factors associated with duration and emotional trauma to children. *Youth and Society, 28,* 109-130.

Platz, S. J. and Hosch, H. M. (1988). Cross-racial/ethnic eyewitness identification: A field study. *Journal of Applied Social Psychology, 18*, 972-984.

Reese, C. M., and Cherry, K. E. (2002). The effects of age, ability, and memory monitoring on prospective memory task performance. *Aging, Neuropsychology, and Cognition, 9*, 98-113.

Russel, S. (January 27, 1997). Virtual fugitives. *Electronic Media, 16(5)*,19.

Sadler, L. L. (1986). Scientific art and the milk carton kids. *Paper presented at the 7th Annual Guild of Scientific Illustrators. Washington D.C.*

Sedlak, A. J., Finkelhor, D., Hammer, H., and Shultz, D. J. (2002, October). National estimates of missing children: An overview. *National Incidence Studies of Missing, Abducted, Runaway, and Thrownaway Children.* Washington D.C.: Office of Juvenile Justice and Delinquency Prevention, U.S. Department of Justice.

Smith, R. E. (2003). The cost of remembering to remember in event-based prospective memory: Investigating the capacity demands of delayed intention performance. *Journal of Experimental Psychology: Learning, Memory, and Cognition, 29*, 347-361.

Smith, R. E., and Bayen, U. J. (2004). A multinomial model of event-based prospective memory. *Journal of Experimental Psychology: Learning, Memory, and Cognition, 30*, 756-777.

Stone, A. (May 6, 2003). Most wanted deck has card dealers flush with orders. *USA Today.* 5a.

Tedisco, J. N. and Paludi, M. A. (1996). *Missing Children: A Psychological Approach to Understanding the Causes and Consequences of Stranger and Non-Stranger Abduction of Children.* State University of New York Press: Albany NY.

USA Today (May 27, 2004). A new kind of terror alert. 12a.

Walmart Foundation (June 21, 2001). Wal-Mart's missing children's boards meet with more success. Walmart Foundation Press Release. Retrieved July 22, 2005, from the World Wide Web: *http://www.walmartstores.com/wmstore/wmstores/Mainnews.jsp?* BV_SessionID=@@@@0634794216.1122048788@@@@andBV_EngineID=cccgaddfdldmdkdcfkfcfkjdgoodglh.0andpagetype=newsandcontentOID=9748andyear=2001andprevPage=NewsShelf.jspandtemplate=NewsArticle.jspandcategoryOID=-8300andcatID=-8248

Wells, G. L. (1978). System variables and estimator variables. *Journal of Personality and Social Psychology, 36*, 1546-1557.

West, R., and Craik, F. I. M., (2001). Influences on the efficiency of prospective memory in younger and older adults. *Psychology and Aging, 16*, 682-696.

Witkin, G. (March, 13, 1995). Forty-five years of bad guys on the run. *U.S. News and World Report, 118(10)*, 15.

Woodside, A. G and Waddle, G. L. (1975). Sales effects of in-store advertising. *Journal of Advertising Research, 15*, 29-33.

Zgoba, K. (2004). The Amber Alert: Appropriate solution to preventing child abduction? *Journal of Psychiatry and Law, 32*, 71-89.

In: Applied Memory
Editor: Matthew R. Kelley

ISBN 978-1-60692-143-2

Chapter 11

REMEMBERING SOCIAL INFORMATION: A FUNCTIONAL ANALYSIS

Matthew B. Reysen
Department of Psychology
University of Mississippi, MS, USA

ABSTRACT

This chapter has three primary goals. The first goal is to review recent research examining the ways that social influences affect participants' memories for events. In particular, such investigations have demonstrated that working with others to reconstruct the past can have a profound impact on later individual memory performance. Next, a potential theoretical explanation for the predisposition towards the encoding, storage, and retrieval of social information is described. This explanation is based on a particular functionalist interpretation of the Social Brain hypothesis, which posits that human intelligence evolved as a result of the need to successfully engage in increasingly complex social interactions. Finally, new empirical evidence supporting such an assertion is presented. In one experiment, participants were exposed to stimulus items which ostensibly originated from either social or nonsocial sources. Participants were able to reconstruct the order of a list of items more accurately if those items were said to have originated from a social source.

INTRODUCTION

Think back to the last time that you had to wait in line to checkout at a grocery store. What sorts of things come to mind? If you are like me, one of your first thoughts may be of the ubiquitous cover pages of gossip themed magazines like *The National Enquirer*. As much as I would like to deny it, the content on such pages is more intrinsically interesting to me than other types of information, such as the new zoning laws that were recently announced in the headline of a local paper. Unfortunately, this is true despite the fact that the new zoning laws are more likely to have an impact on my life than the latest celebrity news. Given the large number of outlets for such information, I certainly am not alone. The question, then, becomes why might I and others like me share a predisposition to focus on information about other people? The central thesis of the current chapter is that the ability to accurately encode, store, and retrieve information about others is essential to successful functioning. In fact, some researchers have proposed that human intelligence evolved, at least in part, as a result of the need to successfully engage in increasingly complex social interactions (e.g., Dunbar, 2007). Consequently, social information may be better remembered than many other types of information.

The present chapter has three primary goals. The first is to provide an overview of some recent areas of investigation into the ways that social influences can affect participants' accounts of events. Next, a potential theoretical explanation for the predisposition towards the encoding, storage, and retrieval of social information will be described. Finally, some new empirical evidence supporting such an assertion will be presented.

IS SOCIALLY-ACQUIRED MISINFORMATION ESPECIALLY HARMFUL?

Recently, there has been a resurgence of interest in the manner in which social influences affect memory performance. The results from such studies are largely, if not entirely, consistent with the hypothesis that social information tends to be better remembered than many other forms of information. Research on the manner in which social influences impact memory performance have approached the issue from at least two directions—each of which has direct real-world implications. Two of these types of applied questions include the following: Is misinformation acquired through social means especially harmful to subsequent individual memory performance, and can social pressure to accept misinformation impact participants' memories?

There are a number of situations in which a person might attempt to remember information with the assistance of others. For example, consider three witnesses who recently experienced an armed bank robbery discussing the events soon after their occurrence. If you were an investigator attempting to gather information about the crime, would you be better off interviewing the witnesses separately or together? Might what one witness says cue another's memory or taint it permanently? The answers to such questions are complicated by the fact that social influences have long been known to impact participants' ability to accurately describe prior events (e.g., Allen and Bragg, 1968; Bless, Strack, and Walther, 2001; Deutsch and Gerard, 1955; Reysen, 2003; Schneider and Watkins, 1996; see Weldon, 2001 for a review).

A number of the studies that have focused on the manner in which social influences affect memory performance have employed either a collaborative inhibition paradigm (e.g., Basden, Basden, Bryner and Thomas, 1997; Weldon and Bellinger, 1997) or a social contagion paradigm (e.g., Roediger, Meade, and Bergman, 2001). In studies examining collaborative inhibition, group members of various sizes are typically exposed to a set of stimulus materials and are then asked to remember the information as a group. More specifically, a group of participants views a set of words or images and then a participant is asked to recall an item from the list. Following this, the first participant is asked to wait while each of her group members recalls an item. This process is repeated until the group's mnemonic resources are exhausted. As the name implies, collaborative inhibition studies have often demonstrated that a group's recall output is typically lower than the pooled recall of an equal number of participants working alone (e.g., Weldon and Bellinger, 1997). One explanation for such a result is that exposure to another participant's recall could interfere with one's ability to remember information (e.g., Wright and Klumpp, 2004). It is possible that some underlying mechanism like output order biases at test (e.g., Basden et al., 1997) could lead directly to such results. Factors such as group size and the number of items to be remembered have been found to influence the extent to which collaborative inhibition occurs (Reysen, 2007).

Despite these observations, it is possible that results like those described above are due less to the act of remembering with others than on other factors such as the relatively impoverished stimulus items typically used or the restrictions on group output, like turn-taking, that are often imposed. In other words, if working with others seriously impairs our ability to remember events, why do we engage in the practice so often? One possible answer to this question can be found in a study on jury deliberations (Pritchard and Keenan, 2002). The study was based on the premise that individual memory errors produced after the course of witnessing a trial could be corrected later following a period of collaboration with others who had viewed the same trial. In the study, participants viewed a scene from a murder trial. After watching the video, participants completed a memory test individually in addition to rendering a verdict. Once this individual test was completed, participants were asked to discuss the evidence presented in the video with several other participants. Following this period of collaboration, participants were asked to complete another memory test. Unlike previous studies (e.g., Basden et al., 1997) in which collaborating groups tended to recall fewer presented words and recalled more words that were not presented (false memories) than an equal number of individuals working alone, Pritchard and Keenan observed an improvement in memory performance following group collaboration and found no evidence of an increase in false memories. Thus, when participants were asked to encode information about other people and the collaboration phase did not involve experimentally imposed restrictions like turn-taking, the results supported the conclusion that group collaboration might improve rather than hinder memory performance (see also, Rajaram and Pereira-Pasarin, 2007; Thorley and Dewhurst, 2007).

In addition to research on collaborative inhibition, another area of investigation into the manner in which social influences impact participants' memories involves the degree to which false information disseminated in groups affects participants' subsequent individual memory reports. In such studies, which employ a social contagion paradigm, participants complete memory tests in the presence of one or more confederates who provide misleading information. Later, participants are tested individually and often incorporate some of the misleading information provided by the confederates into their own versions of events (e.g., Basden, Reysen, and Basden, 2002; Betz, Skowronski, and Ostrom, 1996; Bless et al., 2001; Hoffman, Granhag, See, and Loftus, 2001; Meade and Roediger, 2002; Mudd and Govern, 2004; Roediger et al., 2001). For example, Roediger et al. had participants view pictures of household scenes. After viewing the pictures, the participants were asked to take turns recalling information from the scenes with the help of a confederate. Sometimes, the confederate was instructed to recall information that was not present in the pictures. Roediger et al. demonstrated that participants often recalled false information provided by the confederate, especially when the information was plausible (e.g., saying that a wrench was present in a scene depicting a toolbox when it was not). Thus, similar to the results observed in more traditional studies on misinformation effects (e.g., Loftus, 1993; Loftus and Palmer, 1974), exposure to misinformation from social sources can 'contaminate' participants' own subsequent individual memory reports.

Such a result may not be particularly surprising given that it has been known for years that misinformation from nonsocial sources can affect participants' later individual memory performance. But, if social information is more likely to be encoded, stored, and retrieved than other types of information, one might predict that misinformation obtained from social sources would be more likely to affect participants' subsequent memory performance than information obtained from nonsocial sources. In one study that directly examined this topic, Gabbert, Memon, Allan, and Wright (2004) had participants watch a video of a simulated robbery. Following this, participants were exposed to some events that did not occur in the video either by having participants read a post-event narrative (nonsocial) or through a discussion with a confederate (social). Gabbert et al. observed that participants were more likely to recall the misleading information when it was conveyed in a discussion versus a post-event script. Thus, false information, like veridical information, seems to be more likely to be remembered when conveyed through social means.

Social Pressure can Influence Participants' Memory Reports

Studies employing a social contagion paradigm provide valuable insights into the manner in which participants incorporate memories purportedly produced by others into their own accounts of events. However, despite the fact that many social contagion studies are framed, at least in part, in the context of traditional conformity experiments (e.g., Asch, 1952; Sherif, 1937), researchers have largely ignored the effects of social pressure on memory performance. Essentially, this question concerns whether placing explicit or implicit pressure on participants to remember an event in a certain way can affect their subsequent memory reports. For example, imagine that you are reminiscing with friends and you recall a specific series of events that occurred at a birthday party several years ago. As soon as you mention this, all of your friends clearly remember the events, but insist that they occurred, not at a birthday party, but instead at a New Year's Eve party. Would you be likely to alter your own memory for the event in question based on the assurances of others?

The few studies that have examined the effects of social pressure on memory performance have demonstrated that such pressure can impact performance. For example, Schneider and Watkins (1996) examined the effects of social pressure on recognition judgments. Participants studied a list of words and then completed a recognition test with the assistance of a confederate. For each word on the recognition test, both the participant and the confederate determined whether a target item was on the original list or not. Sometimes the participant responded first, while other times the confederate responded first. When the participant responded second, they presumably faced some degree of implicit pressure to agree with the confederate's response. The confederate's responses were manipulated through subtle cues provided by the experimenter and sometimes the confederate intentionally responded incorrectly. When the participants responded second, they often conformed to the confederate's initial response (see also: Wright, Self, and Justice, 2000).

Whereas the Schneider and Watkins (1996) study provides evidence that participants' recognition performance can be affected by confederate responses, it does not provide clues as to whether social pressure can impact participants' subsequent individual memory reports. To address this issue, Reysen (2005) essentially replicated Schneider and Watkins' (1996) study with the addition of a final individual recognition test following the group test. Using virtual confederates instead of real confederates (see Crutchfield, 1955), participants often conformed to both correct and incorrect responses on an initial group test. In addition, the participants' performance on the final individual recognition test was affected by the initial group interaction. When participants had conformed to incorrect confederate responses on the group test, they were more likely to make subsequent recognition errors when responding in isolation on the final recognition test. Thus, initially working with an incorrect confederate affected the participants' subsequent individual recognition performance. Subsequent research on this topic has demonstrated that both increasing the number of confederates who provide incorrect information and increasing the degree of ambiguity inherent in a situation increases the likelihood of participants reporting incorrect information on individual memory tests following group collaboration (e.g., Reysen, 2007).

A Functionalist Perspective on Memory for Social Information

Although there has recently been an increase in interest in describing the ways that social influences can affect memory performance, less attention has been spent attempting to explain why information obtained from social sources might be especially memorable. In other words, the focus of investigation has been primarily centered on the mechanisms by which information obtained from social sources can impact participants' memory reports. Such a distinction essentially represents the difference between a structuralist approach to such questions and a functionalist approach. Despite the fact that they have been employed less often than other approaches to the study of human memory, such as structuralist approaches, functionalist principles have had a profound impact on the manner in which researchers have investigated the topic (e.g., Anderson, 1996; Anderson and Milson, 1989; Jacoby, Bartz, and Evans, 1978; Mesoudi, Whiten, and Dunbar, 2006; Nairne, Thompson, and Pandeirada 2007; Reysen and Adair, 2008). Whereas a structuralist approach encourages research on the underlying mechanisms of memory systems, a functionalist approach involves shifting the focus of investigation towards the specific problems in the environment that our memory systems have adapted to solve (e.g., Nairne, 2005). Considerations of our mnemonic abilities from a functionalist standpoint involve a focus on the role that those abilities play in overcoming problems in the environment (Klein, Cosmides, Tooby, and Chance, 2002; Nairne, 2005).

Recently, several studies have directly approached the topic of human memory from a functionalist perspective (e.g., Mesoudi et al., 2006; Nairne et al., 2007; Reysen and Adair, 2008; Sharps, Villegas, Nunes, and Barber, 2002). For example, in one such study, Sharps et al. (2002) hypothesized that, given the ancestral importance of hunting, participants' memories for unfamiliar animal tracks might be better than for other comparable stimuli. In their experiments, they had participants study correctly labeled pictorial stimuli from 5 different categories (armored vehicles, sea shells, trees, uncommon cooking utensils and animal tracks). After studying the stimulus items, the pictures were presented without labels and the participants were asked to recall the label that had originally accompanied each image. The main result of the study was that the labels corresponding to the animal tracks were correctly recalled about 30% of the time whereas the correct recall rates were lower than 5% for 3 of the 4 competing categories of stimuli (the uncommon cooking utensils were remembered better than all 4 other categories of stimuli). Although this experiment suffers from the potential for item selection biases, the hypothesis that there may be a mnemonic advantage for animal tracks was at least partially supported. This result led Sharps et al. to suggest that it is at least conceivable that our ability to remember animal tracks is an evolutionary remnant of the pre-agricultural past.

In a similarly motivated study, Nairne et al. (2007) demonstrated that thinking about list items in terms of one's own survival can improve participants' recall better than other well-established deep processing techniques. Nairne et al. had participants study a list of 30 unrelated words after listening to a particular set of processing instructions. The instructions included thinking about items in one of the following ways: Pleasantness, the item's value for assisting with a move, and its' value for survival if stranded alone in a foreign environment. After listing to the instructions, participants rated each list item using a 5-point scale. Nairne et al. observed that participants remembered more studied material after listening to the survival processing instructions than the other types of instructions on both recall and recognition tasks. In a recent follow-up to their original article, Nairne et al. (2008) contrasted free recall results following survival processing with other processing instructions including: Pleasantness, imagery, self-reference, and generation. As in their original article, Nairne et al. oberseved that participants recalled about 10% more of the studied items following survival processing than any of the other forms of processing examined. Thus, a functionally motivated set of processing instructions were capable of leading to better memory performance than some of the best deep processing tasks uncovered to date. Nairne et al. conclude that this mnemonic advantage occurs because their unique processing task taps into a memory system which likely evolved to aid survival, and ultimately fitness (see also: Kang, McDermott and Cohen, in press; Weinstein, Bugg, and Roediger, in press).

Both the Sharps et al. (2002) study and the Nairne et al. papers (2007; 2008) illustrate the types of research questions that can be generated and tested by approaching the topic of human memory from a functionalist perspective. Rather than attempting to examine the specific components of memory systems, both of the aforementioned articles instead sought to explore questions pertaining to the types of information that might be especially well remembered and attempt to provide functionally based explanations to support the hypotheses. As noted above, group interaction involving socially trasmitted information has been found to affect participants' subsequent memory reports. In fact, memories related to our social worlds might be as important, or even more so, to survival and fitness than memories for other types of information. Given this, one might predict a mnemonic advantage for social information versus other types of information. Such a prediction can be based, in part, on a particular functionalist interpretation of human memory involving the Social Brain hypothesis.

The Social Brain Hypothesis

According to the Social Brain hypothesis (e.g., Byrne and Whitten, 1988; Dunbar, 2003), the increase in primate, and more specifically human, intelligence over time may be due, in large part, to the constantly increasing demands of our social worlds. In other words, environmental demands, such as remembering previous interactions with other individuals, may have led to enhancements in our ability to categorize, retrieve, and manipulate information about others. For example, if a person cheated you or stole from you in the past, memories about those previous interactions would likely influence your future dealings with that person. If the Social Brain hypothesis is correct, one might expect social information to be better remembered than other types of information. If today's mnemonic advantage for social information is a result of a long history of adapting to increasing social complexity, then there are likely to be applied implications concerning situations in which indiviudals are asked to process and retreive such information today.

In one study designed to determine whether participants remember social information better than other types of information, Mesoudi et al. (2006) had participants read three short text passages. One passage consisted of factual information about an individual (e.g., Nancy is a 22-year old college student), another described a person who had become pregnant while having an affair with a married college professor (gossip condition), and a third consisted of factual information about the city of Denver (e.g., Denver is the capital of CO). After reading the passages, a first group of participants was asked to recall all of the information they had been asked to process. The output generated by the first group of participants was passed on to a second group. The second group of participants was asked to read and subsequently recall what the first group had written. This process was repeated two more times for a total of 4 "generations" of recall.

The focus of Mesoudi et al.'s (2006) study involved an examination of a possible bias for social concepts in the conveyance of information in human social groups. A propositional analysis determined that participants recalled about 30% more of the studied information from the gossip text than from the other two text passages regardless of the "generation" analyzed. Thus, participants' ability to recall the propositions from the texts appeared to vary as a function of the social nature of the information. These results provide empirical support for the assertion that social information is better remembered than other types of information. However, despite the relatively large differences in recall observed across conditions in Mesoudi et al.'s (2006) study, it is possible that some aspect of the stimulus materials, other than their social or nonsocial nature, could have affected participants' recall levels. More specifically, item selection biases resulting from the differences between the passages, rather than the social or nonsocial nature of the passages, could have affected the outcome.

Reysen and Adair (2008) ran a study designed to determine whether differences in recall for information described as social or nonsocial could be obtained when the experimental stimuli were held constant across conditions. In their experiments, participants studied a list of 30 unrelated words. Following this, participants were given an opportunity to view 5 'critical' words which were selected from the previously studied list. In a 'social' condition, participants were led to believe that the 5 critical words were typed by another participant. In a 'nonsocial' condition, participants were told that the critical words were generated by the computer. After viewing the critical words, participants were asked to complete a free recall test for the original 30 item word list. Despite the fact that the critical words remained constant across conditions, participants recalled about 25% more critical words in the social condition than in the nonsocial condition. Thus, participants were able to recall more critical words when they were led to believe that those words described another person than when they were led to believe that those words were generated by the computer. These results, in accordance with the results of Mesoudi et al.'s (2006) study, suggest that when participants are told that information either describes or originates from another person, it tends to be better recalled than information that originates from nonsocial sources. Thus, as predicted by a set of a priori predictions based on a functional analysis of the Social Brain hypothesis, participants were more inclined to remember information about other people than information believed to be nonsocial in nature.

A Test of the Social Processing Advantage

Taken together, the aforementioned results suggest that people possess an inherent predisposition towards the encoding, storage, and retrieval of social information. This characteristic of human memory appears to be strongly related to both survival, and ultimately fitness, as many successful outcomes result from an interaction between individuals and highly complex social environments. As noted above, previous research has demonstrated that participants recall more information when that information is either social in nature (Mesoudi et al., 2006) or when it is perceived to have originated from a social source (Reysen and Adair, 2008). The purpose of the present experiment is to expand upon these results and determine whether participants' ability to reconstruct the order of a previously viewed stimulus set differs as a function of whether the information is believed to have originated from a social source or not. In other words, can the social processing advantage described above be extended from a recall task to a reconstruction task? If social information is, as predicted, more likely to be remembered than other types of information then one would predict that the social processing advantage described above should extend beyond free recall tasks to include other measures of memory performance.

Method

Participants. Sixty introductory psychology students from the University of Mississippi participated in return for partial course credit.

Design, Materials, and Procedure. Participants arrived at the laboratory in pairs and were seated in front of computer monitors in individual cubicles. The cubicles were arranged in such a manner so that it was not possible for participants to view one another's monitors. After signing an informed consent form, each participant listened to the instructions for the experiment which indicated that they would be studying a number of words in preparation for an upcoming memory test. Participants were told that they would be completing the test either with the help of a group member or with the help of the computer. The participants were then prompted to type their initials and the experiment began.

Despite the initial instructions indicating otherwise, each participant worked alone in one of two conditions. In a 'social' condition, participants were told that they would be working with their group member to remember a list of words. Furthermore, they were told that after viewing a word list, one of them would be asked to recall a few self-descriptive items from the list, while the other participant would be asked to retype some random letter stings. In the 'nonsocial' condition, participants were informed that they would be working on a memory task with the help of the computer. In addition, participants in the nonsocial condition were told that after viewing the word list, they would either be asked to recall some self-descriptive items from the list, or to retype some random letter stings.

After listening to the instructions, all participants viewed a 30 item word list drawn from unique categories from Van Overschelde, Rawson, and Dunloskys' (2004) norms (e.g., apple, chair, eagle, hammer, shirt). The items were presented one at a time in the center of each participant's monitor at a rate of 5 s per item. After viewing the last item in the list, participants in both conditions were asked to retype five 8-character letter sequences composed of randomly selected letters (e.g., "vltkzhdq"). Thus, although all of the participants were asked to complete the retyping task, participants in the social condition were led to believe that while they engaged in that task, their group member was working to recall 5 self-descriptive items from the previously studied list. After the completion of the typing task, participants were provided an opportunity to view five 'critical' words ostensibly either typed by their group member or generated by the computer. In fact, these five critical words were held constant across conditions and were presented one at a time at a rate of 5 s per word in the center of each participant's monitor. Following the presentation of the five critical words, participants were asked to complete a recency control task, which consisted of single digit addition and subtraction problems, for 60 s. Finally, the five critical words were re-presented at the top of each participant's monitor in a new random order and the participants were asked to type the critical words in the order in which they had originally been 'recalled' by either their group member or the computer.

Results

The proportions of critical words that participants placed in the correct serial positions are displayed in Table 1 as a function of instructional condition and serial position. A 2 x 5 mixed ANOVA with instructional condition (social, nonsocial) as a between-subjects factor and serial position (1 through 5) as a within-subjects factor was conducted to determine whether the experimental manipulations affected participants' ability to reconstruct the order of the critical words. The ANOVA revealed statistically significant main effects for both instructional condition $F(1, 58) = 13.21, p < .001$, and serial position, $F(4, 232) = 19.97, p < .0001$. In addition, a statistically significant interaction between instructional condition and serial position was observed, $F(4, 232) = 3.75, p < .01$. Planned comparisons contrasting participants' reconstruction accuracy at each serial position as a function of instructional condition revealed that participants in the social condition achieved higher levels of accuracy in reconstructing the order of the critical words than participants in the nonsocial condition for the second serial position, $t(58) = 2.41, p < .05$, the third serial position, $t(58) = 2.11, p < .05$, the fourth serial position, $t(58) = 3.02, p < .01$, and the fifth serial position, $t(58) = 3.33, p < .01$.

Table 1. The proportions of critical words correctly positioned as a function of instructional condition and serial position

	Serial Position				
Condition	1	2	3	4	5
Social	93 (.25)	87 (.34)	63 (.49)	63 (.49)	73 (.45)
Nonsocial	1.00 (.00)	.60 (.50)	37 (.49)	27 (.45)	33 (.48)

Note: Standard deviations are presented in parentheses.

The interaction between instructional condition and serial position appeared to result primarily from the fact that the difference in accuracy between participants in the social condition and the nonsocial condition was not statistically significant for the first serial position, t (58) = 1.44, p > .05, possibly as a result of a ceiling effect. In addition, the difference between the accuracy rates in the social condition and the nonsocial condition appeared slightly less pronounced for serial positions 2 and 3 (mean difference = .27) than for serial positions 4 and 5 (mean difference = .38).

Overall, the results of present experiment suggest two primary conclusions. First, and perhaps most important, participants in the social condition were, on average, 25% more accurate in reconstructing the order of the critical words in the social condition (M = .76) than in the nonsocial condition (M = .51). Although reconstruction tests are very different than recall tests, this difference is reminiscent of the observation by Reysen and Adair (2008) that participants recalled about 25% more critical words in their social condition than in their nonsocial condition. Second, this result supports the hypothesis that social information is better remembered than nonsocial information and extends prior observations of a social processing advantage for recall (e.g., Mesoudi et al. 2006) to include reconstruction tasks.

CONCLUSION

One purpose of the present chapter was to describe a potential theoretical explanation for participants' predisposition towards remembering social information. This explanation was based on a particular functionalist interpretation of the Social Brain hypothesis, which states that human intelligence may have evolved to adapt to increasing social complexity in our environments. If intelligence more generally, and some mnemonic abilities more specifically, are the result of such a process, then it should be possible to detect a bias in favor of memory for social information versus nonsocial information. Support for such a theory has previously been found for participants' recall of text passages (Mesoudi et al. 2006) and word lists (Reysen and Adair, 2008). In addition to the description of such a theory, a second goal of the current chapter was to provide some new empirical evidence in support of such assertions. The results of the experiment described here lend further support to such a functionalist interpretation of human memory and extend the reach of the social processing advantage to include memory for the order of events.

Although much of the research on this topic has consisted almost exclusively of basic research, it is not difficult to extrapolate beyond such early findings and tentatively foresee applied implications for results such as those presented here. One area of investigation that could prove especially fruitful is the application of functionally based learning strategies to the design of instructional materials. In other words, if it is found to be beneficial to process information in functional terms, such as a consideration of information in a social context, then perhaps better learning outcomes could be achieved by framing information in such a context when it is presented to students.

In conclusion, based on a review of the emerging literature examining the manner in which participants encode, store and retrieve social information, several consistent observations are apparent. Perhaps first and foremost among them is that, as predicted by a particular functionalist interpretation of the Social Brain hypothesis (e.g., Byrne and Whitten, 1988; Dunbar, 2003), participants appear to possess a predisposition towards processing and remembering social information. Taking functionalist principles into consideration seems especially enlightening when analyzing the results of studies focused on applied topics like the manner in which we remember social information. When participants are exposed to information about other people, they tend to remember that information better than other forms of information (e.g., Mesoudi et al., 2006). Furthermore, if people believe that information originates from a social source, they tend to remember it better regardless of whether it is correct (Reysen and Adair, 2008) or incorrect (e.g., Gabbert, Memon, Allan, and Wright, 2004). Taken as a whole, there seems to be a mnemonic advantage for the processing and retrieval of social information that may be explained by the vast array of social complexity that our ancestors faced in the past and that we continue to face today.

Author Note

I thank Stephan A. Adair for his helpful comments on previous versions of this chapter.

References

Allen, V. L., and Bragg, B. W. (1968). Effect of group pressure on memory. *The Journal of Psychology, 69,* 19-32.

Anderson, N. H. (1996). *A functional theory of cognition.* Mahwah, NJ: Erlbaum.

Anderson, J. R., and Milson, R. (1989). Human memory: An adaptive perspective. *Psychological Review, 96,* 703-719.

Asch, S. E. (1952). *Social psychology.* Englewood Cliffs, NJ: Prentice-Hall.

Basden, B. H., Basden, D. R., Bryner, S., and Thomas, R. L. (1997). A comparison of group and individual remembering: Does collaboration disrupt retrieval strategies? *Journal of Experimental Psychology: Learning, Memory, and Cognition, 23,* 1176-1191.

Basden, B. H., Reysen, M. B., and Basden, D. R. (2002). Transmitting false memories in social groups. *American Journal of Psychology, 115,* 211-231.

Betz, A. L., Skowronski, J. J., and Ostrom, T. M. (1996). Shared realities: Social influence and stimulus memory. *Social Cognition, 14,* 113-140.

Bless, H., Strack, F., and Walther, E. (2001). Memory as a target of social influence? Memory distortions as a function of social influence and metacognitive knowledge. In Forgas, J. P.

and Williams, K. D. (Eds.) *Social influence: Direct and indirect processes,* 167-183. New York: Psychology Press.

Byrne, R. W., and Whiten, A. (1988). *Machiavellian Intelligence: Social Expertise and the Evolution of Intellect in Monkeys, Apes and Humans.* Oxford: Clarendon Press.

Crutchfield, R. S. (1955). Conformity and character. *American Psychologist, 10,* 191-198.

Deutsch, M., and Gerard H. B. (1955). A study of normative and informational social influences upon individual judgment. *Journal of Abnormal and Social Psychology, 51,* 629-636.

Dunbar, R. (2007). Evolution of the social brain. In Gangestad, S. W., Simpson, J. A. (Eds.), *The Evolution of the Mind: Fundamental questions and Controversies,* 280-286. New York, NY, US: Guilford Press.

Dunbar, R. I. M. (2003). The social brain: Mind, language, and society in evolutionary perspective. *Annual Review of Anthropology, 32,* 163-181.

Gabbert, F., Memon, A., Allan, K., and Wright, D. B. (2004). Say it to my face: examining the effects of socially encountered misinformation. *Legal and Criminological Psychology, 9,* 215-227.

Hoffman, H. G., Granhag, P. A., See, S. K., and Loftus, E. F. (2001). Social influences on reality monitoring decisions. *Memory and Cognition, 29,* 394-404.

Jacoby, L. L., Bartz, W. H., and Evans, J. D. (1978). A functional approach to levels of processing. *Journal of Experimental Psychology: Human Learning and Memory, 4,* 331-346.

Kang, H. S. K., McDermott, K. B., and Cohen, S. M. (in press). The mnemonic advantage of processing fitness-relevant information. *Memory and Cognition.*

Klein, S. B., Cosmides, L., Tooby, J., and Chance, S. (2002). Decisions and the evolution of memory: Multiple systems, multiple functions. *Psychological Review, 109,* 306-329.

Loftus, E. F. (1993). Made in memory: Distortions in memory after misleading communications. In D. L. Medin (Ed.), *The psychology of learning and motivation: Advances in research and theory, 30,* 187-215. San Diego: Academic Press.

Loftus, E. F., and Palmer, J. C. (1974). Reconstruction of automobile destruction: An example of the interaction between language and memory. *Journal of Verbal Learning and Verbal Behavior,* 13, 585-589.

Meade, M. L., and Roediger, H. L. III. (2002). Explorations in the social contagion of memory. *Memory and Cognition, 30,* 995-1009.

Mesoudi, A., Whiten, A., and Dunbar, R. (2006). A bias for social information in human cultural transmission. *British Journal of Psychology, 97,* 405-423.

Mudd, K., and Govern, J. M. (2004). Conformity to misinformation and time delay negatively affect eyewitness confidence and accuracy. *North American Journal of Psychology, 6,* 227-238.

Nairne, J. S. (2005). The functionalist agenda in memory research. In A. F. Healy (Ed.) *Experimental cognitive psychology and its applications.* 115-126. Washington, DC: American Psychological Association.

Nairne, J. S., Pandeirada, J. N. S., and Thompson, S. R. (2008). The comparative value of survival processing. *Psychological Science, 19,* 176-180.

Nairne, J. S., Thompson, S. R., and Pandeirada, J. N. S. (2007). Adaptive memory: Survival processing enhances retention. *Journal of Experimental Psychology: Learning, Memory, and Cognition, 33,* 263-273.

Pritchard, M. E., and Keenan, J. M. (2002). Does jury deliberation really improve jurors' memories? *Applied Cognitive Psychology,16,* 589-601.

Rajaram, S., and Pereira-Pasarin, L. P. (2007). Collaboration can improve individual recognition memory: Evidence from immediate and delayed tests. *Psychonomic Bulletin and Review, 14,* 95-100.

Reysen, M. B. (2003). The effects of social pressure on group recall. *Memory and Cognition, 31,* 1163-1168.

Reysen, M. B. (2005). The effects of conformity on recognition judgments. *Memory, 13,* 87-94.

Reysen, M. B. (2007). The effects of social pressure on false memories. *Memory and Cognition, 35,* 59-65.

Reysen, M. B., and Adair, S. A. (2008). Social processing improves recall performance. *Psychonomic Bulletin and Review, 15,* 197-201.

Roediger, H. L., III., Meade, M. L., and Bergman, E. T. (2001). Social contagion of memory. *Psychonomic Bulletin and Review, 8,* 365-371.

Schneider, D. M., and Watkins, M. J. (1996). Response conformity in recognition testing. *Psychonomic Bulletin and Review, 3,* 481-485.

Sharps, M. J., Villegas, A. B., Nunes, M. A., and Barber, T. L. (2002). Memory for animal tracks: A possible cognitive artifact of human evolution. *Journal of Psychology: Interdisciplinary and Applied, 136,* 469-492.

Sherif, M. (1937). An experimental approach to the study of attitudes. *Sociometry, 1,* 90-98.

Thorley, C., and Dewhurst, S.A. (2007). Collaborative false recall in the DRM procedure: Effects of group size and group pressure. *European Journal of Cognitive Psychology, 19,* 867-881.

Van Overschelde, J. P., Rawson, K. A., and Dunlosky, J. (2004). Category norms: An updated and expanded version of the Battig and Montague (1969) norms. *Journal of Memory and Language, 50,* 289-335.

Weinstein, Y., Bugg, J. M., and Roediger, H. L. III. (in press). Can the survival recall advantage be explained by basic memory processes? *Memory and Cognition.*

Weldon, M. S. (2001). Remembering as a social process. In D. L. Medin (Ed.) *Psychology of learning and motivation: Advances in research and theory, 40,* 67-120. San Diego, CA: Academic Press.

Weldon, M. S., and Bellinger, K. D. (1997). Collective memory: Collaborative and individual process in remembering. *Journal of Experimental Psychology: Learning, Memory, and Cognition, 23,* 1160-1175.

Wright, D. B., and Klumpp, A. (2004). Collaborative inhibition is due to the product, not the process of recalling in groups. *Psychonomic Bulletin and Review, 11,* 1080-1083.

Wright, D. B., Self, G., and Justice, C. (2000). Memory conformity: Exploring misinformation effects when presented by another person. *British Journal of Psychology, 91,* 189-202.

In: Applied Memory
Editor: Matthew R. Kelley
ISBN 978-1-60692-143-2

Chapter 12

CAN WE DETERMINE THE FUNCTIONS OF EVERYDAY INVOLUNTARY AUTOBIOGRAPHICAL MEMORIES?

***John H. Mace*[*1] *and Elizabeth Atkinson*[2]**
[1] Department of Psychology Eastern Illinois University,Charleston, IL, USA
[2] Department of Psychology, University of New Haven, West Haven, CT, USA

ABSTRACT

Involuntary autobiographical memories (spontaneous recollections of events from one's past) occur daily for most individuals. Long a mystery, in recent years this memory phenomenon has become the focus of a number of memory researchers. An important question to be answered in this area concerns the functional status of these memories. Are involuntary memories merely the accidental by-products of a "restless" autobiographical memory system, occurring for no other reason than pure chance, or do they serve some function? This chapter explores the possibility that involuntary memories serve two major functions. One is a classic survival (adaptation) function which serves to remind us about past dangers that we have experienced so that we might take corrective actions in the future. The other is a self-oriented (identity) function which serves to keep us grounded in our self-perceptions by reminding us of events that contain information related to the self (e.g., one's goals, aspirations, self-image, etc.). The chapter reports the results of three different naturalistic diary studies which present evidence consistent with both of these functions.

INTRODUCTION

Dreaming is a common daily mental experience. Spontaneous recollection of past events (or involuntary memories) is also a common daily mental experience. We know a lot about dreams and dreaming (see Hobson, 2002), and we also know a lot about involuntary memories and involuntary remembering (see Mace, 2007b). However, there is one important question that remains unanswered in both of these areas: What purpose do they serve? We

* Corresponding author.

think that the implications of the functional question in dreams or involuntary memories share many similarities. We have long pondered if dreams have some function (e.g., to disguise the unconscious or to consolidate our experiences of the day into permanent memories), or if they are merely random mental experiences of no functional value, occurring only because we are in an altered state of consciousness (for a review, see Hobson, 2002). The same sort of question can be applied to involuntary memories. Why do we experience them at all? Why do they occur in such a wide variety of circumstances, as reported by numerous involuntary memories studies (e.g., while we are driving, thinking, walking, talking, listening, playing, and so forth, Berntsen, 1996; Mace, 2004, for reviews see Ball, Mace, and Corona, 2007; Berntsen, 2007, Mace, 2007b, c)? Do these memories function as needed reminders of the past in situations of danger or social circumstance, for example? Or are they merely a random, functionless part of the stream of consciousness, occurring only because they happen to coincide with triggers in the environment?

For dreams or for involuntary memories, answers to these questions are important to our understanding of these phenomena. In the case of dreams, one answer tells us that they are random and irrelevant to any human function, while another says they are important because they play a role in the consolidation of long-term memories, having the potential of enhancing our understanding of such concepts as learning, memory, and retention. For involuntary memories the stakes are equally important: They either are irrelevant to everyday life and human functioning, or they have functions in them. If they are functional in one or many ways, this would help us to understand them better, as well as show us another way in which autobiographical memory is functional, just to mention a few of the possibilities.

In memory research, questions regarding functionality are relatively rare because the functions (or at least the main ones) are often quite apparent. For example, to answer the question of functionality in autobiographical or semantic memory, all one need do is imagine life without one or the other. However, if that is not enough to make it clear, then observations of the lives of the densely amnesic or the demented should make it abundantly clear what purposes these types of memories serve. This type of simple analysis of function does not work so easily with involuntary memories. Can we imagine life without involuntary memories or individuals without them (involuntary memory amnesics)? For most people it is probably easy to imagine a functional life or people without involuntary memories, but this obviously does not help us with questions of functionality, because our ease in imagining life without them may simply mean that the magnitude of their function is not as great as function might be in autobiographical or semantic memory, or like dreams, their functions are just not easily gleaned. On the other hand, if involuntary memories are random, functionless memories, then maybe they can be harmful distractors, if, for example, we have too many of them or have them at the wrong times. This adds another dimension to the problem, one which does not appear to exist in the dream question or perhaps in any other area of memory.

In this chapter, we begin the process of answering the question of functionality in involuntary memory. However, it should be stated at the outset that we realize that given the difficulty of establishing functionality (purpose) in any area, we are not claiming to provide definitive answers, only what we think are good clues to the possible answers. Our main goal is simply this. Beyond that, we hope that the study presented here will inspire others to take up what we believe is an important question. Before we describe the nature of our study, we first outline three different viewpoints on the functions of involuntary memories: the *classic functional view*, the *life-situation view*, and the *non-functional view*.

Three Views on the Functionality of Involuntary Memory

The first view, the *classic functional view*, is our view of involuntary memory function. However, we should state that we are not committed to any one position in this paper. We have labeled this view the classic functional view because it is based on traditional notions of adaptation to one's environment (e.g., emphasizing basic survival or utility functions in one situation or another). In this view, involuntary memories are seen as functional because they provide the rememberer with important or useful information in a variety of different situations. We have identified three possible situations and call them practical circumstances, circumstances involving potential danger, and social circumstances. For example, if one is lost in the woods, environmental cues could trigger recent memories which might help in finding the way back. Or in another circumstance, cues in our environment may also tell us something about a past dangerous situation (e.g., as one approaches an intersection in the road, one might instantly remember a recent event in which a car had nearly darted out in front of you). In social contexts, the words of someone's conversation (or one's own thoughts) might trigger memories which are relevant and useful to the situation. One way to think of this view is that involuntary memory production in these situations is telling us "you need to remember this now" or this "memory might be useful to you." Baars and colleagues have advocated a similar view by suggesting that a chief function of involuntary memories is to get the deliberative (or voluntary) process started (i.e., "you need to remember this now" and "you should give this past situation some serious thought", see Baars, Ramamurthy, and Franklin, 2007, and Mace, 2007c).

The next view, the *life-situation view*, was recently proposed by Berntsen (2007). We call this view the life-situation view because this construct is a major tenet of it. In this view, involuntary memories are seen as functional because they may relate to one's current life situation. The life situation is a personhood or sense of self construct which rests on autobiographical memories containing such information (e.g., those related to identity and self-image, personal goals, etc.). Berntsen gives us a detailed account of how this might work:

> The *life-situation* is a personal construct that refers to the individual's current appraisal of his or her recent past and close future. The orientation towards the future can be described as representations of intertwined plans, expectancies, goals -- much similar to the notion of current concerns as described by Klinger (1971). The life situation is also orientated towards the past, however, in terms of ongoing processing of salient past events. The latter is reminiscent of the notion of unfinished personal business as discussed in a psychoanalytic tradition (see Horowitz, 1986), but in the present context it is not delimited to stressful and problematic events. An unproblematic, pleasant conversation with a friend or the reading of an intriguing novel may serve the same function.
>
> My suggestion is that the life-situation --with its past and future orientation --primes clusters of thematically related autobiographical memories and increases the individual's sensitivity to cues with relevance to the life-situation. The immediate situation triggers a particular memory from the pre-activated set if one or more features attended to in the immediate situation overlap critically with the content of one of the pre-activated memories. Memories that are primed by the life-situation but do not possess concrete resemblance to features in the immediate situation are in most cases unlikely to be brought to mind. (p. 41)

Thus, these memories would feature personal life themes (e.g., concerning one's work or important personal relationships, such as friends, family members, or romantic partners) and personal life goals or aspirations (e.g., that one wants to become a psychologist). They should help to maintain one's sense of self or identity and remind us of our personal aspirations and current preoccupations (see Kamiya, 2003, 2007, for a similar functional account).

The last view, the *non-functional view*, is obviously the case against the functionality of involuntary memories. This view states that involuntary memories have no functional value whatsoever and that their occurrence in everyday life is merely accidental or coincidental. Given the vastness and richness of the autobiographical memory base, we should expect involuntary memories to occur from time to time. However, these memories are purely chance occurrences, which occur only because memories in this system happen to coincide with a great number of internal and external cues. Thus, if involuntary memories are brought about by sensible cues under what appears to be useful circumstances, this is merely coincidental. Similarly, if involuntary memories appear to be organized by general principles (thus suggestive of some purpose), this is only because their source is governed by these principles. For example, if involuntary memories show recency (Schlagman, Kvavilashvili, and Schulz, 2007) and priming (Mace, 2005) effects, this is only because these principles govern memories in the autobiographical memory system, and therefore, should not be taken as evidence that involuntary memories are functional.

While the last view is obviously the default, null case, it should be noted that this is not the typical null argument, because it explains how and why involuntary memories are not functional. The first and second views make a case for functionality, however, they differ in that one uses personhood constructs, whereas the other does not (e.g., consider how such constructs are not needed in the driving example given in the classic view). In addition, the classic functional view offers simpler explanations of function (e.g., as in the driving example), whereas the life-situation view is more complex. Nevertheless, despite these differences, it is certainly possible (and indeed plausible) that both the classic and the life-situation views may account for the functional nature of involuntary memories in different situations. Dual-purpose (or multi-purpose) explanations are becoming more commonplace as autobiographical memory research and other approaches are revealing greater complexity to this form of memory than what is typically revealed by more traditional laboratory approaches, such as word-list learning (see, for example, Conway, 2001, 2005). If we can return to our amnesic example above to illustrate, in densely amnesic patients (like the well-known case of patient H.M.), the loss of autobiographical memory functions clearly demonstrates the importance of this system to everyday functioning and survival in the most mundane sense. Less salient, but every bit as real and important, is the loss or impairment of other functions, such as sense of self and person, life purpose, and continuity in space and time (see Bluck, 2003; Conway, 2001, 2005).

Examining Involuntary Memory Function with Naturalistic Diary Studies

In the present study, we used three separate diary recording methods to examine the question of involuntary memory function. Each of the approaches required subjects to record descriptions of their involuntary memories as they experienced them in everyday situations (for reviews of the various diary methods used to study everyday involuntary memories, see Ball and Little, 2006; Berntsen, 1996; Kvavilashvili and Mandler, 2004; Mace, 2004; Schlagman, Schulz, and Kvavilashvili, 2006). Several other items and measures were included, which varied according to the approach and the functional view under examination.

To examine the life-situation view, we had subjects keep a diary of their involuntary memories for 10 days. The diary contained a number of items which attempted to probe life-situation relevance. Recall that the life-situation view argues that involuntary memories are relevant to one's current life focus, which includes both current life events and goals. Accordingly, one of the diary items probed this directly by asking subjects if memories were related to events in their lives, while two other items directly asked if they were related to their personal goals, either short term or more long term. Our reasoning behind these items was fairly straightforward: If involuntary memories have a life focus or purpose according to the life-situation view, then at least some (if not a good number) of them should be related to life events and personal goals. In addition to these direct items, we use two indirect queries. One item asked subjects if the involuntary memories were related to something they were recently thinking about, while another asked if they were related to something they think about frequently. We took "yes" responses to these items and separated them into two categories: mundane thoughts (e.g., thinking about breakfast) versus life-situation thoughts (i.e., thoughts fitting the life-situation view). We then used these responses to assess the life-situation priming prediction. Recall that the life-situation view also predicts that one's life-situation primes clusters of life-situation related memories. If this is true, then the most likely vehicle for such priming is thoughts and preoccupations about events in one's life. There is already good experimental evidence that involuntary memories are primed by recent thoughts and preoccupations (Mace, 2005). Thus, we reasoned that if subjects indicate that their memories are frequently related to life-situation thoughts that they had on their mind, then this would be consistent with the priming prediction of this view. We discuss the priming question in greater detail in the Discussion.

To examine the classic functional view, we used two separate methods. In one approach, we asked subjects to record only one memory (Ball and Little, 2006). Subjects were given an envelope, which they were to open when they had an involuntary memory. The envelope contained a diary page containing questions which asked subjects to indicate if (and how) the memory was useful to them. We reasoned that if any of the memories fit any of the three circumstances specified in the classic view (practically or socially useful, or useful in a situation of potential danger), then subjects should be able to report this. We used the single memory report method because we were concerned that asking subjects such a question repeatedly might contaminate the results with demand characteristics (see Ball and Little, 2006). In the second approach, we compared the involuntary memory descriptions to descriptions of the circumstances in which they occurred, which were recorded over a 14-day period. Here we were looking for evidence that involuntary memories fit our potential danger scenario, and we used a strict criterion for making these decisions. Memories were deemed to fit this aspect of the view only in the event that the memory clearly provided useful information about possible actions or outcomes in obvious situations of potential danger or other clearly adverse circumstances. We held strictly to this criterion because this was the only way that we could be certain about our judgments, not having the benefit of the subject's input (as in the single-record diaries) to reliably assess social or practical relevance.

Method

Participants. A total of 56 participants served in the 10-day (n = 15), 14-day (n = 15), or single-recording diary study (n = 26). The participants were comprised of graduate/undergraduate students and staff from the University of New Haven, as well as some individuals from the community. The participation of these various subject groups was fairly evenly distributed across the three recording methods. The age range of the participants was from 21 to 53 years (M = 24.2), with 37 female and 19 male participants. Participants in the 10- and 14-day diary studies were paid $50.00, whereas participants in the single-record study were paid $5.

Diary designs and procedure. The 10-day and the single-record diary methods were designed specifically for this study, whereas the 14-day method was designed for another study. The 10- and 14-day methods used a pocket-sized diary booklet which contained 50 pages (one page for each memory), whereas the single-record method used a dairy consisting of only one page. Each page in all three of the diaries contained the same five open-ended items which asked subjects to record (1) a brief description of the memory, (2) a brief description of the activity that they were engaged in at the time the memory came to mind, (3) a brief description of the perceived retrieval cue, (4) a brief description of what they were thinking just prior to the memory coming to mind, and (5) their approximate age in the memory (some of these items were not relevant to the focus of this study). Apart from these open-ended items, the 10-day diary contained five closed-ended items which asked subjects if a memory was related to a recently or frequently thought about topic (2 items), to an event in their life (1 item), or to a short- or long-term goal (2 items), with all requiring an explanation in the case of affirmative answers (see Appendix). The single-record diary contained two closed-ended items, one (i.e., the situational usefulness item) which asked subjects if the memory was useful to them in the situation in which it had occurred, and another (i.e., the general usefulness item) which asked if it was useful in some other way, explaining all affirmative answers (see Appendix). We added the general usefulness item to see if a more indirect item would pick up responses consistent with the three classic view situations in the event that the situational usefulness item had failed.

Prior to the start of the diary recording, subjects were given written instructions which defined involuntary and voluntary autobiographical memories, described the requirements for participating in the study, and listed some examples of the types of entries they would be required to make in the diary. All of the participants then met with an investigator either individually or in groups of two or three. The written instructions were reviewed, followed by a question and answer period in which participants were asked to distinguish between an involuntary and a voluntary memory (all were able to make the distinction). Participants in the 10- and 14-day recording studies were given a dairy and told that they were to keep it with them at all times, recording each and every involuntary memory according to the written instructions for the period of time specified (i.e., 10 or 14 days). Participants in the single-record study were given an envelope which contained the single diary page. They, too, were instructed to carry it with them at all times, opening it to answer the questions when they had their first involuntary memory. All participants were given the option of withholding any information that they felt was too private to share.

Results

In the 10-day diary study, subjects recorded a total of 195 involuntary memories ($M = 13$ per subject, 1.3 per day). In the 14-day dairy study, subjects recorded a total of 339 involuntary memories ($M = 23$ per subject, 1.6 per day). These frequencies of occurrences are in line with reported frequencies in past diary studies (e.g., Schlagman, Kvavilashvili and Schulz, 2007; Schlagman, Schulz and Kvavilashvili, 2006). In the single-record study, each of the 26 subjects recorded a single involuntary memory. However, one of these was a prospective memory, which was excluded, thus leaving a total of 25 involuntary memories in this sample. We first present the results of the 10-day study, followed by the 14-day and the single-record studies, which are presented together.

10-day Diary Study. Figure 1 shows the results of the five critical diary items. As can be seen in the figure, subjects frequently answered the items positively (71% of the time, all items combined), indicating that their memories were either related to things they had thought about, life events, or goals. We analyzed subjects' responses on the two thought items. The results of this analysis showed that some of the items were marked as private, while the rest were able to be categorized as either mundane or life situation related. For the recent thought item, most of the responses were categorized as mundane (62% mundane vs. 38% life situation, χ^2 (1) = 5.76, $p<.05$), whereas the reverse was true for the frequent thought item, which showed the life situation category overwhelming outstripping the mundane category (14% mundane vs. 86% life situation, χ^2 (1) = 51.84, $p<.001$). An inspection of the life event responses showed that all of the responses were consistent with life event themes. Similarly, all of the responses entered for the goal items (both long and short term) were deemed as goals.

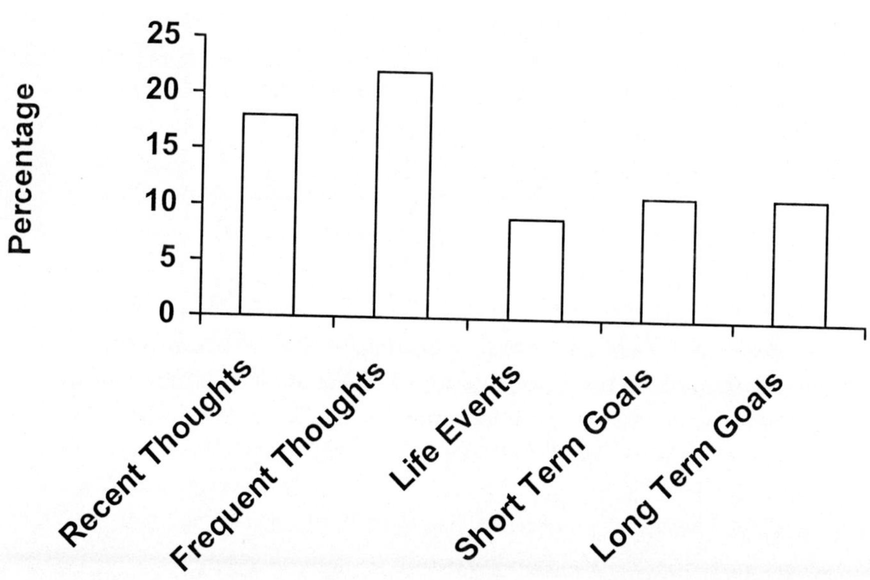

Figure 1. Percentage of "yes" responses on the five items in the 10-day study.

14-day and Single-Record Diary Studies. Unlike the 10-day study which was designed with items that specifically addressed functionality, the 14-day study was originally constituted for a different purpose. As such, it yielded less analyzable data, as the functionality analyses had to be gleamed from two open-ended items (the description of the involuntary memory and the activity that one was engaged in when the memory came to mind). Judgments could not always be made as sometimes the descriptions for these items were either marked private or they were lacking in adequate detail. Our initial inspection of these items in the 14-day diaries revealed that judgments could not be made in 116 (34%) of the 339 recorded memories. Of the 223 that we could render judgments on, we found that 18 (8%) had fit our usefulness criterion (i.e., the potential danger scenario). These memories were distributed across 8 (53%) of the 15 subjects used in this analysis.

Turning to the single-record diaries, we analyzed the two critical items (situational usefulness and general usefulness) in terms of the two possible responses (affirmative or negative) and also in terms of the descriptions given for affirmative responses. An analysis of the responses on the situational usefulness item showed that eight (32%) of the subjects indicated that the memory was useful to the situation in which it had occurred. An inspection of their descriptions for this item showed that two (8%) fit the potential danger criterion that we used for the 14-day study (e.g., that she had tripped in a specific location previously), two (8%) were more mundane, but nonetheless having practical relevance to their immediate situation (e.g., getting lost while driving), while four (16%) had social relevance in that subjects had indicated that they were triggered by and relevant to the conversation that they were engaged in. The analysis of the general usefulness item showed five (20%) of the subjects answering affirmatively. An inspection of the descriptions for this item showed one subject indicating that the memory had positively impacted her mood, three indicating that it had reminded them that they had chosen the right career paths (perhaps consistent with the life-situation view), and one indicating practical relevance or a situation involving future danger or adversity (namely that it reminded her that should stay away from an activity that she had experienced as adverse). We deemed this last response as a situation of potential danger, and Figure 3, then, shows the percentage of responses fitting into the three situational categories.

CONCLUSION

The results of the 10-day diary study showed that nearly one-third of the involuntary memories recorded by these subjects were related to life events and personal goals (31% combined across these three items, see Figure 1), while more than one-third of the memories were related to things that they had on their minds (40%, combined across the thought items, see Figure 1), many of which could be categorized as life-situation thoughts (as high as 86% in the case of frequent thoughts, see Figure 2). Thus, these findings were consistent with the life-situation view. The analysis of the 14-day diary study showed a small percentage (8%) of the involuntary memories fit our strict criterion for usefulness. Regarding the single-record study, nearly one-third of the subjects (representing nearly a third of the memories) indicated on the situational usefulness item that the memory was useful to the circumstance in which it had occurred.

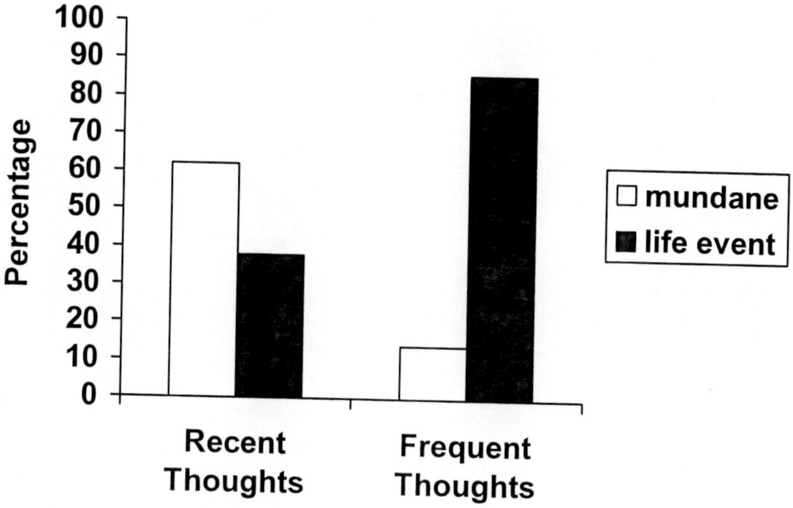

Figure 2. Mundane versus life-situation thoughts in the recent and frequent thought items in the 10-day study.

Some of the descriptions of usefulness fit our potential danger criterion (8%), while others fit the practical or social circumstance usefulness categories (totaling 24% of the memories). The results of the general usefulness item showed some 20% of the subjects (i.e., 20% of the memories) answered this item affirmatively, however, its interpretation was a little less clear. One of the responses may be interpreted as consistent with our strict criterion, some (the emotional ones) appeared to be irrelevant to the classic view (but perhaps fitting some other view, e.g., emotional regulation functions, see Pasupathi, 2003), while some (life path responses) could be interpreted as fitting the life-situation view. In sum, then, a total of 36% fit the three categories of the classic view (see Figure 3).

Apart from these observations, the recent and frequent thought items in the 10-day study produced results consistent with the notion that life-situations prime pools of life-situation relevant memories. Although the results are only suggestive, there is otherwise good evidence that involuntary memories are primed by recent cognitive activity (e.g., preoccupations and reminiscing) in a fashion that is very much akin to associative priming (Mace, 2005). In a study examining this hypothesis, Mace first showed that the contents of involuntary memories recorded in diaries were frequently related to the contents of subjects' current preoccupations (i.e., various life themes), which they noted in a post-diary questionnaire. Following this up with experimental means, other groups of subjects came into the laboratory for voluntary memory priming sessions on one or more occasions while they were keeping a diary of their daily involuntary memories for two weeks. In these sessions, subjects recalled memories from their years in high school, memories from the past year, or other circumscribed temporal periods. At the completion of the diary recording phase, the diaries were inspected for memories from the various time periods. The results showed that subjects had experienced significantly more involuntary memories from the temporal period that they were primed for in the laboratory than relevant control subjects.

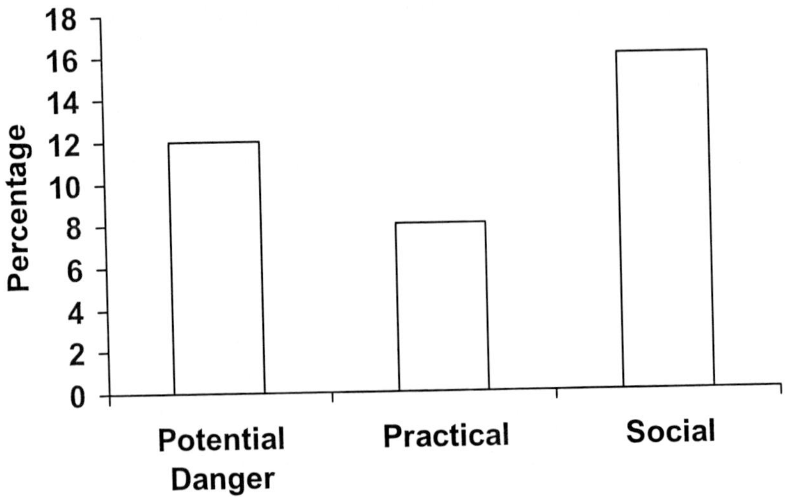

Figure 3. Distribution of memories fitting the three situational categories of the classic functional view in the single-record study.

Mace argued that the results suggest that daily cognitive activity primes (or activates) memories related to the content of such activities, which in turn might result in their activation in everyday life when one encounters relevant cues. Furthermore, if part or all of one's daily involuntary memory productions is associated with recent thoughts and preoccupations, then this would at the very least make them relevant to our current circumstances in a way similar to that articulated in the life-situation view.

Although the results from the thought items in the current study lack the experimental rigor that was present in the Mace (2005) study, they are consistent with the notion that cognitive activity (current, recent, and frequent) is involved in the activation and selection of everyday involuntary memories. More importantly for the purposes of this study, the appearance of life-situation thoughts in these items (particularly the frequent thought item) suggests that this sort of priming might be one means by which life-situation relevant memories come to the fore in everyday involuntary memory production. We believe that this is consistent the priming aspect of the life-situation view, though the view is silent on the specifics of priming.

Thus, how do these results presented here answer the involuntary memory function question? The most obvious interpretation is that they supply us with some suggestive evidence which appears to support both the classic and the life-situation functional views. As noted earlier in this paper, it is logically possible for both of these functional views to be true. Each makes an independent account in which one does not preclude the other (i.e., they cannot be conceived of as mutually exclusive), and such multi-purpose functional views are both sensible and now commonplace in autobiographical memory (e.g., Conway, 2001, 2005). While it is certainly tempting to suggest that both of these views can account for the functional nature of involuntary memory production, we should note that it is also possible that there are other functional accounts which we have not identified. In addition, it is also possible that the non-functional view might account for the appearance of some everyday involuntary memories. That is, the acceptance of any functional view does not preclude the possibility that some involuntary memories are merely accidental, as this view states.

This observation leads us to the question of which function (life-situation, classical, or other) is more prominent in everyday involuntary memories. Although the data presented here may not be able to provide many clues here, it seems reasonable to assume that the relative proportions of each of these functions in everyday life would vary according to a number of factors and circumstances. For example, our subcategory of classical functions, potential danger, had a very low incidence of occurrence in our sample. One might expect this, given that such circumstances should be relatively rare in everyday life. However, there might be occasions, circumstances, or even environments where its frequency of occurrence could adjust rapidly upward. We saw an example of this in our laboratory when a subject participating in a diary study had relatively mundane involuntary memories which changed in both frequency and content when had had returned to a previously experienced dangerous environment. The subject had been in Washington D.C. on the day of the 9/11 event when a jetliner was crashed into the Pentagon. Upon returning sometime later, he experienced in inordinate number of involuntary memories triggered by various environmental cues (so numerous he indicated that he could not capture them all in his diary). The memories fit our potential danger scenario (i.e., this is what happened in this location, and so forth), and this situation illustrates how an environment once associated with danger or some other adverse situation might automatically trigger memories where it previously had not (e.g., one can easily imagine that this subject's previous trips to Washington D.C., a place he frequented, do not produce such involuntary memories, if any at all). We have seen other examples of this in other samples collected in our lab (e.g., one surrounding the Yale Law School bombing in 2003). And, of course, there may be many other situations and factors which might govern or change which functional roles are at work in everyday involuntary memory production (e.g., the relative presence or absence of important life events in one's life, individual differences, and so forth).

However, this study and the conclusions being made suffer from one important limitation, they are unassociated with experimental tests. Despite the encouraging signs for functional perspectives presented here, the lack of true experimental tests of these views would certainly allow for the results to be cast as alternatively fitting the non-functional view. According to this view, the involuntary memories observed in the various samples reported here occurred through sheer accident or coincidence (i.e., as a result of chance encounters with triggering cues or by some other means). Their fit to the two functional views is also coincidental. That is, one would expect involuntary memories to occasionally be related to life events or goals, or to appear useful to us in social or practical circumstances, and therefore, the results presented here may be due to pure chance, rather than causal relation to the functional views. Of course it is difficult to refute such a view, as it does rest on firm logical grounds. However, we offer an alternative to this position, one that critics or future researchers might find helpful.

One solution to this dilemma is to take a weaker position on the functionality question. That is, involuntary memories may not have evolved to have a specific function (or functions), and therefore, may indeed be a random or accidental mental phenomenon, like slips of the tongue. Nevertheless, unlike slips of the tongue, they may still be useful to the rememberer if they provide information that could be relevant or important in the context in which they occur. Such an approach has proven successful with other involuntary memory questions. For example, involuntary memory chaining (the case when one memory spontaneously triggers another) has been shown to occur in everyday involuntary remembering and during voluntary remembering (Mace, 2005, 2006). Mace (2007a) was able to argue that the occurrence of involuntary memory chaining during voluntary recall is functional to the voluntary recall process because chaining frequently brings memories to mind which are relevant to the memories that one intends to recall. This argument would not have been possible if the observations had turned out differently and chaining had produced irrelevant autobiographical memories (perhaps even semantic memories). So, in some ways, then, this could be seen as a test of a functional or usefulness hypothesis, without making any teleological claims on the process of chaining itself. By this reasoning it may not matter if chaining has or does not have an express set of functions, so long as usefulness can be demonstrated (see the use of similar arguments in Bluck, Alea, Habermas, and Rubin, 2005). The same sort of logic can be applied to our observations of everyday involuntary memories. Usefulness was demonstrated, and therefore, as long as these observations can be made, it may not matter if one can establish support for the purposeful nature (or teleology) of everyday involuntary memory production, or even if they should turn out to be random, purposeless mental phenomena. While this type of argument might fit the classic-view results better than the life-situation results, future studies might adopt diary approaches which may be able to satisfy this criterion (e.g., adding items which might probe the usefulness of life-relevant memories).

In conclusion, we have presented results which appear to fit the two functional views put forth in this paper. While it is true that such results cannot rule out the possibility that involuntary memory production is merely an accidental memory phenomenon (e.g., the accidental products of a memory system that is rarely if ever at rest), their apparent usefulness causes us to imagine how such accidentals might serve us in our everyday lives, anyway. Like the question of dream function, we find this question both intrinsically interesting and important to our understanding of this common mental phenomenon. We hope that others will share our interest and take up the questions surrounding the functions of everyday involuntary memories.

Appendix

Closed-ended Items used in the 10-day and Single-Record Diaries

10-day Diary Items

Thought items

Is the memory related to something you were recently thinking?

Yes No If yes, explain

Is the memory related to something you think about a lot?

Yes No If yes, explain

If yes, how often have you thought about this?

Life event item

Is the memory related to events currently in your life?
Yes No If yes, explain

Personal goal items
Is the memory related to a short-term goal?
Yes No If yes, explain
Is the memory related to a long-term goal?
Yes No If yes, explain

Single-Record Diary Items
Situational usefulness item
Did the memory provide you with any information that was useful to your immediate situation (i.e., what you are thinking or doing right now)?
Yes No If yes, explain
General usefulness item
Beyond this, could you say that the memory was useful to you in some other way?
Yes No If yes, explain

REFERENCES

Ball, C. T., and Little, J. C. (2006). A comparison of involuntary autobiographical memory retrievals. *Applied Cognitive Psychology, 20*, 1167-1179.

Ball, C. T., Mace, J. H., and Corona, H. (2007). Cues to the gusts of memory. In J. H. Mace (Ed.), *Involuntary memory* (pp. 113-126). Malden, MA: Blackwell Publishing.

Baars, B. J., Ramamurthy, U., and Franklin, S. (2007). How deliberate, spontaneous, and unwanted memories emerge in a computational model of consciousness. In J. H. Mace (Ed.), *Involuntary memory* (pp. 177-207). Malden, MA: Blackwell Publishing.

Berntsen, D. (1996). Involuntary autobiographical memory. *Applied Cognitive Psychology, 10,* 435-454.

Berntsen, D. (2007). Involuntary autobiographical memories: Speculations, findings and an attempt to integrate them. In J. H. Mace (Ed.), *Involuntary memory* (pp. 20-49). Malden, MA: Blackwell Publishing.

Bluck, S. (2003). Autobiographical memory: Exploring its function in everyday life. *Memory, 11*, 113-123.

Bluck, S., Alea, N., Habermas, T., and Rubin, D. C. (2005). A tale of three functions: The self-reported uses of autobiographical memory. *Social Cognition, 23,* 91-117.

Conway, M. A. (2001). Sensory-perceptual episodic memory and its context: Autobiographical memory. In A. Baddeley, M. Conway, and J. Aggleton (Eds.), *Episodic memory: New directions in research* (pp. 53-70). Oxford: Oxford University Press.

Conway, M. A. (2005). Memory and the self. *Journal of Memory and Language*, 53, 594-628.

Hobson, J. A. (2002). *Dreaming: An introduction to the science of sleep*. New York: Oxford University Press.

Horowitz, M. J. (1986). *Stress response syndromes, 2nd edition*. Northvale NJ: Jason Aronson.

Kamiya, S. (2003). Some observations on the functions of involuntary memory: An analysis of the circumstances surrounding occurrence. *Japanese Journal of Psychology*, 74, 444-451.

Kamiya, S. (2007). Self-confirmative functions of involuntary autobiographical memories. *Japanese Journal of Psychology*, 78, 260-268.

Klinger, E. (1971). *Structure and functions of fantasy.* New York: Wiley.

Kvavilashvili, L., and Mandler, G. (2004). Out of one's mind: A study of involuntary semantic memories. *Cognitive Psychology*, *48*, 47-94.

Mace, J. H. (2004). Involuntary autobiographical memories are highly dependent on abstract cuing: The Proustian view is incorrect. *Applied Cognitive Psychology, 18,* 893-899.

Mace, J. H. (2005). Priming involuntary autobiographical memories. *Memory*, *13*, 874-884.

Mace, J. H. (2006). Episodic remembering creates access to involuntary conscious memory: Demonstrating involuntary recall on a voluntary recall task. *Memory*, *14*, 917-924.

Mace, J. H. (2007a). Does involuntary remembering occur during voluntary remembering? In J. H. Mace (Ed.), *Involuntary memory* (pp. 50-67). Malden, MA: Blackwell Publishing.

Mace, J. H. (Ed.) (2007b). *Involuntary memory*. Malden, MA: Blackwell Publishing.

Mace, J. H. (2007c). Involuntary memory: Concept and theory. In J. H. Mace (Ed.), *Involuntary memory* (pp. 1-19). Malden, MA: Blackwell Publishing.

Pasupathi, M. (2003). Emotion regulation during social remembering: Differences between emotions elicited during an event and emotions elicited when talking about it. *Memory*, *11*, 151-163.

Schlagman, S., Kvavilashvili, L., and Schulz, J. (2007). Effects of age on involuntary autobiographical memories. In J. H. Mace (Ed.), *Involuntary memory* (pp. 87-112). Malden, MA: Blackwell Publishing.

Schlagman, S., Schulz, J., and Kvavilashvili, L. (2006). A content analysis of involuntary autobiographical memories: Examining the positivity effect in old age. *Memory*, 14, 161-175.

In: Applied Memory
Editor: Matthew R. Kelley

ISBN 978-1-60692-143-2

Chapter 13

REMEMBERING WHAT WE DID: HOW SOURCE MISATTRIBUTIONS ARISE FROM VERBALIZATION, MENTAL IMAGERY, AND PICTURES

Linda A. Henkel*[*] *and Michelle Carbuto
Department of Psychology, Fairfield University, Fairfield, CT, USA

ABSTRACT

Memory errors in everyday life are pervasive and can range from being minor inconveniences to having significant consequences. At the root of many memory errors are source misattributions in which a person mistakenly claims that the source of a remembered event was something other than what it actually was (e.g., a person claiming to have performed an action that he or she merely thought about completing; erroneously remembering that he or she saw an event when he or she actually only read about it or saw pictures of it). The present chapter examines how source misattributions can create false beliefs and memories in which people claim that they did things that they actually did not. The role of three different but related everyday experiences in the creation of such memory errors is explored in depth — hearing or talking about various experiences, engaging in mental imagery, and viewing photographs — followed by presentation of a new study examining how photographs can lead to false claims of having committed actions that were not actually performed.

INTRODUCTION

We all have had instances where we swear something happened the way we remember but in reality the original event was quite different than what our memories would have us believe. I have a vivid memory for the time my brother fell off the stage while playing the trombone in 5th grade, despite the fact that I was not actually there when the event occurred. Presumably, I constructed my memory based on stories I had heard about the incident. Such

[*] Corresponding author.

memory errors are sometimes amusing and sometimes embarrassing, such as when you tell a great new joke to the person who told it to you in the first place or you claim at a company meeting that you came up with a terrific new idea when in fact that idea was already presented by a co-worker at a prior meeting. Memory errors can also sometimes be quite troublesome, such as testifying that you actually saw the defendant drive away in a green SUV when in fact you learned about the vehicle from a newspaper report you read.

At the root of many memory errors are *source misattributions* in which a person mistakenly claims that the source of a remembered event was something other than what it really was. Source misattributions include confusions between different external and internal sources: Did Susan or Tim say it? Did you see it on the television or hear it on the radio? Did you actually see it or did you hear someone else talk about it? Did you hear her say that or did you just infer it or imagine it? These errors can have fairly minor consequences (e.g., getting soaked in an afternoon rainstorm because although you thought you remembered putting your umbrella in your briefcase, you actually only thought about doing so) or much more serious consequences (e.g., someone accusing a relative of molesting him or her as a child when the memories were in fact created through hypnosis and imagery work during psychotherapy). The present chapter examines how source misattributions can create false beliefs and memories in which people claim that they did things that they actually did not. The role of three different but related everyday experiences in the creation of such memory errors is explored in depth—hearing or talking about various experiences, engaging in mental imagery, and viewing photographs—followed by presentation of a new study examining how photographs can lead to false claims of having committed actions that were not actually performed.

The Source Monitoring Framework

A highly influential model of constructive memory known as the *source monitoring framework* explains the occurrence of such memory errors in terms of the same cognitive and social processes that produce accurate remembering (Johnson, 2006; Johnson, Hashtroudi, and Lindsay, 1993; Johnson and Raye, 1981; Mitchell and Johnson, 2000). According to the source monitoring framework, people do not typically "tag" memories with their source (e.g., Shannon said this at our department meeting of September 2007). Instead they make attributions using both heuristic and systematic judgments based on the qualitative features of the memory, such as the amount and quality of perceptual and contextual detail, and on other information, such as the plausibility of the event and congruence with other beliefs (e.g., I know I have never been to London, so my memory for what Big Ben looks like must have come from a book or movie). Source judgments can be made with little conscious deliberation, or with more extensive reasoning and evaluation. When a specific memory derived from a source has features that are typical of that source, people will likely correctly attribute the memory to that source. Thus when I have a rich and detailed memory for the first rock concert I attended, I am able to rely on the features of that memory as cues to correctly judge that this was an actual experience, rather than mistakenly attributing it to some other source, such as a dream, a movie, or a review in *Rolling Stone.* Based upon this same principle, when a specific memory derived from one source has features that are more typical of another source, a source misattribution is likely to occur. Thus, when I heard stories about my brother flying off the stage with his trombone, I was able to vividly and easily imagine this event, leaving me with an internally generated memory that had features of a memory that had actually been perceived.

According to the source monitoring framework, source misattributions may also arise when people confuse different instances or versions of similar experiences, engaging in *feature importation* (Henkel and Franklin, 1998; Henkel, Franklin and Johnson, 2000; Henkel, Johnson, and DeLeonardis, 1998; Lyle and Johnson, 2006) and *content borrowing* (Lampinen, Meier, Arnal, and Leding, 2005). For example, people are more likely to mistakenly claim that they saw an object that in fact had been imagined when they earlier had seen a physically similar or conceptually similar object (Henkel and Franklin, 1998). They may confuse features of complex autobiographical events recorded in their diaries, mistakenly claiming that Justin attended a concert with them when in fact Justin had gone to an art show with them and it was Jesse who accompanied them to the concert (Odegard and Lampinen, 2004). In addition, information filled in on the basis of stereotypes (Bayen, Nakamura, Dupuis, and Yang, 2000; Mather, Johnson, and DeLeonardis, 1999) or general knowledge (Bransford and Johnson, 1972; Johnson, Bransford, and Solomon, 1973; McDermott and Chan, 2006) also can lead to inaccurate assessments of a memory's source.

The source monitoring framework posits that source judgments are often based on the qualitative features of memories in conjunction with flexible evaluation processes, that is, source judgments are not based solely on the qualities and features of the memories but also are impacted by the manner in which information is accessed and evaluated. Numerous studies have supported this premise. For instance, source errors occur more frequently when a person uses more lax criteria in evaluating a memory's origin, as when people are more likely to falsely claim that they saw a photograph of an event that they actually read a descriptive passage about when the memory test encourages them to rely on familiarity (e.g., Did you encounter this or not, and if yes, was it seen as a picture?) rather than carefully considering the different potential sources of their memory (e.g., Was this encountered in the text, as a picture, both in the text and as a picture, or neither?) (Dodson and Johnson, 1993). In addition, source errors occur more frequently when an individual has a vested interested in believing a memory came from one rather than another source (Benney and Henkel, 2006; Mather, Shafir, and Johnson, 2003). For example, people are more likely to misattribute a prediction made by an unreliable source to a reliable source if the prediction is about a relatively more desirable outcome (i.e., the "wishful thinking effect"; Gordon, Franklin, and Beck, 2005). Because accurate source monitoring is dependent on the cognitive processes that bind together the complex features of memories and on the processes that reactivate and evaluate those features, variables that disrupt encoding and binding processes impair source attribution accuracy. For example, source monitoring accuracy declines when people are under stress, operating under divided attention or sleep deprivation, and when they focus on their own emotional responses rather than on factual event details (see Mitchell and Johnson, 2000).

Quite often, source judgment processes produce accurate assessments of a memory's origin, but errors do occur. As noted, source misattributions are at the root of many memory errors and distortions that occur in our everyday lives, as well as in settings with clinical and forensic relevance. Using a source monitoring perspective, the present chapter reviews relevant research to better understand what makes people think they did things and experienced events that they did not actually do or experience. What can make you falsely remember grabbing your umbrella on the way out the door? What can make you falsely remember having watched your brother topple from the stage at a school concert? While there are numerous factors that influence the accuracy of source attributions and the frequency of errors, this chapter focuses on situations where information arising from three different sources—verbal information, mental imagery, and photographs—can be mistakenly attributed to actual perceptual experiences, leading people to believe that they actually did things that they did not.

Within this context, this chapter also examines how source misattributions play a critical role in the development of false beliefs and memories for autobiographical events. Several researchers have developed models to explain the formation of false beliefs and memories in which source misattributions are a central component (e.g., Hyman and Kleinknecht, 1999; Hyman and Loftus, 2002; Mazzoni, Loftus, and Kirsch, 2001). According to these models, there are several steps involved in the process of developing such false memories. First, participants need to view the event as something that could have plausibly occurred in their lifetime. This could be based on their preexisting beliefs or on experimental manipulations affecting perceived plausibility. They then must develop a belief that the event happened to them, construct a mental representation of what the event would have been like, and then mistakenly attribute their constructed mental representation to actual experience.

The Role of Verbal Misinformation and Descriptive Narratives in Source Misattributions

Numerous studies illustrating the malleable nature of memory have shown that what people hear about or see after an event can give rise to source misattributions in which they claim this post-event information had been experienced as part of the original event. In the classic misinformation paradigm, incorrect information given to people after an event—by an authority figure questioning them, by another witness, from an article they read in the newspaper—has led people not only to misremember details about the event (e.g., when someone remembers seeing a stop sign when in fact it had been a yield sign) but also to introduce nonexistent elements (e.g., remembering a barn at the side of the road when there were no buildings at all) and even fabricate entire events (e.g., claiming to have spilled a punch bowl at a wedding as a child, when no such event occurred in actuality) (e.g., Davis and Loftus, 2007; Loftus and Palmer, 1974; Loftus, 1975; Toglia, Read, Ross, and Lindsay, 2007; Zaragoza, Belli, and Payment, 2007). The post-event misinformation can appear embedded in questions about the original event. For example, the question, "When the car raced past the barn, how fast was it going?" implants the suggestion that there was a barn at the scene when there was not. The misinformation can also appear in narratives describing the event. For example, if a person reads the sentence "The car raced past the red barn on the country road" in the narrative description of another supposed witness, he or she may incorporate the other witness's faulty report of a barn into his or her own recollection of the event.

Source misattributions occur when people mistakenly claim that the post-event information they came across in narratives or embedded in questions had been part of the original experience. They correctly remember exposure to the information but they incorrectly attribute its source. A number of factors have been found to influence the likelihood of such source misattributions occurring, which is consistent with principles put forth by the source monitoring framework (e.g., Johnson et al., 1993; Mitchell and Johnson, 2000). For instance, the misinformation effect is stronger when the misinformation is provided by an authority figure or a credible source (Davis and Loftus, 2007). Errors are also more likely when the rememberer is less likely to notice discrepancies between the original event and the misinformation, such as when he or she is under stress or has limited attentional resources available at the time (Davis and Loftus, 2007).

Another paradigm used to explore how verbal misinformation and descriptive narratives can lead to memory distortions explored the creation of false memories for childhood experiences. Information was provided by an informant who was a family member of a given participant as to what events occurred and did not occur in that participant's childhood. The adult participants read brief narrative descriptions of events that they were told were actual events from their childhood that had been provided by the familial informant (e.g., Loftus and Pickrell, 1995). Some of the probed events were ones that the informant indicated really did happen to the individual. However, some were in fact ones that the informant indicated did not occur. In both cases, participants were led to believe that the event did really occur to them as children. After reading the narratives and then trying to remember additional details from the various events, 31% of the 374 participants tested in eight different studies were scored as having false memories for the event described in the narrative that the individual's family member claimed did not occur (see Lindsay, Hagen, Read, Wade, and Garry, 2004). Further, the process of verbalizing and describing one's own thoughts can also lead to source misattributions. In one study, participants were asked to describe various hypothetical events that may or may not have occurred in their childhood (Sharman, Manning, and Garry, 2005). The act of verbalizing and describing the events lead to increased confidence that the events were actually experienced as a child.

These findings are similar to those from studies on forced confabulation, in which participants are required to generate responses and details for information that they did not experience. Even though they were fully aware at the time that they were generating their own misinformation in response to the questions, when their memory was tested later for what they had witnessed or experienced, they often stated with high confidence that the confabulated detail did in fact happen (Ackil and Zaragoza, 1998; Lane and Zaragoza, 2007; Pezdek, Sperry, and Owens, 2007).

We encounter verbal sources constantly throughout our everyday lives—in listening to other people's recollections of shared events, in encountering media sources describing events that we never experienced at all, even in creating such misinformation ourselves as we retell the stories of our lives—and the information provided by these sources can shape our memories. Taken together, these studies show that information from a variety of verbal sources describing an action or event can create memories that are easily mistaken for having arisen from actual experience of that action or event.

The Role of Mental Imagery in Source Misattributions

Some verbal descriptions are especially evocative and as such may lead to the creation of accompanying mental imagery. The story I heard about my brother falling off the stage induced auditory images of the sound of the trombone hitting the floor and the audible gasp of the audience. It also invoked a detailed visual image of the surprised look on his face. According to the source monitoring framework of Johnson and colleagues, mental imagery can have a powerful impact on the accuracy of source judgments (Johnson and Raye, 1981; Johnson et al., 1993). We encode into memory not only the things we see, hear, do, and actually experience, but we also encode our thoughts, feelings, imagery, and intentions, and as such, we sometimes confuse those internally generated events (thoughts, feelings, imagery) with externally derived events (perceptual experiences such as seeing a word printed, or hearing someone's voice).

Because people make both heuristic and more systematic evaluations of a memory's source based in part on the phenomenal features that are part of the remembered event, they are more likely to mistakenly attribute internally generated imagined events to perception when the internally generated events are rich, vivid images that are easy to generate and envision. For example, when participants had to create mental images to complete symmetrical geometric shapes, they were more likely to later mistakenly claim that they had seen the shape in its whole form when it was a shape that was easier to imagine as completed than when it was a shape that was difficult to imagine in its completed form (Finke, Johnson, and Shyi, 1988). In another study, after seeing photographs of various scenes, participants were more likely to falsely remember having seen a photo of a scene that they did not in fact see when they had earlier read a short descriptive paragraph of the scene, and they were especially likely to do so when they were less aware they were creating mental images while reading the descriptive passages (Intraub and Hoffman, 1992; see also Foley, Wozniak, and Gillum, 2006). This latter finding that source errors are more likely when imagery is unintentionally generated than when it is intentionally generated is consistent with the source monitoring framework's view that increased cognitive operations associated with a memory can provide cues to its internally generated source.

Even when imagery is intentionally created, this can still lead to source errors, especially when it is especially vivid (Durso and Johnson, 1980) or resembles things that were actually seen (Henkel and Franklin, 1998; Henkel et al., 2000; Lyle and Johnson, 2006). Individual differences in imagery ability also have been linked to source misattributions, with people who self-report more frequent and vivid imagery sometimes showing more errors in attributing internally generated events to the outside world (Dobson and Markham, 1993; Horselenberg, Merckelbach, Muris, Rassin, Sijsenaar, and Spaan, 2000; Johnson, Raye, Wang, and Taylor, 1979; Wilkinson and Hyman, 1998).

The impact of imagination on source accuracy is further illustrated in a series of studies on what has been termed *imagination inflation*. A typical study investigating this phenomenon requires participants to indicate on a questionnaire whether they remember experiencing various events as a child (e.g., Were you ever bitten by a dog? Did you ever find $20 on the street?). They are later asked to imagine experiencing some of these events that they initially said they did not experience. Some events are imagined once, some several times, and some not at all. When probed later, after the imagery task, about what events really happened in their childhood, they reported greater confidence in having experienced the events that they were asked to imagine, with confidence increasing the more times the event had been imagined (e.g., Baran and Niedzwienska, 2002-03; Garry, Manning, Loftus, and Sherman, 1996; Garry and Polaschek, 2000; Heaps and Nash, 1999; Hyman and Billings, 1998: Paddock, Noel, Terranova, Eber, Manning, and Loftus, 1999). People were more likely to exhibit this imagination inflation effect for events that were plausible than those that were implausible (Pezdek, Blandon-Gitlin, and Gabbay, 2006), but even for some relatively unusual events, such as the uncommon medical procedure of having a skin sample taken from one's finger as a child or unusual actions such as proposing marriage to a soda machine, imagination can lead to false beliefs and memories for the event's occurrence (Mazzoni and Memon, 2003; Seamon, Philbin, and Harrison, 2006).

Of course, in this imagine-childhood-events paradigm, imagery may not necessarily be creating false memories as much as it is reactivating veridical memories. Because of this concern, an experimental analogue of the imagination inflation effect was developed to carefully control what events were truly experienced by individuals (Goff and Roediger, 1998; see also Foley and Johnson, 1985; Suengas and Johnson, 1988). People were given various objects and asked to perform or imagine performing different actions (e.g., open the envelope, break the pencil). They later were asked to imagine performing certain events varying numbers of times, with some events imagined once, some three times, some not at all. Later they had to indicate which actions they in fact had performed earlier and which ones had been only imagined. Results showed that the more times they imagined an event, the more likely they were to falsely claim to have performed it.

Other work using this experimental version of the imagination inflation paradigm has found that the imagined actions that were falsely judged as having been performed were subjectively experienced as vivid memories that were confidently held (Thomas, Bulevich, and Loftus, 2003), and that even relatively bizarre imagined actions (e.g., kiss the magnifying glass; sit on the dice) were likely to be misjudged as having been performed (Thomas and Loftus, 2002). In addition, misattributions were more likely to occur when the imagery task made participants focus on sensory and perceptual details (Thomas et al., 2003), consistent with the source monitoring framework's claim that source accuracy declines when imagined events have richer perceptual-like characteristics.

Other studies, both prior to and subsequent to the Goff and Roediger (1998) study, have also demonstrated that people can mistake actions that they imagined performing as ones that they actually did perform (e.g., Hornstein and Mulligan, 2004) and that source misattributions increase as the number of imaginings increase (Lampinen, Odegard, and Bullington, 2003; Seamon, Philbin, and Harrison, 2006). Young children are especially vulnerable to confusions between imagined and performed actions (Foley and Johnson, 1985; Foley and Ratner, 1998; Lindsay, Johnson, and Kwon, 1991; Markham, 1991; Sussman, 2001), as are older adults (Guttentag and Hunt, 1988) and individuals with schizotypal traits (Peters, Smeets, Giesbrecht, Jelicic, and Merckelbach, 2007).

Imagination can also lead to changes in estimates of the number of times one remembers engaging in specific behaviors. After participants estimated the frequency of drinking various beverages in their daily lives including caffeinated ones, they were given a brief imagery task in which they envisioned themselves engaging in consuming a new caffeine-free drink (Thomas, Hannula, and Loftus, 2007). Later when they were asked to estimate how frequently they drank caffeinated beverages, their estimates decreased when they had earlier imagined themselves drinking noncaffeinated ones relative to when they had only read about drinking noncaffeinated beverages or when they imagined someone other than themselves drinking caffeine-free beverages. This work is consistent with earlier work on the source monitoring framework in which it was found that repeated imagination of what an object looked like led to increased reports of having actually seen photographs of that object (Johnson et al., 1979).

In sum, the various findings regarding confusions between the products of imagination and actual perceptual experience illustrate key principles of the source monitoring framework. People engage in both heuristic and strategic evaluations of a memory's source based in part upon the qualitative features of those memories. Vivid imagery that is easy to generate, as when someone repeatedly imagines a scenario, results in mnemonic representations that have features more typical of perceptually derived events, and may therefore be misattributed to perception. Concerns about the possible dangers of memory distortions when imagery-based exercises are used in a psychotherapeutic setting have lead several researchers to urge more education and awareness among mental health practitioners and limitations on the use of such techniques when the validity of memories is an issue (e.g., Arbuthnott, Arbuthnott, and Rossiter, 2001; Lindsay and Read, 1994; Thayer and Lynn, 2006). In addition, caution has been urged in the use of imagery-based techniques when interviewing witnesses in criminal investigations because their use has been linked to increases in erroneous memories (Bekerian, Dennett, Hill, and Hitchcock, 1992), especially when it is part of a hypnotic induction (Mazzoni and Lynn, 2007). Negative consequences of the use of imagery-based techniques advocated in popular interrogation manuals when interrogating suspects in criminal cases have also been brought to light (Henkel and Coffman, 2004).

The Role of Pictures and Photographs in Source Misattributions

The various findings discussed thus far show that both verbal misinformation and visual imagery can apparently "paint a picture in one's mind" that can be confused with actual perception. This begs the question: how might actual pictures influence memory accuracy? Several studies have shown that exposure to pictures also can lead to source misattributions, and this occurs in both forensically relevant and everyday situations. For example, mock crime studies have shown that witnesses are more likely to falsely identify an innocent person if they happened to see that person earlier while viewing mug shots (Deffenbacher, Bornstein, and Penrod, 2006). Other research had participants watch a video of people engaging in commonplace scenarios—such as having a picnic in a park or cleaning and tidying around the house—and then later review photographs of objects and events from the scene. Some of the items and events depicted in the photographs had originally been in the scene and some had not (Koutstaal, Schacter, Johnson, Angell, and Gross, 1988; Koutstaal, Schacter, Johnson, and Galluccio, 1999; Schacter, Koutstaal, Johnson, Gross, and Angell, 1997). Two days later participants were asked to remember what they had originally seen in the video, and results showed that photograph review had both positive and negative effects on memory. People were not only more likely to correctly remember seeing in the video items that they had viewed in the photographs, they were more likely to falsely remember seeing in the video items that appeared in the photographs but had not in fact been in the video. In addition, when they had seen photographs that they later falsely attributed to the video, they were more likely to ascribe high ratings of recollective detail than when they had not seen such photographs.

Reviewing photos that depict our past experiences is one common way in which we encounter and use photographs in our everyday world. Another way is when photographs accompany text that we read, such as with news stories and in textbooks. Pictures promote memory retention because they can guide our understanding and comprehension (Bransford and Johnson, 1972) and serve as valuable retrieval cues (Waddill and McDaniel, 1992; see also Glenberg and Grimes, 1995). However, photos embedded in text can also make a newspaper article seem more believable and affect readers' opinions (see Garry, Strange, Bernstein, and Kinzett, 2007). For instance, when people read a newspaper article about a diplomatic mission during a military conflict, their opinions about topics not directly covered in the story (e.g., estimating how long a war might last or the number of casualties that might be incurred) were biased based upon the nature of the pictures that accompanied the story (e.g., articles with patriotic pictures were associated with lower anticipated casualty rates) (cited in Garry et al., 2007). In addition, the inclusion of photos in newspaper articles can directly lead to false beliefs and erroneous memories. Participants read an article about a hurricane's effect on a coastal region that included a picture of the area either before the hurricane hit or after (Garry et al., 2007). Although the article did not mention personal injury or death, participants who saw the photo of the destruction in the region after the hurricane were more likely to mistakenly claim that the article included information about death and injury.

Modern image-manipulation technology has allowed exploration of the impact of falsified photographs on autobiographical memories in an innovative way. Using photo editing software, researchers doctored actual photos from participants' childhood provided by a family member (Wade, Garry, Read, and Lindsay, 2002). They showed participants actual photographs from their childhood as well as a doctored photograph of the individual as a child taking a hot air balloon ride with a relative. The participants were interviewed several times and asked to try to remember each of the events depicted in the photographs. By the time of the 3rd interview, 50% of the participants claimed to remember at least some details of the hot air balloon ride. Even seeing photos from a given time period in one's childhood—but not directly suggestive of the nonreal event—can produce false beliefs. Adults who viewed a class photo while trying to remember the time that they put a gooey, slimy substance in a teacher's desk (an event that according to their parents had never occurred) were more likely to later say that they remembered the suggested event than those who did not view the class photo (Lindsay et al., 2004). In fact, 70% of the participants were rated as having developed a memory for the fake event. Young children are especially vulnerable to photograph-induced false beliefs and memories (Strange, Hayne, and Garry, 2007), even when the suggested event is relatively implausible (Strange, Sutherland, and Garry, 2006). In addition, photograph-induced false beliefs and memories have been found not only for personal autobiographical experiences, but for past public events as well (Sacchi, Agnoli, and Loftus, 2007), which is important given concerns about digital hoaxes that have appeared in the media.

What is it about the presentation of photographs that leads to the creation of erroneous beliefs and memories? Some have argued that photographs can provide a "cognitive springboard" for participants to generate thoughts, feelings, and images in association with the targeted but fictitious event, and the resulting product of these cognitive processes is similar enough to actually perceived experiences to lead participants to claim that they remember the pseudoevent (Strange et al., 2006; Wade et al., 2002). This interpretation is consistent with the source monitoring framework's claim that people evaluate the various perceptual, contextual, and affective features of a targeted memory in comparison to the constellation of features typically associated with memories derived from a certain source, such as perception, and render an assessment of the memory's source (here, claiming it was something that they remember actually happening to them). Viewing photographs can lead to source misattributions when the individual simply misremembers the source of the mnemonic experience. For example, the vividly detailed representation produced by viewing a picture may not be remembered as having been a picture but misremembered as having been one's actual experience of an event. In addition, the mental representations induced by viewing photographs can be incorporated into one's memory for an event, consistent with studies showing *feature importation* (Henkel and Franklin, 1998; Henkel et al., 2000; Henkel, Johnson, and DeLeonardis, 1998; Lyle and Johnson, 2006) and *content borrowing* (Lampinen et al., 2005).

Interestingly, comparisons of the differential impact of photos and narratives on the creation of memories for suggested events have found that although both pictures and narratives are associated with relatively high rates of false beliefs and memories, narratives are even more effective than are photos in leading participants to claim that they remember events that presumably did not in fact happen (Garry and Wade, 2005; Garry and Gerrie, 2005; Strange, Gerrie, and Garry, 2005). Garry and colleagues argue that narratives promote a stronger sense of familiarity and encourage cognitive operations that are more likely to lead to mental representations that are confused with actual experiences. In particular, photos appear to constrain imagination, with participants sometimes concentrating on the rich details presented in the photo and yet being unable to generate their own associations to them. Narratives, on the other hand, allow participants more room to imagine their own details of events in a fluent manner, and the resulting mental representation is more likely to be mistaken as a memory for a real event (see also Lane and Zaragoza, 2007, for a similar explanation as to why verbal elaboration brings about higher levels of eyewitness suggestibility).

People encounter photographs in many different everyday settings. They may review their own personal photo albums while they reminisce about their trip to the Grand Canyon or try to remember the names of the people that they sat with at a wedding. They may view photos of things they themselves never experienced, such as a friend's trip to Big Sur. People also encounter photos in newspapers and magazines depicting both familiar and novel scenes. Photographs can be used as tools for memory organization and retrieval in a wide variety of settings. They have been found to be beneficial in helping hospital patients remember their experiences (Radley and Taylor, 2003) and in aiding people with Alzheimer's disease in their everyday functioning in an adult day care setting (Nolan, Matthews, and Harrison, 2001; Weiner and Abramowitz, 1997). Photographs can even help children as young as 2 years old remember activities and experiences (Deocampo and Hudson, 2003). Photographs are also used in both clinical and forensically relevant settings. Patients undergoing psychological therapy may be encouraged to bring in family photos as catalysts for discussions of their feelings and memories (Weiser, 2004), and photos are sometimes used in interviewing victims, witnesses, and suspects.

The use of photos as potential memory aids as part of criminal investigations, for instance showing potential witnesses pictures of suspects or even showing them crime scene photos, is controversial because while it can help trigger accurate memories, it can also contaminate what is reported by the individual. The use of crime scene photos in interrogations to elicit confessions is especially controversial. In one widely used training manual by Inbau and colleagues (2001), *Criminal Interrogations and Confessions,* mixed messages are given regarding their use. Some places in the text their use is advocated, whereas in other places the authors suggest some caution. It has been argued that certain interrogation tactics such as showing suspects pictures from a crime scene or describing details of the crime and having the suspect imagine it can contribute to the incidence of false confessions by creating confusion as to the source of one's memories (Henkel and Coffman, 2004).

Laboratory studies have successfully induced people to falsely confess to actions that they did not commit, with people sometimes coming to genuinely believe that they committed the action and offering "remembered" details about it (Blair, 2007; Forrest, Wadkins, and Larson, 2006; Horselenberg, Merckelbach, and Josephs, 2003; Kassin and Kiechel, 1996; Russano, Meissner, Narchet, and Kassin, 2005). The present study used a laboratory approach to examine circumstances under which people claim that they performed an action that they in fact only imagined. Although the actions were relatively simple and not of an illegal nature, this study sheds light on the fundamental cognitive processes by which peoples' memories for their actions can be altered by other information, such as photographs. This study was modeled after the imagination inflation paradigm to examine the role that photographs play in people claiming to remember committing actions that they did not in fact do.

Method

Participants. Participants consisted of 37 undergraduates from Fairfield University, who participated to partially fulfill requirements or for extra credit in their psychology class. Ages ranged from 18 to 22 years ($M = 19.81$, $SD = 1.22$).

Materials and Procedure. Participants were tested individually and were told that the study examined peoples' perceptions of different actions. They were asked to perform and imagine performing a series of 60 distinct actions with objects (e.g., crush the paper cup; imagine breaking the pencil). All of the actions were ones that would leave behind some evidence that the action had been completed. Half of the actions were performed, and half were imagined. Each trial consisted of the experimenter placing the object or objects on the table in front of the participant and reading aloud an action statement indicating whether the participant was to perform the action or imagine themselves performing the action ("Crack the walnut"; "Imagine unwrapping the candy"). Six seconds were allotted for each trial, after which the experimenter removed the object or objects while participants rated how frequently they engaged in the named action in a typical week. Response options were *never, rarely, sometimes*, and *often,* and this was done to increase participants' attention and motivation. This first phase in which actions were performed and imagined took approximately 20 minutes.

Participants were then given a second task in which they viewed a series of photographs with captions on the computer of various actions in completed states (e.g., they would see a picture of a broken pencil with the caption "Break the pencil"). Their task was to indicate whether the caption matched the picture or not. Each photo was presented for 5 seconds. Of the 30 actions that were imagined in Phase 1, 10 were shown as photographs once, 10 were shown three times, and 10 were not shown at all. These were the critical items of interest. All critical imagined events shown as photographs had captions that matched the event depicted. Randomly intermixed were 12 actions that were either originally performed (n = 6) or were new (n = 6), and these were presented 1 or 3 times as well. A subset of these originally performed or new actions had captions that did not match the accompanying photograph. They were not asked to remember the items at this time but rather to just view the photos, under the guise of recording reaction times for deciding whether the caption matched the photos or not.

One week later, participants returned for a surprise source memory test in which they were given a list of individual actions and had to remember whether the named action was one they had actually performed, one they had imagined performing, or whether it was a new action that was neither performed nor imagined. The 60 originally performed and originally imagined action phrases were all presented, randomly intermixed with 15 new action phrases.

Results

An alpha level of .05 was used for all analyses. Recognition accuracy for old events was calculated as the proportion of performed and imagined events that were correctly recognized as old, regardless of whether they were correctly attributed to having been performed or imagined, and false alarm rates were calculated as the proportion of new events erroneously claimed as being old (i.e., either performed or imagined). Even with a 1 week delay, the percentage of actions that participants performed or imagined performing in Phase 1 that were correctly remembered as old was relatively high at 91.1%, and overall false alarm rates were relatively low at 4.7%. This indicates that people indeed paid attention and that the events were memorable and discriminable from new events. Not surprisingly, performed actions had a mnemonic advantage: Events that participants had performed (M = 94.9%) were significantly more likely to be remembered as having been part of Session 1 than were events that participants had only imagined performing (M = 87.3%), $t(36) = 5.90$, $p < .001$.

However, just because people successfully remembered *that* an event happened does not mean that they correctly remembered *how* it happened. Of the events that participants correctly remembered as old, how often did they correctly attribute them to their original source? Overall source accuracy was calculated as the percentage of times that performed actions were correctly remembered as performed and imagined actions were correctly remembered as imagined, given that the actions were correctly recognized as old. Source accuracy was somewhat impaired, though well above chance, with average performance at 88.8%, and did not differ significantly between performed actions (M = 88.7%) and imagined actions (M = 89.0%), $t(36) = 0.14$, $p = .88$.

Of greatest interest was whether people could be induced to claim that they performed actions that they had in fact only imagined performing if they had seen photographs of the actions in their completed state, in essence suggesting that the actions were performed. Specifically, did the number of times that imagined events were viewed as completed actions in photographs influence how often participants falsely claimed to have performed those actions? To determine this, source misattribution rates for originally imagined actions were examined. The percentage of imagined events mistakenly judged as performed was found to be a function of the number of exposures to photographic evidence, $F(2, 72) = 4.73$, $p = .01$. As seen in Figure 1, post hoc Sheffe tests revealed that subjects were significantly more likely to erroneously claim that they performed an action they only imagined when they saw a photo three times than when they did not see a photo at all. Subjects were also significantly more likely to erroneously claim that they performed an imagined action when they saw a photo once than when not seen at all. However, there was no significant difference in source misattributions when photos were seen once versus three times. Thus seeing a photograph at all increased errors, with no systematic increase as a function of number of times the photos were presented. Similar patterns were found when source misattributions were conditionalized out of the number of events correctly recognized as old.

Importantly, these source misattributions were not simply a tendency for people to claim that something that seemed familiar had been performed. Analysis of false alarms to new actions—that is, the percentage of times people claimed that a new action had been part of Phase 1—in fact indicated that they were significantly more likely to claim that they imagined a new action ($M = 4.3\%$) than that they performed a new action ($M = 0.3\%$), $t(36) = 3.90$, $p < .001$.

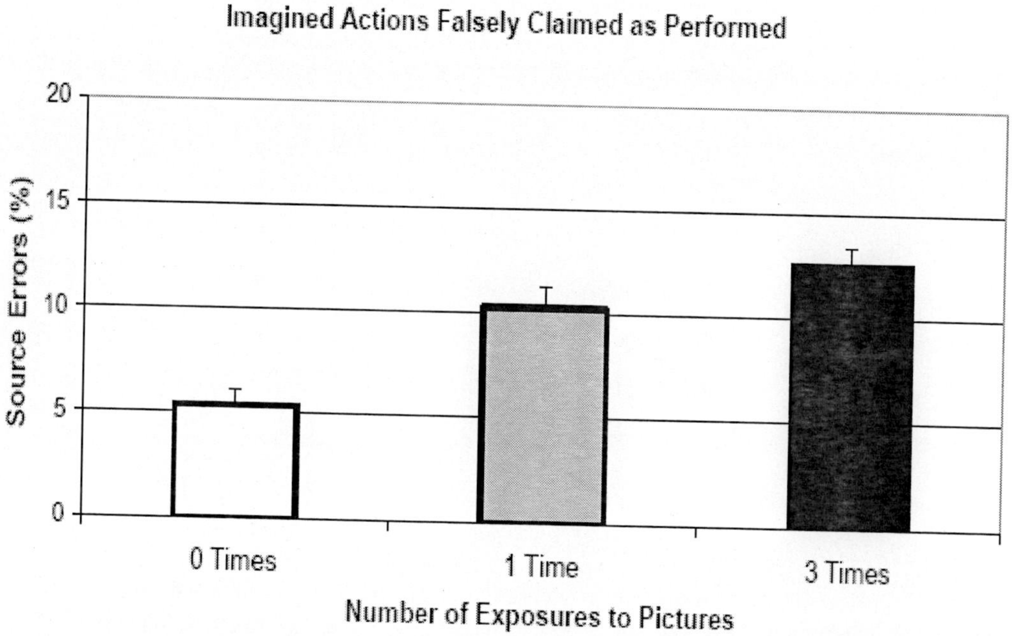

Figure 1. Percentage of imagined events mistakenly judged as performed as a function of number of exposures to photographic evidence.

Discussion and Preliminary Findings from Additional Studies

Results of the present study show that viewing photos of actions that were only imagined can have detrimental effects on memory. After imagining themselves performing various actions, when people saw photographic evidence consistent with an imagined action having been completed, they misattributed their memory to actual performance. The errors were not due to a bias to label questionable memories as "performed" because people were more likely to misattribute new items to imagination rather to performance. Whereas previous studies using the imagination inflation paradigm have found systematic increases in source errors as the number of times events are imagined increases (Goff and Roediger, 1998), the present study did not find such a linear increase in conjunction with the number of times photographs were viewed. It may be that repeated exposure to photographs of originally imagined events produces two opposing effects. On the one hand, exposure to photographs may increase the fluency with which the originally imagined event comes to mind, bringing with it vivid perceptual details that are then mistakenly attributed to having performed event, consistent with the source monitoring framework's basic "recipe" for source misattributions (e.g., see Henkel, 2004). On the other hand, when photographs are presented repeatedly rather than just once, the repetition may create a stronger mental representation for having seen a photograph, which people can then use as an indicator to "override" the familiarity and perceptual details that they would otherwise erroneously attribute to actual experience. This is similar to Garry and colleagues' argument as to why narratives lead to more false beliefs and memories of autobiographical experiences than did photographs (Garry and Wade, 2005; Garry and Gerrie, 2005; Strange, Gerrie, and Garry, 2005).

Nonetheless, results of the present study did provide evidence that that viewing a photograph of completed actions—whether it was viewed once or three times—could lead to false claims of having performed actions that were not in fact performed. Preliminary results from a second study using the same basic design shows that such photo-induced source misattributions increased with the passage of time (Henkel, 2007). Furthermore, even when events were not imagined at all, photos had a detrimental effect on source judgments: People claimed to have performed roughly 12% of the actions that they had only seen as photos, having neither imagined nor performed them at all in the first session, and they held moderately high levels of confidence in their misattributed memories. Confidence levels were as high for imagined actions incorrectly judged as performed as they were for imagined items correctly judged as imagined.

In a third study in this series, participants did not engage in imagery during the first session at all (Henkel, 2007). Instead, they performed a series of actions in the first session, and 1 week later they viewed photographs of completed actions while rating how frequently they engaged in the depicted action in a typical week. Some of the photos depicted events that had been performed in Session 1 and some were new. Individual photos were presented 0, 1, or 4 times. In addition, to determine whether increased rates of falsely claiming to have performed actions were due solely to increased familiarity with the events rather than to photographs per se, participants were also exposed to captions naming additional actions but without an accompanying photograph. Captions appeared 0, 1, or 4 times. Two weeks after the first session, participants were given a surprise source recognition task in which they had to indicate which actions they had actually performed and how confident they were that they had performed them. Preliminary results showed that more false claims of having performed new actions were made when the actions had been shown as pictures than as just captions, and that as the number of exposures increased, so too did error rates. On average participants erroneously claimed to have performed over 35% of the actions that they did not perform but had seen as photographs 4 times, and participants rated most of their misattributed actions as ones with which they were *confident* or *very confident* about. Thus, exposure to photographs of completed actions leads to people falsely claiming to have committed actions that they did not in fact commit.

While these findings are of relevance to understanding confusions between performed and imagined actions, the actions studied did not have the emotional significance of events such as criminal activities, and errors in claiming to have performed the actions do not have severe consequences. Furthermore, the photographs were never presented as evidence that the person did in fact commit the act. The photo viewing task was billed as an unrelated task in which judgments about the photos or captions were of interest (e.g., response time to judge captions; frequency ratings of engagement in that activity). A very clever recently developed paradigm using falsified videotape evidence has been used to better understand the role that photographic evidence may play in creating false beliefs and memories about prohibited actions. Nash and Wade (in press) had participants perform a gambling task in which they wagered money and had to collect from or pay to the bank in accordance with the outcome of the bet. They were videotaped during the task. Upon returning to the lab for a continuation of the study, the experimenter accused them of taking money from the bank when they should have returned money to the bank. They were either told that the evidence of them doing so was on video, or they were actually shown the videotape of them performing the "illegal" act. Unbeknownst to the participants, the videotape had been doctored so that it appeared that they did in fact take money when they had lost the bet. When faced with the seemingly incontrovertible videotaped evidence, extremely high false confession rates were obtained. In fact, when a confederate posing as a new participant asked the accused individual what had happened, many of the individuals made statements suggesting that they truly believed that they committed the act. Given the wonders of modern technology and the ease with which falsified evidence can be created, these results are alarming in that they suggest the high levels of faith that people put on what they assume to be a veridical recording of reality. These findings suggest that photographs and video recordings can have an especially damaging effect on memory accuracy in situations in which people have no reason to question the veracity of the evidence. Even just the allusion to photographic evidence was found in the above study to produce high rates of false confessions. Although police would be unlikely to doctor photographic evidence in criminal investigations, they do engage in the practice of alluding to physical evidence that does not in fact exist in an attempt to elicit confessions from recalcitrant suspects (Leo, 1996; Kassin, Leo, Meissner, Richman, Colwell, Leach, and La Fon, 2007), and the present findings suggest that this practice may lead people who are not in fact guilty to take responsibility for the accused action.

Conclusion

Erroneous judgments about the source of one's memory can lead to false beliefs and false memories about what one experienced and what one did. The source monitoring framework of Johnson and colleagues describes how source attributions are based upon qualitative characteristics of the remembered experience and other information available in memory, such as schemas and world knowledge, as well as on flexible decision processes applied to the activated mental representations (Johnson et al., 1993; Johnson and Raye, 1981; Mitchell and Johnson, 2000). This framework details a number of factors that lead to source misattributions. The present chapter examined how three different but related types of post-event experiences can shape what one remembers, and the research reviewed here shows that source misattributions can arise when people are exposed to verbal misinformation, when they engage in mental imagery, and when they view pictures. All three can lead to the creation of vivid and perceptually rich mental representations that can be easily mistaken as having arisen from having actually experienced the depicted information or event. According to the source monitoring framework, when the internally generated representation derived from verbal descriptions or mental imagery contains features more typically associated with memories derived from actual perception, such as rich perceptual-like detail and reduced cognitive operations, source misattributions are likely to occur. For example, when people encounter verbal misinformation after an experience (e.g., embedded in questions or in a descriptive narrative about the event), they may correctly remember *that* the information was presented, but mistakenly attribute it not to the questions or narrative but to having been part of the actual original experience. When people are instructed to vividly imagine objects or events or spontaneously do so, they may likewise misattribute the resulting perceptually rich mental representation to actual perception, especially when the imagery is easy to create. Such errors can occur for objects that are part of a scene, for actions, and for autobiographical events.

The presentation of pictures and photographs has also been shown to lead to memory misattributions whereby people erroneously claim that they had performed actions they had not performed, or experienced objects or events that they only viewed in pictures. Following principles of the source monitoring framework, such errors arise when people mistakenly attribute the source of their memory for the photograph to an actual experience or event.

The source misattributions examined here illustrate the malleable and reconstructive nature of memory. Although much of the research discussed here is drawn from carefully controlled laboratory studies, these findings highlight the cognitive processes involved in making judgments about the source of our experiences, and as such have implications for the accuracy of memory in a variety of contexts. Erroneous memories are problematic in legal venues, such as when the recollections of eyewitnesses and victims are offered as forensic evidence and when mug shot and crime scene photographs are used in the questioning of witnesses, victims, and even alleged perpetrators. Memory errors and distortions are also problematic in clinical settings, and can occur when mental health clients engage in mental imagery or are encouraged to view photographs as potential memory aids. In addition, the possibility of source misattributions in our everyday remembering and reminiscing is also noteworthy, especially given the pervasiveness of post-event verbal, imagery, and pictorial information in our daily lives.

Author Note

Thanks to Karen Mitchell for her insightful comments on an earlier draft of this chapter.

References

Ackil, J., and Zaragoza, M. (1998). Memorial consequences of forced confabulation: Age differences in susceptibility to false memories. *Developmental Psychology, 34*, 1358-1372.

Arbuthnott, K., Arbuthnott, D., and Rossiter, L. (2001). Guided imagery and memory: Implications for psychotherapists. *Journal of Counseling Psychology, 48*, 123-132.

Baran, B., and Niedzwienska, A. (2002-03). Imagination inflation and implicit memory theories. *Imagination, Cognition and Personality, 22*, 227-289.

Bayen, U., Nakamura, G., Dupuis, S., and Yang, C. (2000). The use of schematic knowledge about sources in source monitoring. *Memory and Cognition, 28*, 480-500.

Bekerian, D., Dennett, J., Hill, K., and Hitchcock, R. (1992). Effects of detailed imagery on simulated witness recall. In F. Losel, D. Bender, and T. Bliesener (Eds.), *Psychology and law: International perspectives* (pp. 302-308). Oxford, England: Walter De Gruyter.

Benney, K. S., and Henkel, L. A. (2006). The role of free choice in memory for past decisions. *Memory, 2006,* 1001-1011.

Blair, J. P. (2007). The roles of interrogation, perception, and individual differences in producing compliant false confessions. *Psychology, Crime, and Law, 13*, 173-186.

Bransford, J., and Johnson, M. (1972). Contextual prerequisites for understanding: Some investigations of comprehension and recall. *Journal of Verbal Learning and Verbal Behavior, 11*, 717-726.

Davis, D., and Loftus, E. (2007). Internal and external sources of misinformation in adult witness memory. In M. Toglia, J. D. Read, D. F. Ross, and R. C. L. Lindsay (Eds.), *The handbook of eyewitness psychology, Vol. I: Memory for events* (pp. 195-237). Mahwah, NJ: Erlbaum.

Deffenbacher, K., Bornstein, B., and Penrod, S. (2006). Mugshot exposure effects: Retroactive interference, mugshot commitment, source confusion, and unconscious transference. *Law and Human Behavior, 30*, 287-307.

Deocampo, J., and Hudson, J. (2003). Reinstatement of 2-year-olds' event memory using photographs. *Memory, 11*, 13-25.

Dobson, M., and Markham, R. (1993). Imagery ability and source monitoring: Implications for eyewitness memory. *British Journal of Psychology, 84*, 111-118.

Dodson, C., and Johnson, M. K. (1993). Rate of false source attributions depends on how questions are asked. *American Journal of Psychology, 106*, 541-557.

Durso, F., and Johnson, M. K. (1980). The effects of orienting tasks on recognition, recall, and modality confusion of pictures and words. *Journal of Verbal Learning and Verbal Behavior, 19*, 416-429.

Finke, R., Johnson, M. K. and Shyi, G. (1988). Memory confusions for real and imagined completions of symmetrical visual patterns. *Memory and Cognition, 16*, 133-137.

Foley, M., and Johnson, M. K. (1985). Confusions between memories for performed and imagined actions: A developmental comparison. *Child Development, 56*, 1145-1155.

Foley, M., and Ratner, H. (1998). Distinguishing between memories for thoughts and deeds: The role of prospective processing in children's source monitoring. *British Journal of Developmental Psychology, 16*, 465-484.

Foley, M., Wozniak, K., and Gillum, A. (2006). Imagination and false memory inductions: Investigating the role of process, content and source of imaginations. *Applied Cognitive Psychology, 20*, 1119-1141.

Forrest, K., Wadkins, T., and Larson, B. (2006). Suspect personality, police interrogations, and false confessions: Maybe it is not just the situation. *Personality and Individual Differences, 40*, 621-628.

Garry, M., and Gerrie, M. (2005). When photographs create false memories. *Current Directions in Psychological Science, 14*, 321-324.

Garry, M., and Polaschek, D. (2000). Imagination and memory. *Current Directions in Psychological Science, 9*, 6-10.

Garry, M., and Wade, K. (2005). Actually, a picture is worth less than 45 words: Narratives produce more false memories than photographs do. *Psychonomic Bulletin and Review, 12*, 359-366.

Garry, M., Manning, C., Loftus, E., and Sherman, S. (1996). Imagination inflation: Imagining a childhood event inflates confidence that it occurred. *Psychonomic Bulletin and Review, 3*, 208-214.

Garry, M., Strange, Bernstein, D. M., and Kinzett, T. (2007). Photographs can distort memory for the news. *Applied Cognitive Psychology, 21,* 995-1004.

Glenberg, A., and Grimes, T. (1995). Memory and faces: Pictures help you remember who said what. *Personality and Social Psychology Bulletin, 21*, 196-206.

Goff, L., and Roediger, H. (1998). Imagination inflation for action events: Repeated imaginings lead to illusory recollections. *Memory and Cognition, 26*, 20-33.

Gordon, R., Franklin, N., and Beck, J. (2005). Wishful thinking and source monitoring. *Memory and Cognition, 33*, 418-429.

Guttentag, R., and Hunt, R. (1988). Adult age differences in memory for imagined and performed actions. *Journals of Gerontology, 43*, 107-108.

Heaps, C., and Nash, M. (1999). Individual differences in imagination inflation. *Psychonomic Bulletin and Review, 6*, 313-318.

Henkel, L. A. (2007). *How photographs distort our memories: Source confusions after seeing pictures of imagined events*. Paper presented at the 48th annual meeting of the Psychonomic Society, Long Beach, CA.

Henkel, L. A., and Coffman, K. (2004). Memory distortions in coerced false confessions: A source monitoring framework analysis. *Applied Cognitive Psychology, 18*, 567-588.

Henkel, L. A., and Franklin, N. (1998). Reality monitoring of physically similar and conceptually related objects. *Memory and Cognition, 26*, 659-673.

Henkel, L. A., Franklin, N., and Johnson, M. K. (2000). Cross-modal source monitoring confusions between perceived and imagined events. *Journal of Experimental Psychology: Learning, Memory, and Cognition, 26*, 321-335.

Henkel, L.A., Johnson, M. K., and De Leonardis, D. M. (1998). Aging and source monitoring: Cognitive processes and neuropsychological correlates. *Journal of Experimental Psychology: General, 127*, 251-268.

Hornstein, S., and Mulligan, N. (2004). Memory for actions: Enactment and source memory. *Psychonomic Bulletin and Review, 11*, 367-372.

Horselenberg, R., Merckelbach, H., and Josephs, S. (2003). Individual differences and false confessions: A conceptual replication of Kassin and Kiechel (1996). *Psychology, Crime and Law, 9*, 1-8.

Horselenberg, R., Merckelbach, H., Muris, P., Rassin, E., Sijsenaar, M., and Spaan, V. (2000). Imagining fictitious childhood events: The role of individual differences in imagination inflation. *Clinical Psychology and Psychotherapy, 7*, 128-137.

Hyman, I., and Billings, F. (1998). Individual differences and the creation of false childhood memories. *Memory, 6*, 1-20.

Hyman, I., and Kleinknecht, E. (1999). False childhood memories: Research, theory, and applications. In L. W. Williams and V. L. Banyard (Eds.), *Trauma and memory* (pp. 175-188). Thousand Oaks, CA: Sage.

Hyman, I., and Loftus, E. (1998). Errors in autobiographical memory. *Clinical Psychology Review, 18*, 933-947.

Hyman, I., and Loftus, E. (2002). False childhood memories and eyewitness memory errors. In M. L. Eisen, J. A. Quas, and G. S. Goodman (Eds.), *Memory and suggestibility in the forensic interview* (pp. 63-84). Mahwah, NJ: Erlbaum.

Inbau, F. E., Reid, J. E., Buckley, J. P., and Jayne, B. C. (2001*). Criminal interrogation and confessions* (4th ed.). Gaithersburg, MD: Aspen.

Intraub, H., and Hoffman, J. (1992). Reading and visual memory: Remembering scenes that were never seen. *American Journal of Psychology, 105*, 101-114.

Johnson, M. K. (2006). Memory and reality. *American Psychologist, 61*, 760-771.

Johnson, M. K., and Raye, C. (1981). Reality monitoring. *Psychological Review, 88*, 67-85.

Johnson, M. K., Bransford, J., and Solomon, S. (1973). Memory for tacit implications of sentences. *Journal of Experimental Psychology, 98*, 203-205.

Johnson, M. K., Hashtroudi, S., and Lindsay, D. (1993). Source monitoring. *Psychological Bulletin, 114*, 3-28.

Johnson, M. K., Raye, C., Wang, A., and Taylor, T. (1979). Fact and fantasy: The roles of accuracy and variability in confusing imaginations with perceptual experiences. *Journal of Experimental Psychology: Human Learning and Memory, 5*, 229-240.

Kassin, S., and Kiechel, K. (1996). The social psychology of false confessions: Compliance, internalization, and confabulation. *Psychological Science, 7*, 125-128.

Kassin, S. M., Leo, R. A., Meissner, C. A., Richman, K. D., Colwell, L. H., Leach, A., La Fon, D. (2007). Police interviewing and interrogation: A self-report survey of police practices and beliefs. *Law and Human Behavior, 31,* 381-400.

Koutstaal, W., Schacter, D., Johnson, M., and Galluccio, L. (1999). Facilitation and impairment of event memory produced by photograph review. *Memory and Cognition, 27*, 478-493.

Koutstaal, W., Schacter, D., Johnson, M., Angell, K., and Gross, M. (1998). Post-event review in older and younger adults: Improving memory accessibility of complex everyday events. *Psychology and Aging, 13*, 277-296.

Lampinen, J., Meier, C., Arnal, J., and Leding, J. (2005). Compelling untruths: Content borrowing and vivid false memories. *Journal of Experimental Psychology: Learning, Memory, and Cognition, 31*, 954-963.

Lampinen, J., Odegard, T., and Bullington, J. (2003). Qualities of memories for performed and imagined actions. *Applied Cognitive Psychology, 17*, 881-893.

Lane, S., and Zaragoza, M. (2007). A little elaboration goes a long way: The role of generation in eyewitness suggestibility. *Memory and Cognition, 35*, 1255-1266.

Leo, R. A. (1996). Inside the interrogation room. *Journal of Criminal Law and Criminology, 86*, 266-303.

Lindsay, D., and Read, J. (1994). Psychotherapy and memories of childhood sexual abuse: A cognitive perspective. *Applied Cognitive Psychology, 8*, 281-338.

Lindsay, D., Hagen, L., Read, J., Wade, K., and Garry, M. (2004). True photographs and false memories. *Psychological Science, 15*, 149-154.

Lindsay, D., Johnson, M., and Kwon, P. (1991). Developmental changes in memory source monitoring. *Journal of Experimental Child Psychology, 52*, 297-318.

Loftus, E. (1975). Leading questions and the eyewitness report. *Cognitive Psychology, 7*, 560-572.

Loftus, E., and Palmer, J. (1974). Reconstruction of automobile destruction: An example of the interaction between language and memory. *Journal of Verbal Learning and Verbal Behavior, 13*, 585-589.

Loftus, E., and Pickrell, J. (1995). The formation of false memories. *Psychiatric Annals, 25*, 720-725.

Lyle, K., and Johnson, M. (2006). Importing perceived features into false memories. *Memory, 14*, 197-213.

Markham, R. (1991). Development of reality monitoring for performed and imagined actions. *Perceptual and Motor Skills, 72*, 1347-1354.

Mather, M., Johnson, M., and De Leonardis, D. (1999). Stereotype reliance in source monitoring: Age differences and neuropsychological test correlates. *Cognitive Neuropsychology, 16*, 437-458.

Mather, M. Shafir, E., and Johnson, M. K. (2003). Remembering chosen and assigned options, *Memory and Cognition, 31*, 422-433.

Mazzoni, G. A. L., Loftus, E. F., and Kirsch, I. (2001). Changing beliefs about implausible autobiographical events: A little plausibility goes a long way. *Journal of Experimental Psychology: Applied, 7*, 51-59.

Mazzoni, G., and Lynn, S. (2007). Using hypnosis in eyewitness memory: Past and current issues. In M. Toglia, J. D. Read, D. F. Ross, and R. C. L. Lindsay (Eds.), *The handbook of eyewitness psychology, Vol. I: Memory for events* (pp. 321-338). Mahwah, NJ: Erlbaum.

Mazzoni, G., and Memon, A. (2003). Imagination can create false autobiographical memories. *Psychological Science, 14*, 186-188.

Mazzoni, G., Loftus, E., and Kirsch, I. (2001). Changing beliefs about implausible autobiographical events: A little plausibility goes a long way. *Journal of Experimental Psychology: Applied, 7*, 51-59.

McDermott, K., and Chan, J. (2006). Effects of repetition on memory for pragmatic inferences. *Memory and Cognition, 34*, 1273-1284.

Mitchell, K., and Johnson, M. K. (2000). Source monitoring: Attributing mental experiences. In E. Tulving and F.I.M. Craik (Eds.), *The Oxford handbook of memory* (pp. 179-195). New York: Oxford University Press.

Nash, R. A., and Wade, K. A. (in press). Innocent but proven guilty: How being told about or seeing (fake) video evidence influences false confessions. *Applied Cognitive Psychology.*

Nolan, B. A., Mathews, R. M., and Harrison, M. (2001). Using external memory aids to increase room finding by older adults with dementia. *American Journal of Alzheimer's Disease, 16*, 251-254.

Odegard, T., and Lampinen, J. (2004). Memory conjunction errors for autobiographical events: More than just familiarity. *Memory, 12*, 288-300.

Paddock, J., Noel, M., Terranova, S., Eber, H., Manning, C., and Loftus, E. (1999). Imagination inflation and the perils of guided visualization. *Journal of Psychology: Interdisciplinary and Applied, 133*, 581-595.

Peters, M., Smeets, T., Giesbrecht, T., Jelicic, M., and Merckelbach, H. (2007). Confusing action and imagination: Action source monitoring in individuals with schizotypal traits. *Journal of Nervous and Mental Disease, 195*, 752-757.

Pezdek, K., Blandon-Gitlin, I., and Gabbay, P. (2006). Imagination and memory: Does imagining implausible events lead to false autobiographical memories? *Psychonomic Bulletin and Review, 13*, 764-769.

Pezdek, K., Sperry, K., and Owens, S. M. (2007). Interviewing witnesses: The effect of forced confabulation on event memory. *Law and Human Behavior, 31*, 463–478.

Radley, A., and Taylor, D. (2003). Remembering one's stay in hospital: A study in photography, recovery and forgetting. *Health: An Interdisciplinary Journal for the Social Study of Health, Illness and Medicine, 7*, 129-159.

Russano, M., Meissner, C., Narchet, F., and Kassin, S. (2005). Investigating true and false confessions within a novel experimental paradigm. *Psychological Science, 16*, 481-486.

Sacchi, D. L. M., Agnoli, F., and Loftus, E. F. (2007). Changing history: Doctored photographs affect memory for past public events. *Applied Cognitive Psychology, 21*, 1005-1022.

Schacter, D., Koutstaal, W., Johnson, M., Gross, M., and Angell, K. (1997, June). False recollection induced by photographs: A comparison of older and younger adults. *Psychology and Aging, 12*, 203-215.

Seamon, J., Philbin, M., and Harrison, L. (2006). Do you remember proposing marriage to the Pepsi machine? False recollections from a campus walk. *Psychonomic Bulletin and Review, 13*, 752-756.

Sharman, S., Manning, C., and Garry, M. (2005). Explain this: Explaining childhood events inflates confidence for those events. *Applied Cognitive Psychology, 19*, 67-74.

Strange, D., Gerrie, M., and Garry, M. (2005). A few seemingly harmless routes to a false memory. *Cognitive Processing, 6*, 237-242.

Strange, D., Hayne, H., and Garry, M. (2007). A photo, a suggestion, a false memory. *Applied Cognitive Psychology, 22*, 587-603.

Strange, D., Sutherland, R., and Garry, M. (2006). Event plausibility does not determine children's false memories. *Memory, 14*, 937-951.

Suengas, A. G., and Johnson, M. K. (1988). Qualitative effects of rehearsal on memories for perceived and imagined complex events. *Journal of Experimental Psychology: General, 117*, 377-389.

Sussman, A. (2001). Reality monitoring of performed and imagined interactive events: Developmental and contextual effects. *Journal of Experimental Child Psychology, 79*, 115-138.

Thayer, A., and Lynn, S. (2006). Guided imagery and recovered memory therapy: Considerations and cautions. *Journal of Forensic Psychology Practice*, *6*, 63-73.

Thomas, A., and Loftus, E. (2002). Creating bizarre false memories through imagination. *Memory and Cognition*, *30*, 423-431.

Thomas, A., Bulevich, J., and Loftus, E. (2003). Exploring the role of repetition and sensory elaboration in the imagination inflation effect. *Memory and Cognition*, *31*, 630-640.

Thomas, A., Hannula, D., and Loftus, E. (2007). How self-relevant imagination affects memory for behaviour. *Applied Cognitive Psychology*, *21*, 69-86.

Toglia, M., Read, J. D., Ross, D. F., and Lindsay, R. C. L.(2007). *The handbook of eyewitness psychology, Vol. I: Memory for events*. Mahwah, NJ: Erlbaum.

Waddill, P., and McDaniel, M. (1992). Pictorial enhancement of text memory: Limitations imposed by picture type and comprehension skill. *Memory and Cognition*, *20*, 472-482.

Wade, K., Garry, M., Read, J., and Lindsay, S. (2002). A picture is worth a thousand lies: Using false photographs to create false childhood memories. *Psychonomic Bulletin and Review*, *9*, 597-603.

Weiner, R. L., and Abramowitz, L. (1997). Use of photographs as therapy for demented elderly. *Activities, Adaptation, and Aging, 21*, 47-51.

Weiser, J. (2004). PhotoTherapy techniques in counseling and therapy--Using ordinary snapshots and photo-interactions to help clients heal their lives. *Canadian Art Therapy Association Journal*, *17*, 23-53.

Wilkinson, C., and Hyman, I. (1998). Individual differences related to two types of memory errors: Word lists may not generalize to autobiographical memory. *Applied Cognitive Psychology*, *12*, 29-46.

Zaragoza, M., Belli, R., and Payment, K. (2007). Misinformation effects and the suggestibility of eyewitness memory. In M. Garry and H. Hayne (Eds.), *Do justice and let the sky fall: Elizabeth Loftus and her contributions to science, law, and academic freedom* (pp. 35-63). Mahwah, NJ: Erlbaum.

In: Applied Memory
Editor: Matthew R. Kelley
ISBN 978-1-60692-143-2

Chapter 14

Children in an Information Society: The Relations Between Source Monitoring, Mental-State Understanding and Knowledge Acquisition in Young Children

***Angela D. Evans*[1] *and Kim P. Roberts*[2*]**
[1] Institute of Child Study University of Toronto, Toronto, ON, Canada
[2] Department of Psychology, Wilfrid Laurier University Waterloo, ON, Canada

Abstract

Children are exposed to information from many sources (e.g., teachers, television, the internet) and they need to know which sources to rely on and which to discount. In the chapter, we argue that using information sources appropriately is related to children's understanding about the mind. Children watched a slide show with an experimenter (the knowledgeable interviewer) and were later asked questions about the slide show by both the knowledgeable interviewer (KI) and a 'naïve' interviewer (NI) who did not see the slideshow. Both interviewers presented some false suggestions and children were later interviewed by a third interviewer. Children were also given two 'theory-of-mind' tests (False Belief, Tunnel) and a source-monitoring test. Children who passed the theory-of-mind tasks incorporated the knowledgeable interviewer's false suggestions into their reports of the show (more than children who failed) and the source-monitoring test revealed that children genuinely believed they actually saw the suggested items during the show. This investigation shows that an understanding of the mind and source monitoring are related, and that children with more sophisticated understanding of the mind can differentiate between knowledge from more and less reliable sources. These results highlight the skills needed to develop before children are able to make appropriate decisions about the information to which they are exposed.

* Corresponding author.

INTRODUCTION

We live in an information society in which information is distributed in many different forms. Our children are exposed to a variety of sources of information (e.g., television, internet, magazines, teachers, and friends) and are faced with the challenging task of determining which sources are reliable both during information delivery and when mentally retrieving information. It is important that children learn to perform these tasks as they attempt to develop a knowledge base about the world and themselves. As children develop their knowledge base, they need to learn which sources of information may be unreliable and thus, should be ignored (i.e., some websites or misleading television commercials) and which sources of information are reliable and should be incorporated (i.e., material from teachers). Being able to remember where we learned something is not only an important skill in the development of a knowledge base but also in the development of autobiographical memory. In order to avoid autobiographical confusion, children must be able to differentiate between things they did themselves and things they just imagined or were told about, as well as distinguishing between multiple, personal episodes (e.g., interactions with friends).

When attempting to recall information or memories, we often rely on a set of cognitive skills. For example, we may ask ourselves simple questions to determine whether an event took place such as "Did I actually do that or did I just think about doing it?" (i.e., monitoring the sources of events) or "Amy said that it happened, but is her perspective reliable?" (i.e., monitoring mental states). As adults we often implicitly use these cognitive skills without awareness, while younger children may struggle to make such distinctions while developing these skills.

Our goal in the present chapter is to outline our theoretical position on how children can use source monitoring and mental-state understanding in knowledge acquisition. We outline, in order, the relationship between source monitoring and knowledge acquisition, the relationship between mental-state understanding and knowledge acquisition, and the relationship between mental-state understanding and source monitoring. We will then present some preliminary data to show the relation between children's source monitoring, mental-state understanding, sensitivity to the credibility of various knowledge sources, and the subsequent effects on their knowledge. We begin by first providing an overview of the source-monitoring framework.

THE SOURCE-MONITORING FRAMEWORK

According to the source-monitoring framework, source monitoring refers to "the set of processes involved in making attributions about the sources of memories, knowledge, and beliefs" (Johnson, Hashtroudi, and Lindsay, 1993, p1.). Source is not retrieved as part of the memory representation but attributed when memory records are retrieved and evaluated. In general, memories from actual experiences typically contain perceptual, contextual, semantic, affective, and temporal information, whereas memories lacking in these characteristics and rich in information about cognitive operations are more typical of imagined experiences. Although this might be a conscious and deliberate process (e.g., when reasoning that you could not have heard a particular fact from a particular person because you have never met them), many decisions are made automatically, effortlessly, and without conscious awareness. Many source attributions are made by some combination of automatic and effortful processing such as when memory records are retrieved and judged according to some schema (e.g., when vivid perceptual information about a woman's voice is retrieved and you reason it was your grandmother rather than your mother who said it because the voice fits your schema of an older woman).

Source misattributions are not exclusively the result of memory errors because often we can remember the sources but have trouble matching the sources to the content of the memories. Lindsay and Johnson (1987) suggest that some sort of metacognitive awareness may be important for making source decisions. Further, because source monitoring is dependent on setting criteria (e.g., on how much perceptual information needs to be present before an attribution of 'experienced event' is made), these judgments are naturally subject to cognitive biases (Johnson et al., 1993). Such biases might include perceptions about how our mind works, which leads us to our interest in how source monitoring is related to children's understanding of the mind, and how this interacts with their acquisition of knowledge about a topic. Perceptions about the credibility of different sources might theoretically be used in setting criteria, using biases, and subsequent source attributions. We chose to investigate these relationships in young children who undergo enormous developments in source monitoring (see Roberts, 2000, for a review) and mental-state understanding (see Flavell, 2004, for a review) thus, an investigation of these processes with preschoolers is an ideal way to understand such development.

The Relationship between Source Monitoring and Knowledge Acquisition

It is well-established that when people are exposed to information from different sources they sometimes blend information from those sources together (see Roberts, 2002 for a review). For example, people can blend memories of television and real-life events (Roberts and Blades, 1999; Thierry and Spence, 2002), film and narrative about film (e.g., Ackil and Zaragoza, 1995), different instances of a similar event (Connolly and Lindsay, 2001; Powell et al., 1999), or real-life and interview questions about the real-life event (Welch-Ross, 1999). One of the explanations for such blending is a deficit in source monitoring. People can forget where they learned about something, genuinely believing they learned the information first-hand; or people may remember that there were multiple sources of information but still be confused as to what information came from which source.

There have been several empirical demonstrations of links between source monitoring and knowledge acquisition. In Ackil and Zaragoza's (1995) study, 5- to 11-year-olds and adults watched a video, listened to a summary of the film that also included misleading details that did not occur in the film, and were later interviewed about the video. Although all age groups mistakenly claimed that some suggested items occurred in the video, there was a developmental decrease in such source errors. In Giles, Gopnik, and Heyman's (2002) study, children watched a silent vignette, listened to a spoken narrative, and were later asked both recall questions and source questions. Children who were asked the source questions first performed better on the subsequent recall questions than children who received the source questions after recall. Leichtman and Ceci (1995) found that asking children whether they actually *saw* the fictitious event occur (i.e., Sam Stone soiling a teddy bear and ripping a book when visiting their classroom) resulted in fewer children inaccurately reporting the event to have occurred. Similar results were found by Roberts and Powell (2006) in a repeated-event study, where encouraging children to identify the source of a false belief (e.g., "Did you *see* the newspaper that day or did I only *tell* you about the newspaper?") helped children retract their inaccurate reports. Taken together, these studies indicate that there seems to be an important relationship between source monitoring and knowledge acquisition such that blending of accurate and inaccurate information happens less when people are encouraged to monitor the sources of information.

However, source monitoring, at least in the explicit way that it has been addressed in the above studies, cannot be the only skill involved in accurately recalling memories. If monitoring sources was sufficient, we would find source training effects for all children. In reality, training effects are only reliably found from about age 7, sometimes at ages 5 or 6, and it currently is not clear whether, and in what circumstances, training can help children aged 3 to 4 (Poole and Lindsay, 2001, 2002; Thierry and Spence, 2002). If this is the case, what else might be involved aside from our explicit monitoring of sources? One possibility is that there may be a relation between source monitoring and knowledge of mental states, such as understanding conflicting mental representations and false beliefs (e.g., Gopnik, 1990; Gopnik and Graf, 1988; Welch-Ross, 1999, 2000). Welch-Ross' Mental-State Reasoning Model (Welch-Ross, 2000) indicates specific relations between source monitoring, theory-of-mind understanding, and suggestibility.

The Relation between Mental-State Understanding and Knowledge Acquisition

The Mental-State Reasoning Model. Welch-Ross' Mental-State Reasoning Model was designed to explain misinformation effects (when misleading post-event information influence one's report of an event). The central tenet of the Mental-State Reasoning Model is that the development of reasoning about mental states reduces misinformation effects and leads to effective source monitoring. Although the model specifically discusses misinformation effects, the research can also be extended to consider children's memory in general (not just suggestibility) because children are exposed to many different sources in life that vary in their credibility.

The Development of Reasoning about Mental States. According to the Mental-State Reasoning Model, there are three aspects of the child's developing theory of mind that may be important for developmental changes in source monitoring and knowledge acquisition. The first aspect involves children's understanding of the connection between experiencing and knowing. An understanding of other people's access to knowledge develops between 3- and 4-years of age and by 5 years of age children know that not all experiences are informative. For example, Ruffman and Olson (1989) found that older children understood that a person who looks inside a box (i.e., had an experience that provided knowledge) knows the contents of the box, whereas someone who has not looked inside the box, does not know the contents.

A second, more complex aspect of mental-state understanding is children's ability to reason about conflicting, counterfactual representations of a single reality. Between 4- and 5-years-old, children begin to understand that mental processes involve representations that may not correspond to actual events or circumstances, and that different representations result from having access to different information. This can be seen in children's performance on the "mistaken-location" false belief task (knowing that a person can hold a false belief about the location of an object if it was moved in their absence), "mistaken-contents" false belief task (knowing that a person can hold a mistaken representation about the content of box based on the label of the box), and "mistaken-identity" or appearance-reality false belief tasks (knowing that an object can look different from what it really is) (Gopnik and Astington, 1988; Flavell, Green, and Flavell, 1986; Wimmer and Perner, 1983). Rather than reasoning about conflicting representations, 3-year-olds appear to "update" their original representation to the newest representation so that the representation is consistent with the current view (e.g., by claiming slime is a rock because it looks like a rock).

The third relevant aspect of mental-state understanding is an awareness that knowledge states originate from specific experiences. Gopnik and Graf (1988) assessed this relation by either showing, telling, or giving a clue to 3-, 4-, and 5-year-olds about the contents of a drawer and asking them to identify the source of their knowledge. While 3-year-olds had difficulty identifying the source of their knowledge, 5-year-olds were able to accurately identify whether they had been shown, told, or guessed the contents of the drawer. Similarly, O'Neill and Gopnik (1991) assessed children's understanding that experiences lead to a belief by either allowing a child to see, feel, or be told the contents of a "toy tunnel". Again, 3-year-olds had difficulty identifying the source of their knowledge while 4- and 5-year-olds did not.

Empirical Research on Mental-State Understanding and Knowledge Acquisition. Welch-Ross, Diecidue, and Miller (1997) conducted a study to assess the relationship between children's reasoning about conflicting mental representations and accurate reporting after a misleading interview. Children aged 3 to 5 were read a story, immediately asked non-misleading or misleading yes/no recognition questions, and interviewed about the event after a delay. Understanding conflicting mental representations did not correlate with non-misled item responses but did correlate negatively with suggestibility. Thus, children who could reason about conflicting mental representations confirmed original event information and rejected suggested information while children who did not have an understanding of conflicting mental representations appeared to update their original event memory with the suggestion. According to the Mental-State Reasoning Model, children who reasoned about conflicting mental representations were able to reject suggestions and reinstate their memories of the event because they understood that the interviewer did not have access to relevant knowledge. Templeton and Wilcox (2000) replicated Welch-Ross' findings while including an additional group of 6-year-olds. In their study, representational ability (as assessed by the mistaken location false-belief task) and general memory ability predicted the degree to which new information was incorporated into the memory representation of the target event. Collectively, these studies demonstrate that mental-state reasoning (specifically understanding conflicting mental representations) is related to the way in which children (and adults) build up and retain memories.

The Relation between Mental-State Understanding and Source Monitoring

The Mental-State Reasoning Model states that mental-state understanding determines the acquisition of knowledge by its connection with source monitoring. Specifically, children who can reason about conflicting mental representations should be less likely to incorporate information that differs from their experience than children without such understanding. Children who can reason about conflicting mental representations may remember the original information and the suggested information, yet they may report the original information (rather than the suggested information) only if they are able to also monitor the sources of their memories. It is possible that children may understand knowledge origins, and remember original and suggested information, but become confused between the two sources. These children will evidence source confusion and the resulting knowledge base will be compromised because there is a higher probability (compared to counterparts with an understanding of conflicting mental representations and intact source monitoring) that new information will be incorporated with the original information.

Empirical support for these proposed mechanisms was provided by Welch-Ross (1999) who found that children with an understanding of conflicting mental representations took longer to respond to forced-choice misleading questions (choice between the original event item and a previously suggested item) than those without an understanding. Welch-Ross reasoned that the reaction times were longer because these children were choosing between two conflicting sources; children without an understanding of conflicting mental representations merely updated the original information with the suggested and thus were faster when answering misleading questions. Although these data provide some support for the idea that children with an understanding of conflicting mental representations were processing the two conflicting sources, the contribution of source-monitoring skills is not apparent because there was no direct measure of source monitoring in Welch-Ross' study.

Robinson and Whitcombe (2003) point out that most research using the misinformation paradigm tests the relation between mental-state reasoning and knowledge acquisition when children are presented with knowledge from an indirect source who has no (known) knowledge of the event. However, like Robinson and Whitcombe, we are interested in a broader understanding of children's knowledge acquisition. In some circumstances, children may be exposed to sources that are *as informed* or *better informed* than children, even if the children have first-hand knowledge of the information. Teachers and parents, for example, may be more knowledgeable about a topic than children and it would be appropriate for children to incorporate information from these sources into their knowledge base (rather than simply rejecting the information, as would be required in a standard misinformation paradigm). In addition, it can be assumed that if young children and adults hold equal access to information, children may believe adults hold more accurate information than themselves. Investigating the relation between children's mental-state reasoning and knowledge acquisition can be comfortably accomplished with a modification to the misinformation paradigm and, indeed, Welch-Ross did this by manipulating interviewers' knowledge.

Specifically, Welch-Ross (1999) assessed how interviewers' knowledge of an event (whether they were naïve or knowledgeable) and children's ability to reason about conflicting mental states related to children's suggestibility. Children were read a story from a video and asked misleading and non-misleading yes/no questions about the story by the same person who initially read the story and is thus a knowledgeable interviewer, and also by a naïve interviewer who claimed to have no knowledge of the story. After a delay, children were asked forced-choice, recognition questions about the items they had been questioned on before (e.g., "Did Sally fall from the jungle gym at the park or did Sally fall from the seesaw at the park?"). Half of the questions were misleading in that children chose between the original item and a suggested item from session 1. The rest were non-misleading questions where children chose between the original item and a novel item. Children completed three mental-state understanding tasks to assess their understanding of knowledge (the see-know task adapted from Ruffman and Olson, 1989, and the mistaken location and mistaken identity false-belief tasks, Wimmer and Perner, 1983; Flavell, Green, and Flavell, 1986). Results indicated that children who could reason about conflicting mental representations (i.e., who passed the false-belief tasks) reported more suggestions delivered by the Knowledgeable interviewer than suggestions from the Naïve interviewer. Conversely, children who did not pass the conflicting mental representations tasks reported suggestions from both types of interviewers (Naïve and Knowledgeable). Welch-Ross reasoned that children who passed the false-belief tasks understood that the knowledgeable interviewer had access to relevant information (i.e., was a credible source). As the false-belief task measures children's ability to reason specifically about mental states related to knowing, Welch-Ross argued that the children who passed the false-belief task processed suggestions from the knowledgeable interviewer more deeply than other items because hearing false information was unexpected.

Implicit in Welch-Ross' arguments is that processing the items more deeply also helped source monitoring, and in Welch-Ross (2000), she outlines three possibilities derived from the Mental-State Reasoning Model. First, an explicit awareness that knowledge originates with particular experience may motivate the encoding and retrieval of source cues. Alternatively, source monitoring may contribute to the awareness that a variety of specific experiences causes the mental state of knowing. A third possibility is that source monitoring and an awareness of origins of knowledge may simply emerge spontaneously due to other factors. However, these claims cannot be tested without a direct measurement of children's source-monitoring abilities in a knowledge acquisition task. Thus, there currently is no published empirical support to test the predictions of the model with respect to source monitoring and its relationship to mental-state understanding and subsequent knowledge acquisition.

The Present Study

The purpose of the present chapter is to investigate the relations between source monitoring, reasoning about mental states, and knowledge acquisition. The main question is whether children's understanding of the mind relates to how they integrate memories of information from different sources. More specifically, what is the contribution of source monitoring to this knowledge acquisition? Based on Welch-Ross' (1999) methods, children watched a video and were then interviewed about the video by both a knowledgeable and naïve interviewer who each asked non-misleading and misleading questions. After a delay children were given a recognition test by a third interviewer, a source-monitoring test, and a series of mental-state understanding tasks.

We expected that, at the final interview, children who had lower levels of mental-state understanding would accept the suggestions from each interviewer equally often due to a lack of understanding of the relation between information access and knowledge acquisition. However, children who were proficient in mental-state understanding were predicted to accept more of the suggestions from the knowledgeable interviewer than the naïve interviewer. We also expected a reinstatement effect such that children proficient in mental-state understanding would be more accurate when questioned about non-misleading details reviewed by the knowledgeable interviewer than those from the naïve interviewer. Children who understand that there is a relation between information access and knowledge acquisition should be more likely to incorporate the knowledgeable interviewer's suggestions into their memories since they understand that the knowledgeable interviewer had access to information, and reject suggestions from the naïve interviewer who they know did not have access to information. In addition, it was hypothesized that children who 'passed' the mental-state understanding tasks would have higher source-monitoring scores than children who 'failed' the mental-state understanding tasks. We expected that those children who passed the mental-state understanding tasks would be able to reason about multiple possible sources (the video and interviewers) because they could reason about conflicting mental representations. Such reasoning combined with an understanding of the information access of the interviewer should predict the ability to accurately attribute knowledge to the interviewers and the video. Conversely, children who do not pass the mental-state understanding tasks (and could not reason about conflicting mental representations or information access) should be more likely to make source misattributions.

Method

Participants, Materials, and Procedure. Seventy-two children between the ages of 3- to 5- years-olds participated (M = 57 months, range 42 to 70 months). Informed consent was obtained from parents and verbal assent from children prior to participation.

Session 1: Initial Interview. A female research assistant, who later served as the Knowledgeable interviewer (KI), read a story about Frankie the Frog getting ready for winter. The story was accompanied by animation (PowerPoint slide show) that was shown on a television. The 10-minute story consisted of 48 target items (e.g., a blue bird, a raccoon, Frankie catching a fly with is tongue). The KI and child then completed a puzzle as a distracter task for 2 minutes.

Next, children were interviewed about the story they had just seen and heard. Half of the children were interviewed by the KI first and the rest were first interviewed by the female Naïve interviewer (NI). Upon completion of the puzzle, children who were initially interviewed by the KI were asked 24 yes-no recognition questions about the frog story. Twelve questions were non-misleading in that they probed items that were present in the story and thus a "yes" answer was correct. Twelve other questions were misleading because they probed items that were not present in the story and thus the correct response was "no". The questions were asked in a random order and were counterbalanced so that each item served equally often as a non-misleading or misleading question. Once the KI asked all of her questions the NI entered the room and was introduced to the child by the KI. The KI explained to the NI that they had just read a story about Frankie the Frog. The KI then excused herself from the room, the NI entered, and the NI then completed a second puzzle with the child. Once the child had completed the second puzzle the NI said, "I've never seen the Frankie the frog video, I don't know anything about it, may I ask you some questions about the video?" The NI then asked the child 24 additional yes-no recognition questions (these 24 questions were different from the questions the KI asked). As with the KI's questions, 12 were non-misleading and 12 were misleading. The questions were counterbalanced between interviewers in a between-subjects design so that all questions were asked by both the KI and NI across the experiment. The order of interviewers was reversed for children who were interviewed by the NI first. Session 1 took approximately 20 minutes to complete.

Session 2: Final Interview and Theory-of-Mind Tasks. A third research assistant, who presented herself as naïve, interviewed the children 5 to 7 days after the initial session. The interview began with a *recognition test* comprising forced-choice questions, one for each of the 24 target items in the frog story (e.g., Did Frankie the Frog see a *blue bird* in the video or did Frankie the Frog see a *yellow bird* in the video?). Twelve of the questions were misleading where the child chose between the original item from the story and the suggested item from the first interview (6 suggestions from the KI and 6 suggestions from the NI). For the 12 non-misleading questions, the child chose between the item that appeared in the story and a novel item (e.g., a *green bird*). For both types of questions half of the questions presented the correct item first. All questions were shuffled and asked in a random order. Prior to being asked the recognition questions children were given practice saying "I don't know" to questions.

Following the recognition questions, children completed a *source-monitoring task* in which they were presented with photographs of the KI, the NI, and the television from Session 1. The photographs were to assist children in identifying the sources of information. The interviewer said, "Some of the children I've been talking to told me that [KI's name] and [NI's name] asked them about things that did NOT happen in the video. So if I ask you about something and you saw it in the story point to this picture of the T.V. and if I ask you about something and you didn't see it in the video but [KI's name] or [NI's name] asked you about it I want you to point to their pictures. Okay?" Children were then given 8 practice questions: For 2 questions the video was the correct answer, 2 questions the KI was the correct answer, 2 questions the NI was the correct answer and 2 questions "no-one" was the correct answer. Children were praised for correct answers and corrected when they gave an incorrect answer. Children were then asked 24 source questions that probed different items to those probed in the previous 24 recognition questions. For twelve of the questions the correct source was the television and for 12 of the questions the correct source was one of the interviewers (6 KI and 6 NI questions). All 48 items were counterbalanced between the recognition questions and source questions.

After the source-monitoring task children completed the *theory-of-mind tasks*. Two False-belief tasks were administered to assess children's ability to hold conflicting mental representations in mind as well as their understanding that representations result from having access to information. The first False-belief task children performed was the *mistaken contents task* (Gopnik and Astington, 1988). The researcher showed the child a Smarties box and asked the child "What do you think is inside this box?" The experimenter then showed the child that there was actually a pencil inside the box. The experimenter closed the box back up with the pencil inside they asked the child "What is inside this box?" (reality control question) followed by, "When you first looked at the box, what did you think was inside?" (former false-belief question). The experimenter then brought out the puppet, Leo the Lion, and said, "Now it is Leo's turn to look at the box, I'm going to show Leo the closed box you first saw. What will Leo think is inside this box?" (false-belief question). Children were given a score out of three for the mistaken contents task. For each of the reality control, former false-belief and false-belief questions they correctly answered they were given one point.

The second False-belief task was the *mistaken identity task* (Flavell, et al., 1986). Children were shown slime that looked like a rock and asked "What is this?" The experimenter then demonstrated to the child that it was really slime and allowed the child to touch it. The experimenter then asked the child two test questions, "When you look at this with your eyes right now, does it look like a rock or does it look like slime?" "What is it really really, is it really really slime or is it really really a rock?" For the second trial children were shown a red strawberry and asked, "What colour is this?" The experimenter then placed a clear green piece of paper in front of the strawberry and asked two test questions, "When you look at this with your eyes right now does it look red or does it look green?" "What colour is it really really is it really really green or is it really really red?" Children received 1 point for each correct answer and so could score a total of 4 for the mistaken identity task.

Finally, children completed the *Tunnel task* based on Whitcombe and Robinson's (2000) modification of O'Neill and Gopnik's (1991) task. The Tunnel task assesses children's source-monitoring skills based on their ability to understand the link between information access and knowledge. The Tunnel task required a box with a window on one side, so that children could see but not feel inside the box, and an opening on the other side with a sock, so that children could feel inside but not see. Six pairs of toys (plus 4 practice pairs) differed in how they looked or how they felt. Three pairs looked different and felt the same (e.g., a red car and a blue car) and three pairs felt different and looked the same (e.g., two bubble bottles one filled with bubbles and one empty – heavy and light). The experimenter explained to the child that all the pairs of toys would either feel different (weight) or look different (colour). All items were hidden behind a screen until each trial began.

Children were then given 4 practice trials, two where the experimenter had more information than the child (e.g., the items were of different colours and the experimenter looked inside the box while the child felt) and two where the child had more information than the experimenter. The order was counterbalanced between subjects. To start each trial, children were shown two toys, asked to identify the difference between the toys, and their labels for the toys were checked. Once the difference (colour or weight) had been identified, the two toys were placed behind a screen. Leo the puppet covered one of the toys (e.g. the blue car) with a cloth and moved it into the box so that neither the experimenter nor the child knew which toy was inside the box. One person looked inside the box and the other person felt inside the box based on the trial. The child was then asked by Leo, "Which car do you think is inside the box, is it the red one or the blue one?" Once the child stated his/her answer, Leo asked the experimenter, "Which car do you think is inside the box?" (the experimenter either was consistent with or contradicted the child's statement based on experimental condition). The puppet then asked the child once more as if confused, "Which car do you think is inside the box?" (*identity question*). Here the child could either change his/her answer to what the experimenter had stated (in contradicting condition) or repeat his/her original answer. Finally, the puppet asked the child, "How do you know "X" is in the box?" (*source question*). If the child did not give a source on his/her own they were given three options from Leo, "Is it because you saw it, because you felt it or because [experimenter's name] told you?" (order of options were counterbalanced within subjects). Children were given feedback during the practice trials on whether or not they were correct as well as why they were correct or incorrect.

Once children completed all 4 practice trials the 6 experimental trials began. In two trials the child was less informed and the experimenter contradicted the child's statement (one see and one feel trial). This was termed the *less informed* condition. In two trials the child was more informed (e.g., the child felt inside the box when the item feels different, such as a treasure chest that is heavy or light, and the experimenter looked) and the experimenter disagreed (one see and one feel trial). This was termed the *more informed* condition. Finally, in two trials the child was less informed and the experimenter agreed (one see and one feel trial). This was termed the *consistent* condition and was included so that the experimenter was not always disagreeing with the child. The consistent trials served no experimental purpose and so will not be considered further. All children received the consistent trials as the third and fourth out of six trials. Observing the experimenter incorrectly contradict the child's answer in the more informed condition might reduce the experimenter's credibility. However, the order of the more informed and less informed trials was counterbalanced between children so that half of the children received the more informed trials first and the less informed trials last and half of the children received the opposite order, and no effects of order were observed. Children's responses were coded based on Whitcombe and Robinson's (2000) coding scheme. If the child correctly identified the item in the tunnel (either by seeing/feeling the item or adjusted his/her answer to what the experimenter said) he/she received one point. Scores were calculated per condition (less informed, more informed) thus identity scores ranged from zero to two per condition, as did source scores.

Results

Children's scores were used to determine whether they 'passed' or 'failed' each theory-of-mind measure. False-belief scores were combined to form a score out of 4 as in Welch-Ross' (1999b). Children were considered to have passed only if they correctly answered all four questions. Twenty-four children passed the false-belief tasks and 48 children failed. Scores on the Tunnel task were considered separately for the *more informed* and the *less informed* conditions. Children were credited with passing if they correctly answered the source question ("How do you know it's a …?") on both trials per condition (i.e., a score of 2/2). Fifty-nine children passed the more informed condition and 13 children failed while only 17 children passed the less informed condition and 55 children failed. We checked to see whether those children who passed the less informed condition said they knew what the object was because the experimenter told them to all 4 trials (2 more informed trials and 2 less informed trials). Only two children were found to have said 'you told me' on all trials.

The results section begins by assessing the relation between theory of mind and recognition accuracy in the initial interview, followed by the final interview. Analyses are then presented on the relationship between theory-of-mind understanding and source monitoring in the final interview.

Initial Interview Recognition Scores. A series of analyses of variance (ANOVAs) were run to assess whether theory-of-mind performance was related to children's ability to resist false information from each of the interviewers. Specifically, each theory-of-mind task was used in a 2 Theory-of-mind performance (Pass, Fail) x 4 Question type (non-misleading question asked by KI, non-misleading question asked by NI, misleading question asked by KI, misleading question asked by NI) ANOVA on the number of questions correct. False-belief, Tunnel task *less informed,* and Tunnel task *more informed* scores each served as the theory-of-mind between-subject factors respectively in each ANOVA.

A main effect of question type was found in all three ANOVAs: $F_{\text{false-belief}}(3, 210) = 5.80$, $p < .05$, $\eta^2 = .08$, $F_{\text{tunnel less-informed}}(3, 210) = 4.40$, $p < .05$, $\eta^2 = .06$, $F_{\text{tunnel more-informed}}(3, 210) = 10.13$, $p < .05$, $\eta^2 = .13$. Follow-up paired samples *t*-tests indicated that children were more accurate in response to non-misleading questions (*M*s = 8.24 and 8.46, *SD*s = 4.19 and 4.02, for KI and NI respectively) than misleading questions (*M*s = 6.22 and 6.58, *SD*s = 3.69 and 3.41 for KI and NI respectively) regardless of whether they passed the theory-of-mind tasks, $t(71) = -2.64$, $p < .05$, Cohen's $d = .51$, and $t(71) = -2.73$, $p < .05$, Cohen's $d = .50$ regarding questions from the knowledgeable and naïve interviewers, respectively. Thus, children were indeed suggestible overall and there were no significant differences between interviewers.

A main effect of task was also found for the false-belief task, $F(1,70) = 8.64$, $p < .05$, $\eta^2 = .11$, and remained significant after covarying age, $F(1,69) = 5.27$, $p < .05$, $\eta^2 = .07$ indicating that those children who passed ($M = 8.24$ out of 12) were significantly more correct than those who failed ($M = 6.94$ out of 12). Thus, recognition scores will be covaried in analyses of the Final Interview responses involving the False Belief task.

Finally, an interaction between children's performance on the Tunnel *more informed* task and question type was found, $F(3, 210) = 3.08$, $p < .05$, $\eta^2 = .04$, and remained significant when age was covaried, $F(3, 207) = 2.73$, $p < .05$ $\eta^2 = .04$. Follow-up Univariate ANCOVAs for each question type only indicated a significant difference in response to misleading questions from the knowledgeable interviewer, $F(1,69) = 7.73$, $p < .05$, $\eta^2 = .13$. Specifically, children who passed ($M = 6.78$, $SD = 3.27$) were significantly more accurate in response to misleading questions from the knowledgeable interviewer than children who failed ($M = 3.68$, $SD = 3.83$). No other significant main effects or interactions were found.

Final Interview: Recognition Scores. As before, a series of 2 Theory-of-mind performance (Pass, Fail) x 4 Question type ANOVAs was performed on the number of questions correct on the final interview. False-belief, tunnel *less informed,* and tunnel *more informed* scores were used as the between-subject variables for each of the ANOVAs respectively, and the number of questions correct served as the dependent variable.

A main effect of question type was found in all three ANOVAs: $F_{\text{false-belief}}(3, 210) = 13.41$, $p < .05$, $\eta^2 = .16$, $F_{\text{tunnel less informed}}(3, 210) = 11.14$, $p < .05$, $\eta^2 = .14$, $F_{\text{tunnel more informed}}(3, 210) = 5.10$, $p < .05$, $\eta^2 = .13$. Follow-up paired samples *t*-tests indicated that children were significantly more accurate at non-misleading questions (*M*s = 3.90 and 4.00, *SD*s = 1.32 and 1.31, for KI and NI respectively) than misleading questions (*M*s = 3.02 and 3.15, *SD*s = 1.26 and 1.41, for KI and NI respectively) regardless of whether they passed the theory-of-mind tasks, $t(71) = 3.71$, $p < .05$, Cohen's $d = .62$, and $t(71) = 4.35$, $p < .05$, Cohen's $d = .67$, for the naïve and knowledgeable interviewers, respectively. There were no significant differences between interviewers. Thus, a suggestibility effect was again observed.

A significant interaction was found regarding the tunnel *less informed* task and question type, $F(3, 210) = 2.66$, $p < .05$, $\eta^2 = .04$, which remained marginally significant after covarying age in months, $F(3, 207) = 2.53$, $p = .056$, $\eta^2 = .04$. Follow-up independent samples *t*-tests for each of the question types indicated that children who passed had significantly lower recognition scores in response to misleading questions posed by the KI ($M = 2.59$, $SD = 1.17$) and non-misleading questions from the NI ($M = 3.47$, $SD = 1.21$) than children who failed (*M*s = 3.18 and 4.16, *SD*s = 1.26 and 1.34, for KI misleading and NI non-misleading, respectively), $t(70) = 1.72$, $p < .05$ (1-tailed), Cohen's $d = .49$, and $t(70) = 1.94$, $p < .05$ (1-tailed), Cohen's $d = .54$, respectively. Thus, children who passed the tunnel *less informed* task accepted false information from the knowledgeable interviewer and resisted true information from the naïve interviewer, as predicted. In addition, a planned paired samples *t*-test comparing non-misleading and misleading questions by interviewer for pass children demonstrated that children who passed were significantly more accurate when responding to the KI non-misleading ($M = 4.29$, $SD = 1.21$) than KI misleading questions ($M = 2.59$, $SD = 1.18$), $t(16) = 5.80$, $p < .001$. No other additional main effects or interactions were found.

Overall, children's performance in the Tunnel task was related to their sensitivity to interviewers' knowledge. Understanding where information comes from in situations where they are not informed (*less informed* trials) was related to an over-reliance on the KI and resistance to information from the NI.

Final Interview: Source-Monitoring Scores. A series of 2 Theory-of-mind performance (Pass, Fail) x 4 item source (KI only, NI only, in video and mentioned by KI, in video and mentioned by NI) ANOVAs on correct source scores were performed to assess the relations between children's source-monitoring and each of the theory-of-mind task scores (false-belief, tunnel *more informed*, tunnel *less informed*).

A main effect of source was found in all three ANOVAs: $F_{\text{false-belief}}(3, 210) = 69.25$, $p < .05$, $\eta^2 = .50$, $F_{\text{tunnel less informed}}(3, 210) = 68.29$, $p < .05$, $\eta^2 = .50$, $F_{\text{tunnel more informed}}(3, 210) = 40.09$, $p < .05$, $\eta^2 = .36$. Follow-up paired samples *t*-tests indicated that children were better at identifying the source of non-misleading items than misleading items, $t(70) = 7.90$, $p < .001$, Cohen's $d = 1.33$, and $t(70) = 10.05$, $p < .001$, Cohen's $d = 1.60$, for knowledgeable and naïve interviewers, respectively. There were no significant differences found between interviewers.

When examining the false-belief task, a significant interaction was found between children's performance and source, $F(3, 210) = 3.21$, $p < .05$, $\eta^2 = .04$. Follow-up independent *t*-tests revealed that children who passed the false-belief task were significantly less accurate at identifying the source of misleading questions asked by the knowledgeable interviewer ($M = .58$, $SD = .94$ out of 6) than children who failed ($M = 1.38$, $SD = 1.59$), $t(70) = 2.69$, $p < .05$, Cohen's $d = .61$. Thus, children who passed the false-belief task seem to genuinely believe they actually saw the suggested details from the KI in the video.

A significant interaction was also found for children's performance on the tunnel *less informed* task and source, $F(3, 210) = 4.93$, $p < .05$, $\eta^2 = .07$, which remained significant after covarying age in months, $F(3, 207) = 2.67$, $p < .05$, $\eta^2 = .04$. Follow-up independent *t*-tests indicated that, consistent with performance on recognition questions, children who passed ($M = .59$, $SD = .94$) were less accurate at identifying the source of misleading questions asked by the knowledgeable interviewer than children who failed ($M = 1.27$, $SD = 1.59$), $t(46.24) = 2.19$, $p < .05$, Cohen's $d = .52$. Conversely, children who passed ($M = 4.29$, $SD = 2.02$) were significantly more accurate at identifying the source of non-misleading questions asked by the naïve interviewer than children who failed ($M = 3.11$, $SD = 1.94$), $t(70) = 2.18$, $p < .05$, Cohen's $d = .59$. Both findings are consistent with our hypotheses.

In general, children who passed the theory-of-mind tasks (false-belief, tunnel *less-informed* task) tended to incorporate the knowledgeable interviewer's suggestions into their reports of the event (as shown by the recognition scores) and believe they actually saw suggested items during the event (as shown by the source-monitoring scores).

CONCLUSION

This chapter investigated the relations between source monitoring, reasoning about mental states, and knowledge acquisition in order to gain a greater understanding of the contribution of source monitoring to knowledge acquisition. This was the first known study to explicitly assess this relation using the Mental-State Reasoning Model, and the first to specifically assess the relation using the tunnel task which measures an understanding of the relation between specific perceptual experiences and the reliability of knowledge sources.

Consistent with our predictions, we found that in general, children who passed the mental-state reasoning tasks exhibited a reinstatement effect in that they were more accurate in answering non-misleading recognition questions from the knowledgeable interviewer than the naïve interviewer. Thus, children who understand that experience leads to knowledge incorporated the knowledgeable interviewer's statements into their memories, knowing that the knowledgeable interviewer had access to information about the event. Conversely they rejected statements from the naïve interviewer who they knew did not have access to information about the event, even when she was giving accurate descriptions of what occurred. Thus, children's sensitivity to differential knowledge access determined their acceptance of information from diverse sources even more than the actual content of the information. These findings are not only consistent with our predictions but are also consistent with the literature on children's use of a speaker's previous accuracy to trust current statements. For example Koenig and Harris (2005) found that preschoolers tend to believe the name of a novel object if it is provided by a speaker who previously accurately named familiar objects over a speaker who inaccurately named familiar objects. Although children in the current study are not basing their decisions on the interviewer's previous accuracy they are treating the KI as reliable in the global sense based on their access to knowledge.

We also predicted that children who 'failed' to exhibit an understanding of mental states would accept suggestions equally from both interviewers while children who were proficient in demonstrating mental-state understanding were more likely to accept suggestions from the knowledgeable interviewer than the naïve interviewer. Again, we found clear support for this prediction because children who passed the tunnel *less-informed* task were more likely to incorporate the knowledgeable interviewer's suggestions into their memories than children who did not demonstrate such understanding. These findings are consistent with Welch-Ross' (1999) and Templeton and Wilcox's (2000) findings in that mental-state understanding was related to knowledge acquisition. The novel finding here, however, is that a specific aspect of mental-state understanding (linking specific experience to specific knowledge, as assessed by the tunnel task) was related to knowledge acquisition.

In general, it appears as though children who demonstrated an understanding of mental states relied on the statements made by the knowledgeable interviewer regardless of the accuracy of those statements. At the same time, these children may have rejected the statements made by the naïve interviewer knowing that the naïve interviewer could not have any information about the event. These data show that young children (at least those who showed advanced understanding of mental states) were not naïve consumers of information; rather, they selectively incorporated knowledge only from credible sources. These children did not treat all experimenter utterances as reliable.

It is noteworthy that the predicted effects were observed after the 5- to 7-day delay. In the initial interview, although there was a clear suggestibility effect, children who passed the mental-state understanding tasks also resisted information from the knowledgeable interviewer. By the final interview, however, these same children not only accepted the knowledgeable interviewer's suggestions more than did children who failed the tasks, but were unable to accurately attribute the source of the false information to the knowledgeable interviewer.

Finally, we predicted that children who demonstrated an understanding of mental states would be likely to have higher source-monitoring scores than children who failed to demonstrate an understanding. The results partially supported this prediction. Children who demonstrated an understanding of mental states (passing either the false-belief or the tunnel less-informed tasks) were better at identifying the source of their knowledge for non-misleading items from the naïve interviewer than children who failed to demonstrate such understanding. However, these same children were *worse* than children who failed the mental-state tasks at identifying the source of misleading items suggested by the knowledgeable interviewer. Thus, if children who demonstrated an understanding of mental states were truly able to monitor the source of their knowledge, they would have been able to identify the knowledgeable interviewer as the source of their beliefs regardless of knowing she had knowledge about the event. Clearly, they could not.

One possible explanation for this finding is that children are in a transitional phase in which they have developed an understanding of theory of mind, and are on their way to having the ability to monitor the sources of information, but have yet to completely develop the skill in all circumstances. Thus, they are able to identify the extent of others' knowledge, but lose source-specifying information when they integrate information from a reliable source into their memories. A future study is required to test this hypothesis with older children (e.g., 7- to 9-year-olds) so that we can test the relations with a sample that would include those who have developed the ability to identify the sources of their knowledge in addition to an understanding of mental states.

Traditionally, poor source memory is considered to be a hindrance (e.g., in the case of eyewitness testimony). Other researchers have demonstrated how source monitoring can sometimes be traded for educational gains. For example, in Ratner and Foley's work, young children learn during collaborative activities more when they confuse their own actions with those of their collaborators (e.g., Ratner, Foley, and Gimpert, 2000). Ratner and Foley consider this an aspect of 'appropriation' where children think about how an expert feels when performing a task and eventually internalize the expert's thoughts and actions. This can result in confusion over who carried out which aspects of the task, but benefits the learner because expert actions become incorporated into the learner's knowledge base. Extracting expert content and losing source information may indeed be an efficient way to learn – expert skill is retained while no cognitive resources need be expended on source monitoring. It might be more worthwhile to maintain knowledge of the source from less credible sources (e.g., non-experts) than credible sources so incredible information can be continually gated out.

In general, when presented with information from multiple sources children need to be able to know which sources to rely on, and which to discount. With an understanding of the reliability of sources, children can make judgments of what to integrate into their knowledge base and what not to integrate. However, there seems to be a cost of integrating information from a reliable source into our knowledge base, in that the ability to attribute knowledge to the appropriate source may be lost. Perhaps, as children become older they will be able to attribute the source of the integrated information. Since children must determine how likely it is that a source has access to accurate information prior to deciding to integrate the information into their knowledge base, children may later be able to decode how they know certain pieces of information. The ability to decode such information would be an important skill for children to develop as we often have to re-evaluate our current knowledge in light of new information. Being able to determine the original source of information in order to compare it to the new source would be helpful in determining whether to hold on to the new information or disregard it.

By understanding how children determine whether to integrate information into their knowledge base, educators can assist children in the learning process. Educators can help children make explicit decisions about whether a source is reliable or not as well as whether they should integrate this information into their knowledge base. As educators, we should also be aware that young children cannot make the distinction between reliable and unreliable sources of information and ensure we are at least scaffolding these decisions for them. Future research is required to gain a greater understanding of how these skills develop as well as how we can assist children in utilizing such skills.

ACKNOWLEDGEMENTS

We are grateful to the children, headteachers, and staff of OWL daycares, Emmanuel at Brighton daycare and Sandhills Public School in Waterloo, Ontario Canada. We are also grateful to the research assistants, Jessica Gilbert and Leanne Best for their assistance on this project. We would also like to extend our gratitude to Elizabeth Robinson for her feedback on earlier drafts of this chapter. This study was presented at the Cognitive Development Society Biannual meeting in San Diego, California in October 2005. Support for the research is gratefully acknowledged through a National Sciences and Engineering Research Council Discovery Grant awarded to Kim Roberts.

REFERENCES

Ackil, J. K., and Zaragoza, M. S. (1995). Developmental differences in eyewitness suggestibility and memory for source. *Journal of Experimental Child Psychology, 60,* 57-83.

Connolly, D. A., and Lindsay, D. S. (2001). The influence of suggestions on children's reports of a unique experience versus an instance of a repeated experience. *Applied Cognitive Development, 15,* 205-223.

Flavell. J. H. (2004). Theory-of-mind development: retrospective and prospective. *Merrill-Palmer Quarterly, 50,* 274-290.

Flavell, J. H., Green, F. L., and Flavell, E. R. (1986). Development of knowledge about the appearance-reality distinction. *Monographs of the Society for Research in Child Development, 60,* 201-213.

Giles, J. W., Gopnik, A., and Heyman, G. D. (2002). Source monitoring reduces the suggestibility of preschool children. *Psychological Science, 13,* 288-291.

Gopnik, A. (1990). Developing the idea of intentionality: Children's theories of mind. *Canadian Journal of Philosophy, 20,* 89-114.

Gopnik, A., and Astington, J. W. (1988). Children's understanding of representational change and its relation to the understanding of False-belief and the appearance-reality distinction. *Child Development, 59,* 26-37.

Gopnik, A., and Graf, P. (1988). Knowing how you know: Young children's ability to identify and remember the sources of their beliefs. *Child Development, 59,* 1366-1371.

Johnson, M. K., Hashtroudi, S., and Lindsay, D. S. (1993). Source Monitoring. *Psychological Bulletin, 114,* 3-28.

Koenig, M. A., and Harris, P. L. (2005). Preschoolers mistrust ignorant and inaccurate speakers. *Child Development, 76,* 1261-1277.

Lindsay, D. S., and Johnson, M. K. (1987). Reality monitoring and suggestibility: Children's ability to discriminate among memories from different sources. In S. J. Ceci, M. P. Toglia, and D. F. Ross (Eds.) *Children's eyewitness memory* (pp.92-121). New York: Springer-Verlag.

Leichtman, M. D., and Ceci, S. J. (1995). The effect of stereotypes and suggestions on preschoolers' reports. *Developmental Psychology, 31,* 568-578.

O'Neill, D. K., and Gopnik, A. (1991). Young children's ability to identify the sources of their beliefs. *Developmental Psychology, 27,* 390-397.

Poole, D. A., and Lindsay, D. S. (2001). Children's eyewitness reports after exposure to misinformation from parents. *Journal of Experimental Psychology: Applied, 7,* 27-50.

Poole, D. A., and Lindsay, D. S. (2002). Reducing child witness's False reports of misinformation from parents. *Journal of Experimental Child Psychology, 81,* 117-140.

Powell, M. B, Roberts, K. P., Ceci, S. J., Hembrooke, H. (1999). The effects of repeated experience on children's suggestibility. *Developmental Psychology, 35,* 1462-1477.

Ratner, H. H., Foley, M. A., and Gimpert, N. (2000). Person perspective on children's memory and learning: What do source-monitoring failures reveal? In. K. P. Roberts, and M. Blades (Eds.), *Children's source monitoring* (pp.85-114). Mahwah, New Jersey, London: Lawrence Erlbaum Associates, Publishers.

Roberts, K. P. (2002) Children's ability to distinguish between memories from multiple sources: Implications for the quality and accuracy of eyewitness statements. *Developmental Review, 22,* 403-435.

Roberts, K. P. (2000). An overview of theory and research on children's source monitoring. . In. K. P. Roberts, and M. Blades (Eds.), *Children's source monitoring* (pp.11-57). Mahwah, New Jersey, London: Lawrence Erlbaum Associates, Publishers.

Roberts, K. P., and Blades, M. (1999). Children's memory and source monitoring of real-life and televised events. *Journal of Applied Developmental Psychology, 35,* 1462-1477.

Roberts, K. P., and Powell, M. (2006). The role of prior experience and the timing of misinformation presentation on young children's event memories. *Child Development, 78,* 1137-1152.

Robinson, E. J., and Whitcombe, E. L. (2003). Children's suggestibility in relation to their understanding about sources of knowledge. *Child Development, 74,* 48-62.

Ruffman, T. K., and Olson, D. R. (1989). Children's ascription of knowledge to others. *Developmental Psychology, 25,* 601-606.

Templeton, L. M., and Wilcox, S. A. (2000). A tale of two representations: The misinformation effect and children's developing theory of mind. *Child Development, 71,* 402-416.

Thierry, K. L., and Spence, M. J. (2002). Source-monitoring training facilitates preschoolers' eyewitness memory performance. *Developmental Psychology, 38,* 428-437.

Welch-Ross, M. K. (1999). Interviewer knowledge and preschoolers' reasoning about knowledge states moderate suggestibility. *Cognitive Development, 14,* 423-442.

Welch-Ross, M. K. (2000). A Mental-State Reasoning Model of suggestibility and memory source monitoring. In. K. P. Roberts, and M. Blades (Eds.), *Children's source monitoring* (pp.227-256). Mahwah, New Jersey, London: Lawrence Erlbaum Associates, Publishers.

Welch-Ross, M. K., Diecidue, K., and Miller, S. A. (1997). Young children's understanding of conflicting mental representations predicts suggestibility. *Developmental Psychology, 33,* 43-53.

Whitcombe, E. L., and Robinson, E. J. (2000). Children's decisions about what to believe and their ability to report the source of their beliefs. *Cognitive Development, 15,* 329-346.

Wimmer, H., and Perner, J. (1983). Beliefs about beliefs: Representation and constraining function of wrong beliefs in young children's understanding of deception. *Cognition, 13,* 103-128.

In: Applied Memory
Editor: Matthew R. Kelley

ISBN 978-1-60692-143-2

Chapter 15

CHILDREN'S STRATEGIC REGULATION OF MEMORY ACCURACY

Thomas Roderer and Claudia M. Roebers[13]
Department of Psychology,University of Bern, Switzerland

ABSTRACT

The current chapter introduces a contemporary view on children's memory development during middle childhood. Traditionally, the memory development literature was dominated by research on either capacity development, strategy development, development of domain-specific knowledge, or metacognitive development. More recently, however, researchers have taken an integrative perspective, looking at memory development as a continuously changing interplay of these four components (e.g., Koriat and Goldsmith, 1996). This perspective change has enabled researchers to look at memory reports in real life, including school learning, test behaviour in school and children's eyewitness memory.

Previous research using adults has shown that, under a strict response criterion, individuals withhold uncertain answers to the benefit of memory accuracy, while under a very liberal response criterion, strategic regulation of memory performance implies to provide answers that are likely to be incorrect. The present chapter presents and discusses developmental studies of strategic regulation of memory performance in which the response criterion was either increased or decreased. Although children aged around 6 years appear to be able to withhold uncertain answers in order to increase overall accuracy of their memory reports, effectiveness and precision of regulation activities continue to improve until late childhood. Moreover, the nature and the quality of the underlying memory representation have been found to substantially affect strategic regulation of memory performance. Inter-individual differences in strategic memory regulation abilities can partly been explained through individual working memory capacities indicating that these processes are resource demanding cognitive operations.

[13] Corresponding author.

INTRODUCTION

Traditionally, empirical research on human memory and on memory development has implicitly focused on the *quantitative aspects* of memory performance. For instance, participants of all ages have been asked to recall as many items as possible from a list of words that had been presented to them earlier (i.e., free recall). Typically, participants master such a free-recall task without repeating items already recalled and with fewer commission (adding new items) than omission (leaving out items) errors (Koriat, Ben-Zur, and Sheffer, 1988). In many cases, researchers have not considered the influence of the memory monitoring and control processes that are applied by the participants in an effort to meet what they believe are the researchers` expectations (e.g., considering questions, such as: "Have I reported this item already?" or "How sure am I that this item was on the list?").

In many everyday life situations, the *qualitative aspect* of memory performance is more important than the amount of information recalled. For example, witnesses in court are asked "to tell the truth, the whole truth, and nothing but the truth" thereby strongly emphazising the accuracy of a report and instructing the witness to withhold any information about which he or she is not absolutely sure that it is correct. Again, memory accuracy of such a witness will be influenced by the effectiveness of memory monitoring (confidence judgments) and control processes (withholding uncertain details of the witnessed event). Many achievement tests in school or college trigger monitoring and control processes as well. For instance, if students have the option to choose only a subset of questions in the test, it will be essential for them to select the right questions. Or, if the scoring procedure of a test punishes wrong answers more than omitted answers, test achievement will highly depend on an individual's ability to screen out uncertain answers.

Empirical research on human memory as well as on memory development has changed substantially since the 1990s, by responding to the socially important and applied question of accuracy and reliability of eyewitness testimony. Although studies on memory remain part of mainstream cognitive psychology and understanding memory development is still essential for understanding cognitive development (Bjorklund, 2004), the issue of memory accuracy has challenged the memory quantity focus of experimental work, at least to some extent. In this accuracy-oriented approach, memory is being evaluated in terms of its correspondence with the information originally encoded, with memory retrieval and monitoring processes being inseparably intertwined (Koriat, Goldsmith, and Pansky, 2000).

Koriat and Goldsmith (1996, 1998) have argued that despite the existence of countless studies on human memory, surprisingly little is known about the influence of metamemorial monitoring and control processes on memory performance in terms of quantity and quality. Therefore, they outlined a model of the strategic regulation of memory performance that specifies the interplay between memory retrieval processes and metamemory monitoring and control. The framework makes disparate predictions about memory performance in terms of *quantity* and *quality*. Moreover, the model also includes subjective and objective demands of the task and the social situation in which a memory report is sought. Subjective and objective demands will affect an individual's response criterion in a given situation and will determine whether information is provided or withheld.

At the most general level, strategic regulation of test performance is only possible and can only be effective if an individual has the choice to decide which pieces of information to provide and which to withhold when accuracy of performance is emphasized more strongly than quantity. This is the case, for example, in most verbal interview situations, in written tests with open questions or in cloze tests (e.g., *"The capital of Switzerland is ________."* - *"Bern"* as correct answer needs to be filled in). In situations in which an answer to every question must be given, in contrast, memory accuracy cannot be regulated because monitoring and control processes are inhibited by the test format. At the same time, there are test formats (e.g., free recall) that allow profound strategic decisions, such as which perspective and/or degree of detail to adopt. In such tasks, strategic regulation processes cannot be studied because they are confounded with the test format. In the present chapter, we will review work that has been done addressing the interplay of retrieval, monitoring, and control processes in free versus forced report situations, with both children and adults. Before turning to the empirical findings on the strategic regulation of memory performance, we will describe in more detail the theoretical background including the processes involved in strategic memory reporting.

THEORETICAL BACKGROUND

Consider the following examples: a test is administered that consists of 50 questions. Individual A answers 25 questions correctly and 25 incorrectly, while individual B answers 25 questions correctly but leaves 25 questions unanswered. If *quantity* is the main indicator for evaluating test performance, both test persons would achieve at an identical level (50% correct answers). However, if *quality* of test performance is being regarded as most important, individual A would score substantially lower (50% accuracy of answers) compared to individual B (100% accuracy, because all 25 answers given turned out to be correct). In the context of forensic interviewing, to provide another example, one single question that is answered incorrectly by the eyewitness may – in the worst of all cases - lead to the erroneous conviction of a suspect.

These examples illustrate that different approaches to evaluating memory performance can yield different results. Moreover, the examples allow a researcher to describe the cognitive processes involved in individuals` strategic regulation of memory (test) performance. To begin, there are retrieval processes that are triggered through the questions asked and/or cues given. Then, the upcoming answer must be evaluated in terms of the likelihood that it is correct using metacognitive monitoring processes. Next, control or executive processes will operate on the outcome of retrieval and monitoring tasks, which will inform the decision whether to provide or withhold that answer (e.g., omit an answer from a written test; respond with an "I don't know" in an interview). Finally, the task demands—for example, the social situation (a cross examination in court versus an informal exchange of autobiographical memories) or the scoring system of a test (e.g., more penalties for incorrect than for missing answers)—will set the threshold for the decision of providing or withholding the best candidate answer.

These four components are all involved in the strategic control of memory reports and, according to Koriat and Goldsmith's (1996) model, the interplay between these components predicts that when the threshold to provide an answer is low (e.g., when credits are given for correct answers without penalty for incorrect answers), the quantity of information is high but accuracy is relatively low because individuals are more likely to provide uncertain answers. Conversely, when the threshold to provide an answer is high (e.g., when incorrect responses lead to a loss of credits), participants provide fewer answers (low quantity), but the accuracy of these answers is typically high because individuals are more likely to provide only certain answers.

Koriat and Goldsmith (1996) tested their model with adult participants by applying different scoring systems to knowledge tests. In their studies, participants in the different experimental conditions were told how much money they would earn for correct answers and whether and how much money they would have to pay for incorrect responding. In short, the experimental findings confirmed Koriat and Goldsmith's (1996) predictions. That is, increasing incentives for correct responding without penalties for false answers led to an increase in the number of questions answered, but not to an increase of memory accuracy. However, when the bonus-to-penalty ratio strongly emphasized memory accuracy (e.g., when participants had to pay 2 dollars for every incorrect answer and earned only half a dollar for a correct response), memory accuracy increased compared to a control group. At the same time, memory quantity (total number of questions answered) decreased significantly.

Moreover, extreme manipulation of the threshold led to extreme differences in quantity and accuracy, the *quantity-quality trade-off*—a very strict response criterion (e.g., "You'll loose all your credits if you provide one single incorrect answer!") leads to floor effects in answers provided, but to ceiling effects in terms of accuracy (Koriat and Goldsmith, 1996). Alternatively, a very low response criterion (e.g., "You have to provide an answer to every question, even if you have to guess!") consequently leads to high levels of quantity and low levels of accuracy of performance (Koriat and Goldsmith, 1996). In sum, effective strategic regulation of memory reports depends on individual's ability to (a) search in long-term memory for the requested information, (b) precisely evaluate the retrieved information in terms of the likelihood to be correct, (c) adequately perceive the situational and task demands in which the memory report is given, and (d) efficiently coordinate and control retrieval, monitoring and response behavior in a given situation.

Developmental Progression of the Processes Involved in the Strategic Regulation of Memory Accuracy

Before turning to empirical studies on the development of strategic regulation abilities, we will briefly review developmental progression for the four involved components. Each process undergoes substantial changes over the primary school years and, as will be reviewed later, development in one of the component affects the interplay with the others.

Regarding the ability to retrieve requested information from long-term memory, pronounced age-related changes take place during the primary school years. Both for episodic and for semantic material, it has been shown that children become increasingly able to use externally provided cues for activating the correct parts of the underlying memory representation (e.g., Kobasigawa, 1974). At the same time, children become increasingly skilled in generating effective retrieval cues themselves (e.g., Fivush, 1993; Roebers and Schneider, 2001).

Metacognitive monitoring and control processes have also been shown to improve significantly during the elementary school years, with an earlier development of monitoring compared to a protracted improvement in the related control processes (for a review see Schneider and Pressley,1997). For instance, around the ages of 6 to 8, children become relatively competent at evaluating their learning progress (i.e., judgments-of-learning, Schneider, Visé, Lockl, and Nelson, 2000), can adequately distinguish in their confidence judgments between answers that turn out to be correct versus incorrect (Pressley, Levin, Ghatala, and Ahmad, 1987; Roebers, 2002), and make rather good predictions about which pieces of momentarily inaccessible information will later be correctly recognized (i.e., feeling-of-knowing judgments, Lockl and Schneider, 2002; von der Linden and Roebers, 2006). Despite the early onset of these monitoring skills, further improvements in terms of more accurate confidence judgments and better differentiation are typically observed over the later elementary school years (Roebers and Howie, 2003; Roebers, von der Linden, and Howie, 2007).

Interestingly, the control processes that influence the allocation of study time as a function of judgment-of-learning (Lockl and Schneider, 2004) or "I don't know" responses instead of incorrect answers when confidence is low (Roebers, 2002) appear to develop approximately 2 years later than the corresponding monitoring processes. During a transitional period of time, children appear to have some difficulty in transposing monitoring into metamemorial control. That is, while judgments-of-learning discriminate well between already learned and not yet sufficiently learned items in a paired-associate task (Lockl and Schneider, 2004), or, confidence judgments after incorrect answers are less optimistic than after correct answers (Roebers and Howie, 2003), children do not act on this monitoring adequately by allocating more study time on the difficult items or by reliably giving "I don't know" answers when unsure.

Finally, in regards to children's responsiveness to demands inherent either in the social situation in which the memory report is given or in the task instructions, empirical studies point to an early onset of social-communicative skills on the one side and further slow improvements with increasing age and experience on the other side (Saywitz and Geiselman, 1998). In verbal interviews about observed or experienced events, children aged 6 years and older have been shown to be sensitive to the person of the interviewer, that is, give different answers when interviewed by their own mother compared to a stranger (Goodman, Sharma, Thomas, and Considine, 1995; Jackson and Crockenberg, 1998). Moreover, the status of and the familiarity with the interviewer (Bjorklund, Cassel, Bjorklund, Brown, Park, and Ernst, 2000; Cassel and Bjorklund, 1995), question repetitions (Howie, Sheehan, Mojarrad, and Wrzesisnska, 2004; Poole and White, 1991), and question wording (Gee, Gregory, and Pipe, 1999) substantially affect children's answering behavior. However, more demanding social interactive skills, such as adequately reacting to unanswerable (Roebers and Fernandez, 2002) and to nonsensical questions (Waterman, Blades, and Spencer, 2000), or maintaining memory accuracy in the face of social influence (Schwarz and Roebers, 2006), continue to improve into late childhood.

Given the continued development in memory retrieval, in metamemory monitoring and control competencies, and in social-interactive and social-communicative skills in 6 to 10 year old children, it is both theoretically interesting and practically important to examine the emergence and interplay of these collaborating processes. In order to strategically regulate memory accuracy during an interview or an achievement test, these different functions have to operate simultaneously, have to be coordinated with each other, and information from retrieval and monitoring has to be integrated into adequate response behavior. One can envision that the interplay between these processes could take many forms. For instance, the functioning of the operating cognitive processes could be compensatory—that is, when monitoring is imprecise, control processes could take the vagueness of monitoring into account. Alternatively, the interplay could be cumulative, meaning that control processes building on deficient monitoring will be even more problematic and will result in inferior memory performance (Roebers and Schneider, 2005).

To complicate the issue of strategic regulation of memory accuracy in children, frequencies of "I don't know" responses are hard to interpret in children. This type of response is typically seen as one key indicator of true strategic regulation activities (Koriat and Goldsmith, 1996; Roebers et al., 2007), but age-related changes in the frequencies of "I don't know" responses are not consistently found. This is because on the one hand side, older children remember more information than younger children and should therefore answer less often with "I don't know". On the other hand side, uncertainty monitoring and the related control processes are known to improve with increasing age potentially resulting in an increased readiness to admit lack of knowledge or recollection, that is, in an increased number of "I don't know" responses (Roebers and Schneider, 2005).

Strategic Regulation of Memory Accuracy in Children

Given that the importance of an accuracy-oriented approach to memory reports was first recognized in applied situations (i.e., in the context of adults` and children's eyewitness testimony), early empirical studies on children's ability to strategically regulate their memory performance to the benefit of memory accuracy were conducted in the context of event recall using episodic stimulus material. In the first study based on the theoretical framework of Koriat and Goldsmith (1996), Roebers, Moga, and Schneider (2001) showed children aged 6, 7, and 8 years, as well as adults, a video about a conflict between two groups of children. Three weeks later, participants were individually questioned about the episode using 27 open-ended questions (e.g., "How much money was in the boy's pocket?"; "How could the boy get his money back?"; "What did the gang leader look like?"). Depending on the experimental condition (threshold manipulations), participants either (a) were not given the possibility to skip a question and its answer and also not given any incentives for correct responding (i.e., forced report condition), (b) were instructed to answer the questions as accurately as possible and were given the option to answer with "I don't know" when uncertain (i.e., free report condition), or (c) were given one token (gold coin) for every correct and were taken away one token for every incorrect answer (i.e., incentives condition; adults were given monetary rewards and penalties; Roebers et al., 2001).

Figure 1 presents the main finding from that first study in terms of accuracy of recall as a function of age and threshold manipulation for the entire set of 27 open-ended questions. Results revealed the expected age differences in quantity and quality of recall.

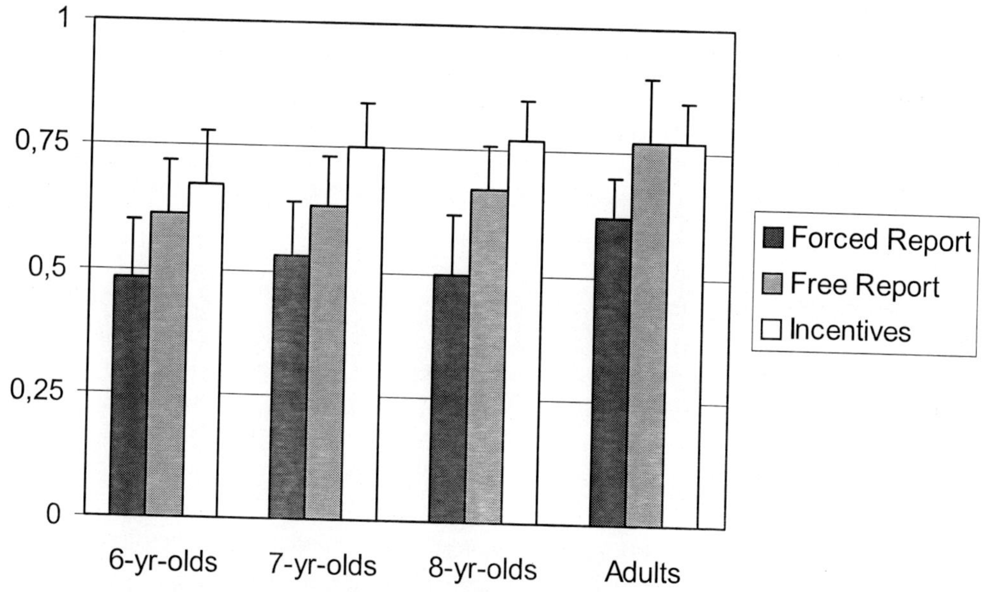

Figure 1. Mean Accuracy Scores when Answering Open-ended Questions about an Observed Event as a Function of Age and Response Threshold; adapted from Roebers, Moga, and Schneider (2001).

More importantly, however, the threshold manipulations were effective in stimulating strategic regulation operations for the accuracy of individuals` memory performance in all age groups. While the different conditions did not affect the number of correct answers (i.e., no effect on memory quantity), participants in the incentives condition produced significantly higher overall memory accuracy scores. Interestingly, the effect of the threshold manipulation was significant in all four age groups and there was no interaction between age and experimental condition that would point to disproportionately better strategic regulation skills in older compared to younger individuals (Roebers et al., 2001).

Also of interest was the finding that all three conditions yielded different outcomes showing that even 6-year-old children sensibly augmented their response criterion in response to the instructions. Further analyses revealed that the enhanced memory accuracy in the free report and in the incentives condition, compared to the forced report condition, was achieved by both, a decrease in incorrect and an increase in "I don't know" responses, independent of age. Thus, although we had anticipated that effective strategic regulation skills are not necessarily fully developed in kindergarten children based on the metacognitive development literature, this first investigation yielded encouraging results. The study documented that even younger children can adequately adjust their answering behavior in response to situational or task demands and can increase the accuracy of their episodic memory reports in the face of explicit, obvious and straightforward communication rules (Roebers et al., 2001).

In order to challenge younger children's strategic regulation skills without penalizing them for wrong answers (because it had proved somewhat hard to take away gold coins from them because, for example, they had not yet earned many or any gold coins, looked upset etc.), the incentives condition in the follow-up study (Roebers and Fernandez, 2002) included one token for every correct but no penalty for an incorrect answer (1:0 bonus-to-penalty ratio). Memory accuracy in the incentives condition was contrasted with a forced (no "I don't know" option) and a free report condition (accuracy instructions plus "I don't know" option). Again, 6-, 7-, and 8-year-olds as well as adults participated in the study. With respect to the included open-ended questions, results of the study confirmed that children were able to regulate their memory performance—to the benefit of accuracy—when incentives were given. Participants in the incentives condition achieved higher memory scores in terms of quality compared to the free and the forced interview conditions, again, independent of age (Roebers and Fernandez, 2002).

Roebers and Schneider (2005; Study 2) explored how the ongoing developmental advancements affected the interplay among the four involved components (see above). In a large-scale study including four age groups (6-, 7-, and 8-year-olds, and adults) being interviewed about an observed event, the incentives condition yielded substantially higher accuracy scores compared to a free report, a feedback-only, and a reward-only condition. Interestingly, detailed analyses on how these increases in accuracy were achieved revealed that the threshold manipulations had no impact on the frequencies of "I don't know" responses. Rather, participants in all four age groups were able to increase overall accuracy by giving significantly *less incorrect* and at the same time *more correct* answers.

Taken together, children have repeatedly been shown to be able to increase the accuracy of their memory reports when the threshold to provide an answer is augmented. Typically, children achieve these benefits by withholding incorrect responses, which suggests that the underlying metacognitive monitoring and control processes are sufficiently developed and can function efficiently under explicit task and social demands. Notwithstanding these metacognitive skills, incentives for correct responding can also lead to increased retrieval effort resulting in remembering even more information, some of which will in fact be correct.

STRATEGIC MEMORY REGULATION UNDER MISLEADING QUESTIONING

In forensic interviews with children, misleading questions are the rule rather than the exception and children typically appear to be extremely vulnerable to follow a false lead (Lamb, Orbach, Sternberg, Esplin, and Hershkowitz, 2002). One explanation for children's susceptibility to misleading questions is that they might misunderstand the expectations of the interviewer. That is, instead of correctly rejecting such hypothetical or probing questions, children may try to please the interviewer by agreeing to the suggestions. To explore this hypothesis, Roebers and Fernandez (2002) asked children a series of open-ended and misleading questions while explicitly manipulating situational demands on the children. Transparent and explicit interview instructions (that included giving incentives for accurate responding) were contrasted with the "usual" accuracy instructions given to children in forensic interviews (e.g., "Try the best you can to give me only correct answers!; If you are not sure what the right answer is, simply answer with "I don't know"!; That's ok, nobody can remember everything!"). In order to avoid any response bias to the misleading questions (i.e., questions suggesting an incorrect response and that are therefore only correctly answered when a "no" – response is provided, e.g. "The boys hiked to the farmhouse, didn't they?" – in the video the boys came with their bikes), open-ended and misleading questions were mixed with positive leading questions (i.e., questions that are correctly answered with "yes"; e.g., "The children slept in the barn, didn't they?" – in the video the children sleep in the barn) within the interview (i.e., question format—open-ended versus misleading—was a within-subject factor; the positive leading questions served as filler questions).

When comparing participants` answers to misleading questions across the three conditions, large effects of the threshold manipulations emerged. While both the liberal (forced report) and the strict response criterion (incentives condition) led to similar amounts of correct answers with children not performing above chance level (52% correct answers to the misleading questions), fewer incorrect (yielding) answers were found in the incentives condition (26%) than in the forced report condition (48%). Moreover, the interaction between age and condition revealed that younger children more strongly benefited from the incentives for accurate answers compared to older children and adults when misleading questions were asked (Roebers and Fernandez, 2002).

Although strategic regulation abilities under misleading questions were confirmed in Roebers and Schneider (2005, Study 2), the investigation did not reveal a stronger effect of the threshold manipulation in younger compared to older children. Moreover, although the model predicts more "I don't know" answers under a strict response criterion because uncertain answers are withheld, Roebers and Schneider (2005) found no effect of the experimental conditions on the frequencies of "I don't know" responses. It should be noted, however, that misleading questions can be answered by either saying "yes" or "no" and technically resemble a recognition task. Indeed, Koriat and Goldsmith (1996) showed that the recognition test format impeded strategic regulation abilities. Hence, the absence of threshold effects on "I don't know" answers in Roebers and Schneider (2005) are not surprising. Taken together, children's vulnerability to give answers to misleading questions appears to stem, at least in part, from a misperception of the interviewer's goals. Although children are given the instruction to be as accurate as possible when answering the questions, and to rely exclusively on their own recollection, they seem unable to consider these accuracy instructions when confronted with social pressure inherent in misleading questions.

The Influence of the Underlying Knowledge for the Strategic Regulation of Memory Accuracy

Of particular interest in this realm of research are the systematic comparisons between central versus peripheral information of the targeted event. In Roebers et al. (2001), two subsets of open-ended questions about the observed event were created. While one group of questions tapped the most central information of the event, the other group mainly focused on peripheral details, such as the appearances of the actors and other miscellaneous details (e.g., color of the bicycle that was stolen). Figure 2 illustrates the influence of question type (central vs. peripheral), age, and experimental condition on memory accuracy.

Analyses revealed that participants abilities to strategically regulate their memory performance was dependent on their recollection: when considering only the central questions, for which 6-year-olds' recall was moderate to good, memory accuracy scores in that age group were higher in the incentives condition than in the two conditions with more liberal response criteria (free report and forced report).

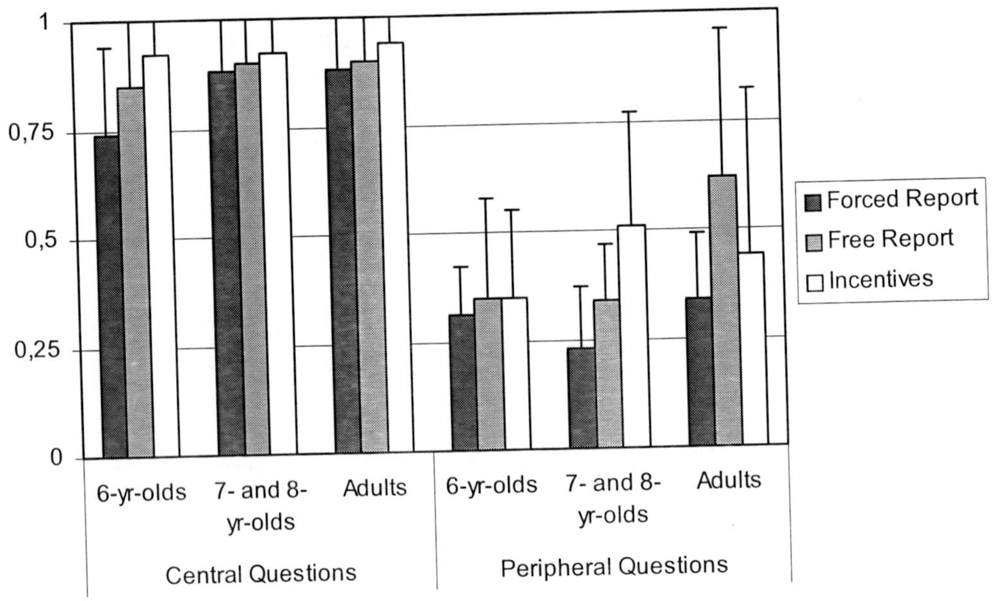

Figure 2. Mean Accuracy Scores in Response to the Central and Peripheral Questions about an Observed Event as a Function of Age and Response Threshold; adapted from Roebers, Moga, and Schneider (2001).

At the same time, there was no evidence for strategic regulation activities in the older children when these central questions were considered for which their recall was at ceiling.

In contrast, when considering the peripheral questions, analyses revealed that there were no indications of strategic regulation of memory accuracy in the 6-year-olds, while in the older age groups, memory accuracy was significantly higher in the incentives condition compared to the other two conditions (see Figure 2 for an illustration of that interaction). With respect to recall, 6-year-olds gave only a few correct answers to this subset of difficult questions. The findings may be interpreted as showing that strategic regulation processes do not occur with "too weak" nor with "too well established" underlying memory representations. While a very solid recollection supersedes strategic regulation for obtaining an accurate report, weak memory representations are likely to lead to low levels of certainty. Uncertainty compared to certainty monitoring has been shown to pose additional demands on children and to develop even later in life (von der Linden and Roebers, 2006) and may thus hinder strategic regulation processes.

Another means to explore the effects of the underlying memory representation on children's strategic regulation skills is to compare their answering behavior in response to answerable versus unanswerable questions (i.e., questions that cannot be answered based on encoding because the requested information was never presented) under different response criteria. Roebers and Fernandez (2002) included unanswerable questions in both open-ended and a misleading question formats in the verbal interviews. Compared to a more liberal response criterion, children aged 6 years and older in the strict condition were able to identify more of these unanswerable questions by more frequently answering with "I don't know" to this kind of question. When comparing the effect sizes of the threshold manipulations for answerable and unanswerable questions, the consequences of the different response criteria on the control processes were larger for the answerable than for the unanswerable questions. This difference may indicate that effortful retrieval processes resulting in the selection of a best candidate answer positively influence metacognitive control processes. When unanswerable questions are asked, retrieval processes within the memory representation of the targeted event will not be successful and thus may not be informative for the subsequent control processes.

Taken together, these studies offer some evidence that the underlying knowledge structure and the quality of the memory representation of the to-be-remembered information strongly influences strategic regulation processes. The findings may be also interpreted as showing that differences in the underlying memory can explain age-related improvement in the strategic regulation of memory accuracy. As children get older, encoding processes improve resulting in more coherent and solid memory representations on which monitoring and strategic control processes are built.

CHILDREN'S STRATEGIC REGULATION SKILLS IN THE CONTEXT OF SEMANTIC KNOWLEDGE TESTS

Thus far, we have focused on strategic memory regulation processes in the context of one everyday memory task—event recall. Another important applied context in which the strategic regulation processes can substantially influence memory performance is achievement testing in school, college, or university. School learning and school careers necessarily employ achievement tests and the quantity and the quality of acquired knowledge are frequently being tested. Reconsider the example, provided earlier when discussing Koriat and Goldsmith's (1996) model, with the two individuals—one who omits uncertain answers and one who provides uncertain answers that turn out to be incorrect. Pronounced differences in terms of test performance can emerge depending on individual's tendency to provide or withhold answers.

From a developmental perspective, the ability to strategically regulate memory performance of semantic knowledge tests should emerge later in life than of event recall (Schneider and Bjorklund, 1998). Children's ability to reminisce past events develops relatively early in life, fostered by frequent parent-child conversations, the majority of which deal with autobiographical memories (Fivush and Nelson, 2004). By doing so, parents teach their children which perspective to adopt, how to search in memory for more relevant information, how to structure their reports in a coherent way, and which degree of detail to choose (Fivush, 1993; Hamond and Fivush, 1991; Ornstein and Haden, 2001; Reese, Newcombe, and Bird, 2006). These skills, once acquired, can be used in any situation in which episodic memories are being recalled. In comparison, retrieval of semantic knowledge from long-term memory is known be more difficult because of the underlying memory representation, because of the only slowly emerging hierarchical structure of children's knowledge base, and because of less practice with retrieving semantic knowledge from long-term memory. It was therefore expected that strategic regulation of memory accuracy in the context of a semantic knowledge test would be observable only in older children and would be less effective than in event recall.

In one recent study, children's ability to strategically regulate their memory accuracy as a function of induced response threshold was investigated for semantic knowledge (Roebers, 2006). As in the previous studies using this experimental paradigm, children were shown a video (i.e., on the production of sugar from sugar beets) and were individually questioned about the video one week later. No convincing evidence for successful strategic control was found in the group of 7-year-olds. However, 9-year-olds significantly improved their memory accuracy when interviewed under a strict response criterion compared to age mates interviewed with liberal response criterion (no incentives or penalties). These gains in the quality of 9-year-olds` memory reports were achieved through more correct, more "I don't know", and fewer incorrect answers. Interestingly, even in this older age group, no differences in memory accuracy emerged between the 1:0 and the 1:1 bonus-to-penalty condition. That is, 9-year-olds were not able to make fine-tuned adjustments in their answering behavior depending on whether they were anticipating and receiving penalties for incorrect answers or not (Roebers, 2006).

Thus, although strategic regulation in the context of semantic knowledge testing is being observed in the later elementary school years, these skills nevertheless appear to be open for further improvements. In comparison to the competencies documented in event recall tasks, semantic knowledge testing appears to pose additional demands on the individual, resulting in both later general development and less precise control behavior under mild threshold manipulations.

THE PRESENT STUDY

As we have outlined earlier in this chapter, there is a protracted development of metacognitive control skills compared to the related monitoring processes. While in the previous studies we have not directly assessed monitoring processes involved in strategic regulation, that is, we have so far not yet included confidence judgments in the experimental procedures, participants in the current study were asked to give confidence judgments after recall. We expected that the deficits in children's differentiated, fine-tuned monitoring of uncertainty, the most important prerequisite for control processes (von der Linden and Roebers, 2006), would show up in the confidence judgments for provided but incorrect answers. An overly confident rating of correctness for these answers could explain inefficient strategic control processes.

Alternatively, some developmentalists suggest an (yet unspecified) influence of working memory capacity for the transformation of monitoring processes into adequate control processes. This developmental dissociation between monitoring and control may in part be explained by a lack of available cognitive resources for performing these operations (Roebers, von der Linden, and Howie, 2006). Such theoretical considerations (see also Towse and Cowan, 2005) are in fact fueled by recent empirical evidence indicating that individual differences in working memory can explain differences in a variety of complex cognitive operations within relative homogenous age groups and developmental progression in these areas, at least to some extent (Barrouillet and Lepine, 2005; De Bruin, Rikers, and Schmidt, 2005; Gaultney, Kipp, and Kirk, 2005; Schneider, Kron, Hünnerkopf, and Krajewski, 2004). Thus, it is likely that metacognitive monitoring processes require and absorb individuals' working memory capacity. The present study therefore included working memory tasks for explaining individual differences in strategic memory regulation activities and memory performance.

In order to increase ecological validity of the experimental paradigm and generalizability to applied (school) settings, we tested children's knowledge of the educational film on sugar production with a cloze test. Cloze tests are frequently used in school settings. In cloze tests, a text is provided with some key terms missing and children's task is to fill in the keywords in the blanks (e.g., *"Before harvesting the sugar beets, the ________ are cut off."* – fill in *"leaves"*). The cognitive demands of a cloze test are comparable to a cued recall test. From the perspective of the test format and from considering the level of recall found in 9-year-olds in the previous study using this stimulus material (Roebers, 2006), a cloze test should enable strategic regulation processes. This is because the cued recall task of a cloze test allows participants to leave out answers, a necessary prerequisite for strategic regulation, and between 50 – 60% correct recall of 9-year-olds in the previous study indicate that the resulting recollection is sufficient to allow strategic regulation processes from that age on.

Method

For the present study, a 2 (age groups: 9 and 11- year olds) x 3 (experimental conditions: bonus-to-penalty ratios) factorial design was employed. The experiment used 4 phases: 2 encoding phases (a school lesson on sugar production and a video presentation on sugar production in order to ensure sufficient knowledge acquisition; Michel and Roebers, in press), a recall phase (cloze test with confidence judgments for each answer), and a working memory assessment.

A total of 120 children (53% female) completed the study. There were 62 9-year-olds (mean age = 9 years; 6 months, SD = 5 months) and 58 11-year-olds (mean age = 11 years and 5 months; SD = 6 months). Boys and girls were randomly assigned to one of three experimental conditions (bonus-to-penalty ratios: 1:1; 1:3; control) resulting in cell sizes of 18 to 22 participants. Children were recruited from schools in and around the city of Bern, Switzerland, and came from predominantly middle class background. Parents gave written informed consent prior to the study; children gave oral consent to participate.

In order to ensure sufficient knowledge acquisition for later recall, the to-be-remembered material was presented twice to the participants, that is, in a school lesson and by a video presentation (Michel, Roebers, and Schneider, 2007). For the *school lesson*, the experimenter went into the classes and introduced herself. Accompanied by photos (taken from the video, see below), she explained the stages of sugar production from sugar beets. The production includes washing, cutting, cooking, filtering, centrifuging, vaccinating, drying, and wrapping of sugar beets and/or sugar. The lesson took about 20 min. per class. During the session, production steps were demonstrated with real kitchen equipment (e.g., washing, brushing, cutting, filtering) and children were allowed to touch the items.

For the *presentation of the video*, the same experimenter visited the classes 7 - 9 days later again. On the same day as the video presentation, small groups of 5 to 6 children from one class were taken into a separate room in their school. The children were told that now the experimenter would want to find out how much the children have learned about the production of sugar. At this point, the experimental manipulation was implemented.

For the *control condition*, the experimenter explained that she wanted to find out how much children remembered about the production of sugar. She asked them to try the best they can to give correct answers, however, if they were not sure what the correct answer is, they should simply skip it by leaving the space in the cloze test empty (Free Report). In addition, they were also allowed to cross out answers, if they doubted them to be correct. For the *1:1 bonus-to-penalty condition*, children were told that the experimenter would later check their answers and give them one point credit for every correct answer and one point deduction for every incorrect answer. Thus, they should try the best they can in order to get as many points as possible. Children with many points would later get a nice surprise. (Of course, all children were later allowed to select a surprise because they had "so many points"). Children assigned to the *1:3 bonus-to-penalty condition* were also told that the experimenter would later check their answers. She explained that for each correct answer they would get one point, for each incorrect answer, however, 3 points would be taken away from them. The raised cost for wrong answers should motivate the children even more than in the 1:1 condition to avoid reporting uncertain or incorrect answers.

After these instructions, small booklets, each containing 18 questions with an item difficulty between .27 and .85 and 6 very easy filler questions were distributed. Independent of experimental condition, the experimenter read the sentences aloud to the children and gave them time for filling in the answers before proceeding to the next item. After all children had completed the cloze test, a part of each page that had been folded to the back was unfolded, making the confidence scale visible. The confidence scale ranged from very unsure to very sure (7 point Likert scale) that the according answer was correct. Before children were allowed to give confidence judgments to each answer written into the spaces in the cloze test, the experimenter explained the rationale and usage of the confidence scale, provided examples, asked example questions, and requested confidence judgments for provided answers (see Roebers, 2002; Roebers and Howie, 2003, for more details). Children learned the use of the scale with ease and then went on and filled in their confidence judgments beside the answers of the cloze test.

Another week later, the children's working memory skills were tested individually in a quiet room at their school. Three different working memory tasks from the WMTB-C (Pickering and Gathercole, 2001) were administered according to the test manual: The *digit recall* consisted of presentation and recall of digits. For the *backwards digit recall* task, the presented digits have to be recalled in reversed order. For the *listening recall* task, children were presented orally with sentences and were asked to evaluate for each sentence whether it makes sense or not (e.g., "*Lions have 4 legs*", "*Pineapples play soccer*"). When asked to recall, the last word of each sentence in a trial (ranging from 1 to 6) was to be recalled (independent of whether the sentence made sense or not) in the order of presentation.

Results and Discussion

Preliminary data analyses revealed no differences between girls and boys. Data was therefore collapsed across gender. Level of significance was set to $p < .05$ and Eta^2 - values are reported as estimators of effect size.

Table 1 presents the mean percentages of correct, incorrect, and left out answers as well as accuracy of recall as a function of age and experimental condition.

Table 1. Mean percentages of correct, incorrect, left out and crossed-out answers in recall (cloze test) as a function of age and experimental condition (Standard deviations in parentheses)

	Control	1:1	1:3
9-yr-olds			
Correct	55 (13)	53 (15)	47 (13)
Incorrect	27 (16)	25 (11)	24 (12)
Left Out	18 (12)	22 (15)	29 (18)
Accuracy	.68 (.15)	.68 (.14)	.67 (.14)
11-yr-olds			
Correct	65 (12)	54 (15)	60 (12)
Incorrect	26 (11)	27 (14)	19 (9)
Left Out	9 (10)	19 (15)	21 (12)
Accuracy	.71 (.11)	.67 (.13)	.76 (.10)

An analysis of variance was conducted on the *percentages of correct answers* with age and condition as between-subjects factor and revealed a main effect of age, $F(1, 114) = 9.43$, $\eta^2 = .07$, with the 11-yr-olds giving significantly more correct answers [59%] than the 9-yr-olds [52%]. There was also a main effect of condition, $F(2, 114) = 3.13$, $\eta^2 = .05$, with the two experimental conditions (1:1 and 1:3) yielding to significantly fewer correct answers [both 53%] than the control group [60%]. There was no interaction between age and experimental condition. This somewhat surprising result can be explained with the overall amount of answers given in the different conditions: While the children in the control group answered 86% of all questions, children in the 1:1 or 1:3 experimental conditions provided only 79% and 74% answers. This apparently more conservative answering behavior may have resulted in withholding not only incorrect answers but also some that would have been answered correctly and provides a first hint to inefficient monitoring processes.

The ANOVA on *the percentages of incorrect answers* with age and condition as between-subjects factor revealed no main effects of age and/or response threshold and no interaction indicating that neither 9- nor 11-year-old`s higher motivation to avoid incorrect answers leads to reporting of less incorrect information.

The ANOVA on the *percentages of answers that were left or crossed-out* revealed main effects of age, $F(1, 114) = 7.11$, $\eta^2 = .06$, with 9-yr-olds [21%] leaving more answers open than 11-yr-olds [15%], and of condition, $F(2, 114) = 7.10$, $\eta^2 = .11$, where post-hoc tests following the Student-Newman-Keuls procedure showed that there were fewer answers left out in the control condition [14%] than in the 1:1 [21%] and in the 1:3 bonus-to-penalty condition [26%] with the latter two conditions not differing significantly from each other. There was again no interaction between age and experimental condition.

Since 11-year-old children can be expected to recall more information than 9-year-olds, there is a smaller probability to leave spaces empty in the cloze test. Thus, the seemingly better strategic regulation in younger children (leaving more spaces empty) might in fact be based on memory gaps. The effect of condition suggests that children who anticipate a reward for good performance activate strategies to reduce incorrect answers. Unfortunately, however, the strategy to reduce the number of answers provided in order to avoid incorrect answers did not lead to better discrimination in the present study.

Although somewhat redundant, mean accuracy of recall was also entered into an analysis of variance with age and experimental condition as between-subjects factors. Results revealed no main effect and no interaction. Inspection of Table 1 reveals that accuracy of recall was somewhat higher in the condition with the highest response criterion compared to the other conditions, but this was only true in the 11-year-olds. The missing effect of condition was not surprising given the inefficient regulation processes (not only incorrect but also potentially correct answers were not provided). Not expected was the finding that, overall, older children would achieve higher memory accuracy than younger children.

Comparing the experimental conditions, both the 1:1 and the 1:3 conditions differed from the control condition in terms of even fewer correct statements and more left-out answers. Assuming that there were no systematic recall differences between the groups, these differences may be attributed to participants' attempt to apply a conservative strategy of holding back more uncertain answers. Unfortunately, this resulted in withholding more correct answers while there were no differences between conditions for the frequencies of incorrect answers. Thus, our expectations of children's less efficient reporting strategies and protracted development in strategic regulation skills compared to event recall were confirmed. The age effects in the different analysis can be mostly attributed to better recall performance in older children mirrored by a higher amount of correct answers while at the same time there were less uncertain answers.

In addition, even in the control condition, in which children were not given incentives or penalties for their answers but in which the experimenters simply intended to find out how much children remembered, many spaces in the cloze test were left empty. In other words, children appeared to apply a relatively strict response criterion for themselves in the first place by withholding many answers. As a consequence, the different scoring schemes aiming to induce even more conservative response thresholds might have been somewhat less effective.

Nevertheless, the children adjusted their response behavior in a school-like test setting in accordance to the scoring scheme applied and withheld even more answers when anticipating penalties for incorrect answers. The findings underline the necessity of making test scoring transparent for students and to encourage and allow strategic regulation processes. In the context of the ongoing discussion about self-regulated learning (Boekaerts, 1999), strategic regulation processes may have a positive long-term effect on learning achievements by allowing students to precisely monitor their retrieval processes and activating appropriate control processes ("come back to that difficult question later," "think harder about the answer to that question before writing anything down," "search for more information, include other sources").

Table 2 presents the mean confidence judgments for the answers given in the cloze test as a function of correctness of answers, age and experimental condition. Results revealed a strong main effect of correctness of answer, $F(1, 101) = 166.56$, $\eta^2 = .59$, but no main effects of age or condition, and no interaction. As can be seen in Table 2, children of both age groups and in all three conditions gave significantly lower confidence judgments for answers that turned out to be incorrect compared to correct answers. Despite the strong main effect of correctness of answers, that is, despite the obvious ability to discriminate between correct and incorrect answers in metacognitive judgments, inspection of the mean level of confidence in Table 2 reveals overall optimistic ratings of answers that all turned out to be incorrect.

Table 2. Mean confidence judgments (min = 1; max = 7) as a function of correctness of answer, trial, experimental condition, and age (Standard deviations in parentheses)

	1:1	1:3	control
9-yr-olds			
Correct answer	6.0 (.7)	5.6 (1.0)	5.9 (.6)
Incorrect answer	4.6 (1.3)	4.4 (1.0)	4.5 (1.0)
11-yr-olds			
Correct answer	6.0 (.6)	6.1 (.6)	5.6 (.8)
Incorrect answer	5.1 (.8)	4.6 (1.2)	4.3 (1.0)

In other words, the mean level of confidence for incorrect answers is still very high and above the scale's middle category pointing to a pronounced overconfidence in recall. However, it is important to keep in mind that children provided only confidence judgments to answers they thought to be correct. In fact, of all judgments, only 12% fell into one of the "unsure" categories, whereas 25% were undecided judgments (neither sure nor unsure), and the majority (63%) were "sure that the answer is correct" judgments. The possibility to withhold answers in a test setting therefore resulted in very high confidence judgments for provided answers. This pre-selection of answers might have led to a ceiling effect consequently preventing any age or condition effects from reaching significance levels (Roebers, von der Linden, and Howie, 2007). Yet, the strong effect of correctness of answer indicates that 9- and 11- year old children are able to discriminate possible incorrect answers from potentially correct answers.

Monitoring accuracy was also assessed by computing gamma correlations between confidence judgments and recall for each item within individuals. Table 3 presents the mean gamma correlations as a function of age and experimental condition. The ANOVA with age and condition as between subject factor did not yield any main effects nor an interaction. Independent of age and experimental condition, monitoring accuracy was moderate and significant, albeit not perfect. The children's confidence judgments of an answer as sure or unsure turned indeed out to be in many cases correct or incorrect respectively. It is sound to assume that the gamma correlations would have been higher under a forced report condition, since the confidence judgments belonging to the withheld answers would have been lower. The increased range from very low to high confidence judgments would certainly lead to higher gamma correlations.

As measure of individual differences in cognitive capacity, working memory was included because this theoretical concept was assumed to be related to and/or involved in strategic regulation processes.

In order to examine whether children's working memory capacity has an influence on their long-term recall and/or on their metacognitive monitoring abilities, the working memory sum score was correlated with measures of recall and monitoring. Because of conceptual communalities and significant intercorrelations among the three working memory tasks ($r = .49$, $p < .001$), an average score was used for the analyses.

Working memory capacity was significantly related to correct recall *quantity* in the cloze test (long-term memory) with $r = .28$, $p < .01$, independent of children's age ($r = .29$, $p < .05$ and $r = .33$, $p < .02$, for the 9- and 11-yr-olds, respectively).

Table 3. Mean gamma correlations as an indicator for monitoring accuracy as a function of age and experimental condition (Standard deviations in parentheses)

	1:1	1:3	control
9-yr-olds	.52 (.47)	.55 (.43)	.49 (.46)
11-yr-olds	.50 (.39)	.60 (.43)	.46 (.51)

There was no substantial correlation with either the number of overall ($r = -.16$, $p = .09$) or the younger children's withheld answers ($r = -.02$, $p = .n.s.$). On the other hand, higher working memory scores in older children were correlated with less answers withheld and thus more answers provided ($r = -.38$, $p < .01$). The results so far simply seem to state that children with better working memory skills recall more correct items.

Working memory capacity was also substantially associated with recall *accuracy*, $r = .21$, $p < .05$, with that association being higher and significant in the younger age group, $r = .34$, $p < .01$, compared to the older age group in which the correlation was non-significant, $r = .05$, n.s.. This result implies that 9-year-old children with a larger working memory capacity achieved higher memory accuracy. Thus, working memory skills in younger children might be linked to the ability to strategically regulate memory accuracy, and this effect was not due to superior recall quantity. This finding supports the idea that increased working memory capacity in young children fuels developmental progressions in strategic regulation skills (Roebers, et al., 2007; Towse and Cowan, 2005). In older children, working memory seemed to be more closely linked to the quantity rather than to the quality of provided answers.

No significant relation between gamma correlations, the indicator of metamemory accuracy and working memory was found. There was no correlation for the total sample $r = .14$, n.s., nor for the younger $r = .14$, n.s., or the older $r = .15$, n.s., age group.

In sum, although children participating in the study tried to adapt to threshold manipulations of the response criterion by withholding more answers, they appeared to use inefficient strategic regulation processes as reflected in the high frequencies of incorrect answers provided in all conditions. These inefficient strategies are probably based on suboptimal monitoring processes and a marked overconfidence in the answers that turned out to be incorrect. While children's age has no obvious effect on monitoring or strategic regulation skills, higher working memory capacity seemed to help children in their regulation of recall, at least in the younger age group, as working memory was positively correlated with recall accuracy in this age group.

Conclusion

In this chapter, we have presented and discussed a research program realized in Germany and Switzerland over the last years dealing with the development of strategic regulation abilities of elementary school children. Children's competence to efficiently control the accuracy of their memory report in response to different social situations and different scoring schemes was assessed in several investigations. In many everyday life situations, including eyewitness testimony and achievement tests in school, memory accuracy is more important than quantitative measures of memory performance. In such situations, individuals have to make decisions about which pieces of information to provide and which to withhold in order to avoid false statements.

The interplay of retrieval, metamemory monitoring, social-communicative skills and metacognitive control processes will determine to what extent an individual can adjust memory performance in terms of quantity and quality to the social situation and the task demands. Overall, results consistently revealed that even 6-year-olds can regulate their answering behavior in response to explicit communication rules. When rewarded for accurate responses, children in their early primary school years can increase correct and decrease incorrect answers. Moreover, when given token for accurate reporting, children were shown to be able to substantially reduce their tendency to give yielding answers to misleading questions and to increase the frequencies of adequate "I don't know" answers to unanswerable questions. Despite the relatively early onset of these skills, the studies also documented slow but continuous improvements until later childhood in terms of effectiveness and flexibility of these higher-order cognitive operations. The underlying memory representation was shown to significantly influence strategic regulation processes, fuelling the ongoing debate about the reciprocal relationship between monitoring and retrieval (Koriat and Bjork, 2006).

Future work in this line of research will need to address monitoring processes preceding the strategic control processes in more detail. First, evidence suggests that the most important and influential memory evaluations take place very early in the process of retrieval and may not easily be accessible for investigations. Once a question is provided, confirmation biases and other influences operate on the metacognitive judgments (Koriat, Lichtenstein, and Fischhoff, 1980). When looking at confidence judgments a person openly provides after having provided an answer to a question, potential biases may have been already at work and thus these confidence judgments may not tell us the whole story about ongoing monitoring processes and may not match accurately with the early, fast, recall preceding monitoring outcomes.

Additionally, an individual differences approach to the study of strategic regulation processes may provide important insights. Typically, within homogenous age groups significant amounts of inter-individual differences are found in the ability to efficiently control memory reports in terms of accuracy. There are first hints that working memory capacity contributes to the success of these higher order memory processes. This is not surprising given the multiple domains in which working memory capacity has been shown to be influential (Barrouillet and Lépine, 2005; Towse and Cowan, 2005; De Bruin, Rikers, and Schmidt, 2005; Gaultney, Kipp, and Kirk, 2005). Knowledge of factors explaining significant amounts of variance in strategic regulation abilities can also be informative concerning the question of influences leading to intra-individual improvements over time.

Acknowledgement

Preparation of this chapter and the reported study were realized while the second author was financially supported by the Swiss National Research Foundation (SNF; Grant No. 100014-112492). We would like to thank Sarah Helfenberger for her help with the data collection.

References

Barrouillet, P., and Lépine, R. (2005). Working memory and children's use of retrieval to solve addition problems. *Journal of Experimental Child Psychology, 91*, 183-204.

Bjorklund, D. F. (2004). Memory development in the new millennium. *Developmental Review, 24*, 343-346.

Bjorklund, D. F., Cassel, W. S., Bjorklund, B. R., Brown, R. D., Park, C. L., and Ernst, K. (2000). Social demand characteristics in children's and adults` eyewitness memory an suggestibility: The effect of different interviewers on free recall and recognition. *Applied Cognitive Psychology, 14*, 421-433.

Boekaerts, M. (1999). Self-regulated learning: Where we are today. *International Journal of Educational Research, 31*, 445-475.

Cassel, W. S., and Bjorklund, D. F. (1995). Developmental patterns of eyewitness memory and suggestibility: An ecologically based short-term longitudinal study. *Law and Human Behavior, 19*, 507-530.

De Bruin, A. B. H., Rikers, R. M. J. P., and Schmidt, H. G. (2005). Monitoring accuracy and self-regulation when learning to play a chess endgame. *Applied Cognitive Psychology, 19*, 167-181.

Fivush, R. (1993). Developmental perspectives on autobiographical recall. In G. S. Goodman and B. L. Bottoms (Eds.), *Child Victims, Child Witnesses: Understanding and Improving Testimony* (pp. 1-24). New York: Guilford.

Fivush, R., and Nelson, K. (2004). Culture and language in the emergence of autobiographical memory. *Psychological Science, 15*, 573-577.

Gaultney, J. F., Kipp, K., and Kirk, G. (2005). Utilization deficiency and working memory capacity in adult memory performance: Not just for children anymore. *Cognitive Development, 20*, 205-213.

Gee, S., Gregory, M., and Pipe, M.-E. (1999). "What colour is your pet dinosaur?" The impact of pre-interview training and question type on children's answers. *Legal and Criminological Psychology, 4*, 111-128.

Goldsmith, M., and Koriat, A. (2008). The strategic regulation of memory accuracy and informativeness. In A. Benjamin and B. Ross (Eds.), *Psychology of Learning and Motivation, Vol. 48: Adrances in Research and Theory*. New York: Academic Press.

Goodman, G. S., Sharma, A., Thomas, F. S., and Considine, M. (1995). Mother knows best: Effects of relationship status and interviewer bias on children's memory. *Journal of Experimental Child Psychology, 60*, 195-228.

Hamond, N. R., and Fivush, R. (1991). Memories of Mickey Mouse: Young children recount their trip to Disneyworld. *Cognitive Development, 6*, 433-448.

Howie, P., Sheehan, M., Mojarrad, T., and Wrzesinska, M. (2004). "Undesirable" and "desirable" shifts in children's responses to repeated questions: Age differences in the effect of providing a rationale for repetition. *Applied Cognitive Psychology, 18*, 1161-1180.

Jackson, S., and Crockenberg, S. (1998). A comparison of suggestibility in 4-years-old girls in response to parental or stranger misinformation. *Journal of Applied Developmental Psychology, 19*, 527-542.

Kobasigawa, A. (1974). Utilization of retrieval cues by children in recall. *Child Development, 45*, 127-134.

Koriat, A., Ben- Zur, H., and Sheffer, D. (1988). Telling the same story twice: Output monitoring and age. *Journal of Memory and Language, 27*, 23-39.

Koriat, A., and Bjork, R. A. (2006). Mending metacognitive illusions: A comparison of mnemonic-based and theory-based procedures. *Journal of Experimental Psychology: Learning, Memory, and Cognition, 32*, 1133-1145.

Koriat, A., and Goldsmith, M. (1996). Monitoring and control processes in the strategic regulation of memory accuracy. *Psychological Review, 103*, 490-517.

Koriat, A., and Goldsmith, M. (1998). The role of metacognitive processes in the regulation of memory performance. In G. Mazzoni and T. O. Nelson (Eds.), *Metacognition and Cognitive Neuropsychology: Monitoring and Control Processes.* (pp. 97-118). London: Lawrence Erlbaum Associates Publishers.

Koriat, A., Goldsmith, M., and Pansky, A. (2000). Toward a psychology of memory accuracy. *Annual Review Psychology, 51*, 481-537.

Koriat, A., Lichtenstein, S., and Fischhoff, B. (1980). Reasons for confidence. *Journal of Experimental Psychology: Human Learning and Memory, 6*, 107-118.

Lamb, M. E., Orbach, Y., Sternberg, K. J., Esplin, P. W., and Hershkowitz, I. (2002). The effects of forensic interview practices on the quality of information provided by alleged victims of child abuse. In H. L. Westcott, G. M. Davies and R. H. C. Bull (Eds.), *Children`s testimony: A handbook of psychological research and forensic practice* (pp. 131-145). Chichester, UK: John Wiley and Sons Ltd.

Lockl, K., and Schneider, W. (2002). Developmental trends in children's feeling-of-knowing judgements. *International Journal of Behavioral Development, 26*, 327-333.

Lockl, K., and Schneider, W. (2004). The effects of incentives and instructions on children's allocation of study time. *European Journal of Developmental Psychology, 1*, 153-169.

Michel, E. and Roebers, C. (in press). Children's Knowledge Acquisition through Educational Films: Influence of Program Characteristics. *Applied Cognitive Psychology.*

Michel, E., Roebers, C. M., and Schneider, W. (2007). Educational films in the classroom: Increasing the benefit. *Learning and Instruction, 17*, 172-183.

Ornstein, P. A., and Haden, C. A. (2001). Memory development or the development of memory? *Current Directions in Psychological Science, 10*, 202-205.

Pickering, S. and Gathercole, S. (2001). *The Working Memory Test Battery for Children.* The Psychological Corporation.

Poole, D. A., and White, L. T. (1991). Effects of question repetition on eyewitness testimony of children and adults. *Developmental Psychology, 27*, 975-986.

Pressley, M., Levin, J. R., Ghatala, E. S., and Ahmad, M. (1987). Test monitoring in young grade school children. *Journal of Experimental Child Psychology, 43*, 96-111.

Reese, E., Newcombe, R., and Bird, A. (2006). The emergence of autobiographical memory: Cognitive, social, and emotional factors. In C. M. Flinn- Fletcher and G. M. Gaberman (Eds.), *Cognition and language: Perspectives from New Zealand* (pp. 177-189). Bowen Hills, QLD, Australia: Australian Academic Press.

Roebers, C. M. (2002). Confidence judgments in children's and adults event recall and suggestibility. *Developmental Psychology, 38*, 1052-1067.

Roebers, C. M. (2006). Developmental progression in children's strategic memory regulation. *Swiss Journal of Psychology, 65*, 193-200.

Roebers, C. M., and Fernandez, O. (2002). The effects of accuracy motivation on children's and adults' event recall, suggestibility and their answers to unanswerable questions. *Journal of Cognition and Development, 3*, 415-443.

Roebers, C. M., and Howie, P. (2003). Confidence judgments in event recall: Developmental progression in the impact of question format. *Journal of Experimental Child Psychology, 27*, 477-493.

Roebers, C. M., Moga, N., and Schneider, W. (2001). The role of accuracy motivation on children's and adults event recall. *Journal of Experimental Child Psychology, 78*, 313-329.

Roebers, C. M., and Schneider, W. (2001). Individual differences in children's eyewitness recall: The effect of intelligence and shyness. *Applied Developmental Science, 5*, 9-20.

Roebers, C. M., and Schneider, W. (2005). The strategic regulation of children's memory performance and suggestibility. *Journal of Experimental Child Psychology, 92*, 24-44.

Roebers, C. M., von der Linden, N., and Howie, P. (2007). Favourable and unfavourable conditions for children's confidence judgments. *British Journal of Developmental Psychology, 25*, 109-134.

Saywitz, K. J., and Geiselman, R. E. (1998). Interviewing the child witness: Maximizing completeness and minimizing error. In S. J. Lynn and K. M. McConkey (Eds.), *Truth in memory* (pp. 190-223). New York: Guilford Press.

Schneider, W., and Bjorklund, D. F. (1998). Memory. In W. Damon (Ed.), *Handbook of child psychology: Volume 2: Cognition, perception, and language* (pp. 467-521). New York, US: John Wiley and Sons.

Schneider, W., Kron, V., Hünnerkopf, M., and Krajewski, K. (2004). The development of young children's memory strategies: First findings from the Wurzburg Longitudinal Memory Study. *Journal of Experimental Child Psychology, 88*, 193-209.

Schneider, W., and Pressley, M. (1997). *Memory development between two and twenty* (2 ed.). Mahwah, NJ, US: Lawrence Erlbaum Associates

Schneider, W., Visé, M., Lockl, K., and Nelson, T. O. (2000). Developmental trends in children's memory monitoring: Evidence from a judgment-of-learning task. *Cognitive Development, 15*, 115-134.

Schwarz, S., and Roebers, C. M. (2006). Age differences in the effects of social influence on children's eyewitness performance and their metacognitive monitoring. *Journal of Experimental Child Psychology, 94*, 229-248.

Towse, J. N., and Cowan, N. (2005). Working memory and its relevance for cognitive development. In W. Schneider, R. Schumann-Hengsteler and B. Sodian (Eds.), *Young children's cognitive development: Interrelationships among executive functioning, working memory, verbal ability, and theory of mind*. Mahwah, New York: Erlbaum.

Von der Linden, N., and Roebers, C. M. (2006). Developmental changes in uncertainty monitoring during an event recall task. *Metacognition and Learning, 1*, 213-228.

Waterman, A. H., Blades, M., and Spencer, C. (2000). Do children try to answer nonsensical questions? *British Journal of Developmental Psychology, 18*, 211-225.

In: Applied Memory
Editor: Matthew R. Kelley

ISBN 978-1-60692-143-2

Chapter 16

APPLYING MEMORY THEORY TO DREAM RECALL: ARE DREAMS AND WAKING MEMORIES THE SAME?

Caroline L. Horton
Psychology, Faculty of Health, Leeds Metropolitan University,
Leeds, England

ABSTRACT

In order to understand and investigate dreams, a report of the dream needs to be elicited. This process relies upon autobiographical memory – memory for one's own experiences (Conway, 1990; 2001). The present chapter aimed to characterize the profile of dreams as memories in relation to waking experiences. Previous investigations have found dream memories to be less rich in detail and in sensory-perceptual information than waking event memories. However, questions remain as to whether dream memories would be recallable and recognizable over time. Twenty-five participants generated dreams and waking events, later recalled them, and subsequently completed a recognition task. Experiment 1 required the generation of retrospective dream and event memories; that is, reporting any experiences that came to mind that had occurred over the lifespan. Experiment 2 compared dream memories with waking experiences that were reported within a day of their occurrence using a diary paradigm. Experiment 1 found dream recall to be significantly poorer than the recall of waking event memories; recognition performance, however, was comparable. Experiment 2 yielded similar performances across dreams and events for both recall and recognition. These data suggest that dream memories are similar to waking memories in accessibility, recallability, and recognizability. Older dreams may lose their recallability, likely due to a lack of rehearsal over time. Dream memories therefore share a similar profile to waking memories, provided that they are reported or rehearsed upon waking, in order to encode initially the experience to memory.

INTRODUCTION

The study of dreams relies upon memory for dream experiences, as there is (as yet) no method of measuring dreams objectively. Hence, in order to investigate dreams, it is necessary to comprehend the processes involved in remembering them. If much detail of a dream memory is lost, it is difficult to ascertain the validity of the original dream experience. Applying knowledge of waking memory to dream memories enables an understanding of the extent to which we can trust reports of dream experiences.

The continuity hypothesis (Schredl and Hoffman, 2003) broadly claims that there is overlap between dreaming and waking. This can be conceived of in terms of content (thoughts or memories appearing in dreams and waking; Botman and Crovitz, 1989-90), cognitive style (individual differences such as personality or rumination; Horton, Conway and Moulin, *in prep*; Schredl and Montasser, 1996-7) and cognitive processes (the kinds of thoughts able to be manipulated, for instance meta-cognitions; Wolman and Kozmova, 2007; or counterfactual thinking; McNamara, 2000). The assumptions of this hypothesis imply not only that characteristics of memories for dreaming and waking experiences would be similar, but also that the encoding and retrieval processes involved in their production would be comparable. The present paper focuses upon memories for dreams specifically, as opposed to dreams more generally, in terms of the experience whilst it is occurring.

Few studies acknowledge the mediating role of memory when investigating dreams. There have been some investigations and theories that conceptualize the state of the sleeping brain and the cognitive processes active within it when considering the production of dreams. These theories, implicitly, make assumptions about the subsequent memories of dreams. Foulkes (1982) proposed that the dreaming brain is in a "reflective only" state, dwelling upon previous thoughts and events. In contrast, the waking brain is purported to be able to switch between this mode and an encoding mode. This implies that the reflections (thoughts) active in the dreaming mind are less easily encoded than waking thoughts and experiences. Foulkes' ideas assume that there is continuity between the sleeping and waking mind in terms of content, thus being in agreement with the basic principle of the continuity hypothesis (Schredl and Hoffman, 2003). Similarly, Domhoff (e.g., 2002) argues that current concerns are activated and present in dreams (the "repetition principle"). Domhoff (2001) demonstrates the development and maturation of dreaming over the lifespan, which is taken as evidence of the cognitive processes involved in dreaming and, perhaps, remembering dreams.

Memories of dreams can be compared to memories for waking experiences. Dream memories are episodic memories (Tulving, 1983): specific memories for an experience or an event. Episodic memories often arise from experiences that we are conscious of whilst they are occurring. Whether a person is reading an e-mail, studying for an exam, or considering what needs to be purchased in order to prepare a particular meal, that person can choose to attend to and encode certain information in an effort to facilitate later retrieval. Some memories, such as memories for dreams, concern experiences that we were not aware of whilst they are occurring. Dreams differ from waking episodic experiences in that we are rarely aware that we are dreaming whilst we are dreaming, with the exception of lucid dreams, which occur in approximately 3% of cases (Cicogna and Bosinelli, 2001). There is therefore reason to believe that the characteristics of dream and waking memories differ, implying some underlying difference between dreams and waking experiences. The present paper focuses upon dreams as memories in comparison to episodic memories for waking events.

Dreams are experientially unique. They are especially incoherent (Hobson, Pace-Schott, and Stickgold, 2000), making it difficult for them to be manipulated into a meaningful memory. One could argue that dream memories may be similar to sensory-perceptual episodic memories (Conway, 2001). Indeed, a number of studies have reported that emotions are especially prevalent in dreams and that they are more sentient and experiential in nature (Hicks, Bautista and Hicks, 1999; Schredl and Doll, 1998). This would assume that dream memories are at least as detailed as episodic memories for waking experiences. However, there is evidence to suggest that dream memories and waking memories are not particularly alike (see "Characteristics of Dream Memories", below), in which case dream memories may be more comparable to general autobiographical memories (Conway, 1990; 2005), which may lack such feelings and experiences. Autobiographical memories, memories for one's own experiences, form part of the self, like a life-story or an autobiography (Conway, 1990; 2005; Conway and Pleydell-Pearce, 2000; Conway, Singer and Tagini, 2004).

This chapter introduces the profile of dreams as unique memories, applying current knowledge of long-term autobiographical memory functioning to dreams. Systematic and direct comparisons between the recallability of dream memories and waking memories had not been undertaken before. Two experiments are described, comparing the retrieval of dream memories to the retrieval of waking event memories. Participants were asked to generate dream and waking memories, which were subsequently recalled and recognized in separate tasks. Experiment 1 investigated retrospective memories—memories for experiences (dreams and waking) that had occurred throughout the lifespan—while Experiment 2 investigated experiences as they were occurring, in a diary paradigm. Findings demonstrate the overlap between memories for dreams and waking experiences, broadly supporting the continuity hypothesis and more specifically characterizing the profile of dream memories.

Theories of Dream Recall and its Failure

Dream recall seems notoriously poor and most individuals accept that, whilst they dream nightly, they rarely recall their dreams (e.g., Reed, 1974). Laboratory investigations, in which dreamers are systematically awakened in different stages of sleep, have provided information about the characteristics of dreams that would have been forgotten under normal circumstances. Approximately 80% of dreams can be recalled from rapid eye-movement (REM) sleep, and approximately 50% of dreams from non-REM sleep (Foulkes, 1962, 1979; Neilson, 2000). On average, 3-6 dreams can be gathered from an individual who is awakened in every REM phase per night (Meier, Ruef and Ziegler, 1968). Dreams have thus been demonstrated to be accessible, to some extent, when individuals are awakened immediately from sleep and when adequate resources are allocated to their retrieval.

In the majority of everyday circumstances, individuals wake less abruptly than when in a lab. Physiological changes occur over the period of awakening. During sleep, the brain is not active in the same way as when awake. Many regions are less active while some, such as the amygdala, are especially active (Maquet, 2000). The frontal lobes are largely attenuated during sleep (Maquet, 2000), accounting for a relative lack of control and inhibition processes and executive functioning (Hobson et al., 2000). One potential consequence of these differences is that dreams may not be encoded for subsequent remembering as well as some other experiences. Moreover, while asleep, memories continue to be activated and brought to mind, albeit in a sometimes discontinuous or apparently incoherent manner.

These changes in physiology of the brain over the sleep-wake cycle have been proposed to account for the difficulty of recalling dreams. The *arousal-retrieval hypothesis* (Koulack and Goodenough, 1974) assumes that short term memory functioning and storage capabilities vary over the sleep-wake cycle. In particular, there are difficulties associated with the allocation of resources, such as attention or repetition of material, in order to facilitate encoding. This results in a difficulty for dreams to be passed through an initial storage stage to reach long term memory while asleep and immediately upon waking from sleep. Given the difficulty for dream memories to be encoded beyond short-term memory and into long-term memory, the context within which dreams are best recalled is immediately upon waking when the dream memory is still in short- as opposed to long-term stores, thus accounting for high recall rates from laboratory settings. The *functional state-shift mode*l (Koukkou and Lehmann, 1983) built upon these ideas by acknowledging that for dream recall to be successful, the context in which it is retrieved should match the context in which it was encoded. This mirrors state- and context-dependent memory effects which are well documented in the memory literature (e.g. Godden and Baddeley, 1975).

Changes in the cognitive profile of the brain over the sleep-wake cycle have also been proposed to account for the difficulty of recalling dreams. Two cognitive models of dream recall, which rely upon knowledge and functioning of the waking memory systems, compliment the physiological views of the dreaming brain. Cohen and his colleagues claimed that dreams are generally less salient than waking memories (Cohen and MacNeilage, 1974) and that waking memories interfere with, and sometimes replace, these dream memories (Cohen and Wolfe, 1973). Koulack and Goodenough's arousal-retrieval model (1974) can account for interference effects (Cohen and Wolfe, 1973) as short-term memory functioning is claimed to become increasingly functional upon awakening, thus favoring waking memories over and above the less salient dream memories (Cohen and MacNeilage, 1974). Empirical support for dream memories being less salient than waking memories has been found in a variety of studies (e.g., Kemp and Burt, 2006; Kemp, Burt and Sheen, 2003).

The idea that dreams may be less salient than waking memories is central to the processes of reality monitoring (Johnson, 1988) and source monitoring (Johnson, Hashtroudi and Lindsay, 1993). These frameworks rely upon the feature that internally sourced memories are less characteristically detailed than memories for events that have actually occurred (Johnson, Suengas, Foley and Raye, 1988), in order to facilitate distinguishing between such experiences. A dream is an example of an internally sourced memory. In this manner dreams are memories, just like episodic memories for waking events, albeit weaker ones in terms of characteristics and detail. One could argue that if a dream memory is not especially detailed, it may not contain enough information to be considered truly "episodic" (Tulving, 1983). Dream memories may therefore be more appropriately considered to be autobiographical memories, although no systematic explorations of this have been previously conducted.

These differences between dreaming and waking memories are claimed to be easily identifiable (Johnson, 1988; Johnson, Kahan and Raye, 1984; Johnson et al., 1988). Thus, there seems to be a need to explore these discrepancies between the characteristics of dreams and waking autobiographical memories. Dreams may lack the contextual detail characteristic of episodic memories. Dream memories undoubtedly will involve a degree of reconstruction at retrieval; in this way dreams rely more greatly on autobiographical memory retrieval processes.

Characteristics of Dream Memories

In general, authors emphasizing the strong characteristics of dreams, such as emotionality or bizarreness, tend to focus on dreams only without comparing them to waking episodic memories (e.g. Cipolli, Bolzani, Cornoldi, De Beni and Fagioli, 1993; Schredl and Doll, 1998). The few studies that have directly compared the characteristics of dream and waking event memories have done so in a reality monitoring framework (Johnson, Kahan and Raye, 1984; Kemp and Burt, 2006; Kemp et al., 2003). That is, they have generally found that dreams contain less perceptual and contextual detail than memories for actual experiences, which facilitates accurate reality monitoring judgments. The extent to which dreams contain cognitive operations can be questioned, though, in that the neurophysiology of dreaming does not lend itself well to an awareness of cognitive operations at the time of experiencing the dream. This may mean that the characteristic difference between dreams and memories are especially profound.

Indeed, Johnson et al. (1984) suggest that dreams are unique in not featuring conscious cognitive operations. Moreover, they found that dream memories could become detailed and salient if sufficient cues and time to recall were provided. Pairs of subjects woke and gave each other reports of real dreams and made-up pseudo-dreams. Later, the subjects could distinguish between the pseudo-dreams they had made up when awake and real dream reports because the latter lacked traces of constructive processes. Although they are distinguishable in Johnson's view, dreams, imaginings, and real memories are all products of the same cognitive system but vary in the contribution of different subsystems. Dreams are generated primarily by the reflective subsystem. It is assumed that when individuals have to make reality monitoring decisions between internally self-generated items and externally other-generated items, the role of cognitive operations is a more reliable source when making the reality monitoring judgment than mere characteristic comparisons. This is because one would probably try to recall more effortful processes along with the recall of the episodic memory for that event or item itself. Johnson et al. (1984) also included a cued recall task. As this is one of the few studies comparing characteristics of dream and waking memories, I employed a similar methodology in the experiments in the present chapter. Additionally a recognition task for the previously generated dreams and events was included. Comparisons of memory retrieval in context have never been previously investigated, although more ecologically valid and episodically rich measures of autobiographical memory are increasingly in use (e.g., use of SenseCam, which captures images from an individual's daily life and can be used as a rich cue in a recall task (Hodges et al., 2006).

Kemp et al. (2003) also found self-rated differences between dreams and "actual" experiences (memories for waking events), in that dreams were rated as significantly less memorable than the "actual" experiences. Dreams were generally rated as significantly less vivid and salient than the events, and more negatively emotional. Diary' ratings for dreams were significantly more fragmented, less coherent, and less characterised by visual and auditory imagery. In fact, dreams were significantly less detailed than the events along 15 of the 16 dimensions in the administered questionnaire (based on Rubin, Schrauf and Greenberg, 2003). Furthermore, the ratings decreased between the times of reporting and subsequent testing.

Kemp et al. (2003) also discovered that remembering dreams and waking experiences differed in terms of recall and recognition. That is, dreams were particularly difficult to recall, yet they were still recognizable. This is not particularly surprising, given the wealth of evidence showing that recognizing an item typically is easier than freely recalling it, due to the presence of an increased number of cues from encoding, at retrieval (e.g., see Tulving, 1983). One could predict, then, that the same should be true for dream memories, given their inherently autobiographical nature. However, it is unclear as to whether dreams and waking experiences display the same trends in this respect. That is, are dreams similarly more recognizable than recallable than events, or more so? As work from our own laboratory (Horton, Conway and Moulin, *in prep*) has demonstrated that dreams are significantly more difficult to freely recall than waking events, it is not clear as to whether the dream memory trace has vanished entirely, implying that recognition of dreams would be problematic also, or whether the memory trace exists and is simply difficult to retrieve. Kemp et al. did not investigate recall and recognition clearly. The experiments described in the present chapter, therefore, aimed to investigate the nature of retrieving dreams and waking events employing a systematic assessment of recall and recognition of dreams.

There appears to be mixed evidence concerning the comparability of dreams and autobiographical memories. Grenier et al. (2005) found that the identifiable autobiographical memories appearing in dreams followed a comparable distribution of loss over time compared to waking autobiographical memories. In a similar vein, Botman and Crovitz (1989-90) found that a retention function, a mathematical depiction of the typical number of recallable memories from any given period in the lifespan, was also reflected in the recall of dreams. Taken together, this seems to support the idea of overlap between the dreaming and autobiographical systems. As has been discussed dreams are, in theory, autobiographical, yet they are internally generated and are experienced independently of a more general waking life context. In addition to the characteristic differences between dream and waking memories, the self, placed centrally as a defining characteristics of autobiographical memory (Conway, 2005; Conway and Pleydell-Pearce, 2000; Conway, Singer and Tagini, 2004), has been argued by some researchers not to be able to appear in dreams (Hartmann, 2000; Hobson and McCarley, 1977; Kahan, LaBerge, Levitan and Zimbardo, 1997).

DIRECT INVESTIGATIONS OF DREAM RECALL

The investigations described above focused upon the comparisons of rated characteristics of dream and waking memories. Comparisons of objective measures of dream recall and recognition have not been conducted previously (with the exception of Kemp et al's (2003) study, discussed above). Johnson et al.'s (1984) experiments involved comparing the recognition of one's own dreams with one's partner's dreams. The work of Montangero and colleagues has expanded upon the understanding of dream memory retrieval processes, although not in direct comparison to waking autobiographical events.

Montangero, Pasche and Willequet (1996) examined the improvement in dream recall when recall cues were provided upon awakening, and Montangero, Ivani and de Saint-Hilaire (2003) directly compared the recallability, as well as the characteristics, of dreams and waking memories (although non-autobiographical ones). Waking memories were manipulated to be comparable to dreams in that dream-like films were created and presented to individuals when awoken at specific times in a sleep lab, so to be as similar to dreams as possible. Thus, dreams and the "events" (films) were compared appropriately, as the films were presented to participants in the night (after they had been awakened 10 minutes after the second onset of REM sleep), when arousal levels and brain activity would be as comparable to the dreaming brain as possible. In addition, the films were viewed and recalled by the participants, being similar to experiencing a dream and then recalling it.

This methodology attempted to make the waking memories deliberately dream-like, which allowed an objective record of the original experience (the film) to be compared to the recalled memory of it. The dream-like films differed from waking memories in terms of style, content and coherence. As De Witt (1988) has argued against what he calls the "hallucinatory movie" view that characterizes dreaming as a passive sensory experience so that dreaming is like watching a movie, Montanero et al's . films may not reflect memory processes involved in remembering waking experiences. Specifically the films may have not have involved a participant's self, as the subsequently reported memories were for experiences in which they were not directly involved. Autobiographical memory is recognized to involve the self (Conway, 1990; 2005; Conway and Pleydell-Pearce, 2000; Conway, Singer and Tagini, 2004). Nevertheless, Montangero et al.'s study is the only one that has attempted to compare dream recall with event recall directly. Measures were taken to ensure that the films would be comparable to dream memories, thus comparing waking events to dreams also illustrates the comparability of these two types of memories. The morning after dreams and film reports had been collected from participants (over the course of separate nights in a sleep lab, using a counterbalanced design) a recall test was administered. The general findings were that more information was recalled in the morning, than when the original experience was recalled in the night. In the case of the films, the validity of the memories of the extra information could be verified, and was found to be accurate in most instances (86%).

The findings of Montangero et al.'s (2003) experiment implied that dream memories are accessible. This is largely contrary to many other studies on dream recall. However, Montangero et al. provided suitable memory cues in the form of event specific knowledge about the dreams and films, and their recent occurrence may have contributed to the dreams being more recallable than older dreams. Indeed, Johnson et al. (1984) found that recent experiences contain more contextual detail than older memories, thus facilitating accurate reality monitoring decisions.

Diaries in Memory Research

Diaries have been used as an autobiographical memory research tool (e.g., Linton, 1982; Odegard and Lampinen, 2004) and also as a means of recording or improving recall for dream memories. They allow experiences to be recorded shortly after they have occurred, providing a detailed and valid measure for subsequent recall tasks. Odegard and Lampinen (2004) used a diary style paradigm to investigate whether people would falsely remember events that shared features with actual autobiographical memories, but the whole episode had not actually occurred. They built upon the design used by Barclay and Wellman (1986) and Conway, Gathercole, Collins and Anderson (1996), which involved later presenting participants with elements of their diary for recall and recognition tests. In the Conway et al. (1996) study, participants recorded false as well as true memories, and these subsequently appeared in the recognition task (along with new material, as well). The Barclay and Wellman (1986) and the Odegard and Lampinen (2004) studies involved altering the actual memories slightly in order to create false event descriptions. This was done in order to create memory conjunction errors; the false recognition of a false memory, which includes features from at least two previously experienced items. The Conway et al. (1996) procedure involved creating false memories (as well as reporting actual events) over a period of 5 months. Reality monitoring and recognition tests were employed after 7 months. Foil items for the recognition tests were created in line with Barclay and Wellman's procedures; that is, altering records of events and thoughts (changing a detail of a memory so that it is plausible, though never happened) and false records of thoughts and events (although still remaining plausible). These studies used autobiographical lures in recognition tests for the first time. Applying this methodology and rationale to dream work affords the opportunity to make direct comparisons between the different types of memories.

In summary, it is widely recognized that memory for dreams is relatively poor (e.g., Reed, 1974) and that theories of dream recall tend to focus upon recall failure (Cohen and Wolfe, 1973; Freud, 1900; Koukkou and Lehmann, 1983; Koulack and Goodenough, 1974). The salience hypothesis (Cohen and MacNeilage, 1974) relies upon some dreams to be characteristically more detailed than others, thus increasing their chance of being recalled. This, coupled with the evidence that dreams and waking memories differ characteristically (e,g., waking memories being more detailed) leads to the idea that dreams are likely to be less well recalled than waking autobiographical memories.

The experiments in the present chapter investigated the characteristics, recallability, and recognizability of dreams as systematically compared to autobiographical memories. The waking memories were referred to as "events" due to their episodic nature, however, they can be conceived as generally autobiographical as the memories being investigated were reported after they had occurred so they are likely to have been reconstructed in memory, presumably to form part of one's life story. Such reconstruction is characteristic of autobiographical memories (Conway and Pleydell-Pearce, 2000; Conway, Singer and Tagini, 2004). While autobiographical memories have been investigated in detail, the characteristics and processes involved in remembering dreams have not (with the exception of studies by Domhoff, 2002; Foulkes, 1982; Montangero et al., 1996; Montangero et al., 2003). Experiment 1 explored the retrieval of dreams and events that have occurred throughout the lifespan. Experiment 2 employed a diary paradigm, allowing for currently-occurring dreams and events to be recorded shortly after they have occurred. Experiment 2 replicated the design of Experiment 1, with the exception that Experiment 2 investigated dreams and events as they occurred as opposed to relying upon potentially rehearsed and altered retrospective accounts. Both experiments assessed the continuity (Schredl and Hoffman, 2003) between autobiographical memories for waking events and dreams, in terms of retrieval modes and characteristics. These were tested in a quasi-experimental study which involved 3 phases—a diary phase in which dreams and events were recorded (Phase 1), a recall task (Phase 2), and a recognition task (Phase 3).

EXPERIMENT 1

Method

Participants. Students at the University of Leeds were asked to participate in a "dream diary study." Participants were informed that they would be required to recall and report their dreams. They were asked if they usually recalled their dreams. Some participants reported that they struggled with recall, but would engage with the study nonetheless. Initially, 63 participants were recruited. Thirty-seven people managed to record their dreams and events (26 people were unable to recall at least 5 dreams). Only 25 completed the full tasks for both experiments. Sample attrition was likely due to the length of the study and due to some unexpected difficulties encountered when completing diaries at home. Specifically, some participants found it difficult to report their dreams, and some admitted that diary completion was troublesome to incorporate into a morning routine. This resulted in a sample consisting of 4 males and 21 females. The mean age was 19 years. Participants were awarded with participant pool credits and were paid £10 upon successful full completion. The analyses reported here are for the 25 individuals who completed the entire study.

Materials. In the first phase of the study, participants were required to recall dream and waking memories. A standard template was used for each report (see Appendix A). Participants were given a pack of 30 templates (for up to 15 dream and 15 event reports to be recorded). These templates included space for the memory to be handwritten, 4 rating scales (emotionality, comprehensibility, personal importance/salience, and surprise), as well as information about when and where the memory occurred. Characters involved in the memory were listed. For the second phase (recall task), 10 reports were randomly selected consisting of 5 dreams and 5 events. The titles of these reports were presented to the participant as a recall cue. They were then instructed to write as much as they could recall about that event. For the third phase (recognition task), the same 10 reports were selected and from each of these, 4 sentences were generated, with 40 sentences in all. Details of each phase can be found below. All tasks were completed in pen and paper form.

Phase 1. Participants were asked to participate in a study investigating dreaming. They were given materials and asked to recall as many "old" dreams as they could. It was explained that "old" meant they could have occurred at any time in the participants' lives, as long as the memories were at least a week old. Fifteen templates were distributed and participants were instructed to recall as many as possible, with a minimum of five. In addition, participants were asked to complete event templates in the same way, although they only needed to complete as many templates as they had completed dream templates. Participants were reminded that the events did not need to relate to the dreams in any way. Relating the memories would have affected the accessibility comparisons between the dream and event memories. Further instructions on the particulars of completion of the templates (including definitions of the characteristics, etc.) were given verbally. Participants completed these paper templates in their own time and were encouraged to do this in one sitting.

Phase 2. Once these materials had been returned by post, there was an intervening period of about 10 days before phase 2 could begin (the maximum of 21 days was employed for a couple of participants who were unavailable for the next phase until that time). The recall task included the 10 titles of the dream and event reports. The report's title acted as a cue in the recall task. An example of a recall task can be seen in Figure 1.

The participant was instructed to identify whether the report referred to a dream or an event, in a source monitoring task. This was followed by a large box in which the participant was instructed to record their memory of the experience in as much detail as they could. The order of the titles (dream/event) was randomized.

Phase 3. After another latency period of circa 10 days, the recognition task was distributed to participants. There were 10 non-related control sentences in each task, which were the same across all the participants (see Appendix B). These sentences were matched along the dimensions of emotionality, comprehensibility, personal importance/salience, and surprise as they typically appeared for each memory type (as based upon findings from pilot studies from our lab; Horton *et al*., in prep). That is, the dreams were more negatively emotional and surprising, although less comprehensible and salient than the events. The remaining 30 of the 40 items in this task were unique to each participant. Table 1 details the structure of these tasks. The experimental sentences were the first two sentences that had been used in the dream/event reports. The related controls were sentences that had been constructed to relate to the title of the report so to create an experience that was believable and typical of a dream or event. Order of presentation of all items was randomized. Examples of experimental and lure sentences are shown in Table 2. The order of the sentences was randomized. Figure 2 shows the items included in this task for each sentence. Participants were instructed to identify whether each presented sentence had appeared in one of their reports or not. In addition they had to indicate the extent to which they recalled recording the event or dream in question.

Scoring Criteria. There were a number of dependent variables of interest, including the characteristic ratings as well as word counts of reports, the proportion of correctly recalled reports at Phase 2, and proportion of correct identifications of sentences in the recognition task (Phase 3). Detail and episodic richness scores were assigned to the memories as based upon the ratings of the Autobiographical Memory Interview (AMI; Kopelman, Wilson and Baddeley, 1989). The definitions of these are shown in Table 3.

At least 5 dreams had to be recalled for inclusion in each experiment. Participants were encouraged to recall as many events as dreams thus the design was matched in terms of numbers of memories generated. If more than 5 of each type of report were recalled, 5 of these were randomly selected for the subsequent recall and recognition tasks.

Participants had to wait for a period of at least 10 days (and no longer than 21 days) between phases 1 and 2, and 2 and 3. This was to ensure that long term memory of both the recent (current) as well as the retrospective dreams and events was being investigated and to prevent recency effects to aid memory for some of these experiences.

Title: socialising

Dream ☐ Event ☐

When do you think this occurred? ______________________

How much detail can you recall?

All the details ☐ Most of the details ☐ Some of the details ☐
A few of the details ☐ None of the details ☐

Figure 1. Sample item in the recall task.

Table 1. Origins of sentences included in the recognition tasks

	Yes = correct recognition	No = correct recognition
Dream	2 targets	2 control (one related, one not)
Event	2 targets	2 control (one related, one not)

Table 2. Sample stimuli (sentences) included in the recognition task

An Example of a dream experimental sentence: *The garden was very strange and things seemed to be out of proportion.*
Example of an event experimental sentence: *Gave first oral presentation at conference, in Coventry.*
Example of a related control sentence (related to the title, "violin at Albert Hall") *It was amazing to be playing my violin at such a place - the audience was huge.*

1. This sentence appeared in one of your dream/event reports:

I saved Sami (boyfriend) from an accident involving a low-flying aeroplane.

True ☐ False ☐

If true, please indicate the extent to which you recollect the actual event happening:

R ☐ K ☐ F ☐ G ☐

If true, please indicate the extent to which you remember reporting the event:

R ☐ K ☐ F ☐ G ☐

If true, please indicate the extent to which you have thought or talked about the event since its occurrence:

Not at all ☐ not really ☐ moderately ☐ a lot ☐ all the time ☐

Do you think this was a Dream ☐ or an event ☐ ?

Figure 2. Sample item in the recognition task.

Table 3. Definitions of the detail and episodic richness ratings, as outlined in the AMI

Detail (general AMI rating) 3 points: A detailed personal memory that is specific in place and time. 2 points: A specific personal memory with few or no details; OR a less specific event in which time and place are recalled. 1 point: A vague personal memory; OR an incident that occurred on multiple occasions but no single instance is recalled. 0 points: A response based on general knowledge; OR no response.
Episodic richness 3 points: Response is rich in detail, containing at least 2 elaborations, and evokes an impression of true re-experiencing. 2 points: Response has moderate detail and contains at least 2 elaborations. 1 point: Limited detail and/or limited elaboration of events. 0 points: No episodic information. The episodic richness score is a basic extension of the detail score, although refers to the specificity of the occurrence. Elaborations almost always contained sensory-perceptual information.

Results

A mean of 9.72 dreams and 8.28 events were reported. Only the dreams and events from the 25 participants who completed all parts of the study were analyzed.

Phase 1: Characteristics. Table 4 details the characteristics of dreams and events. Events were significantly more salient, emotional (positively), comprehensible and containing more familiar characters than the dreams, which themselves contained significantly more unfamiliar characters than the events.

Phases 2 and 3: Recall and Recognition. As there were many variables of interest in this experiment, recall was operationalized according to a number of variables. A report was deemed to have been recalled if it received a response other than remember "none of the details" to the "how much detail can you recall?" question, and a score of 1, 2 or 3 (so not 0) for both the detail and episodic richness ratings. In addition, the recall task itself should have involved writing down something relating to the original memory itself. Vague responses such as, "…something about going shopping…" were not considered to depict episodic recall. The validity of the recall report was compared with the original report to ensure accurate recall. The numbers of reports fitting these criteria were calculated, producing a recall score for each participant. Significantly more events (90%) were recalled than dreams (83.3%, $t(23) = -2.33$, $p<0.05$).

In order to ascertain how much information of the original reports had been recalled, length (word count), detail, and episodic richness ratings were collected and compared for the original reports and at recall. A series of 2 x 2 repeated measures ANOVAs were conducted on these data measuring the main effects of time (original vs. recalled reports), memory type (dream vs. event) and the time x type interactions. Descriptive statistics for these are detailed in Table 5. Original reports (58.44) were significantly longer then recalled reports (46.95), $F(1, 24) = 7.64$, $p < 0.05$.

Table 4. Experiment 1: Comparisons of the characteristics of dream and event reports

	Mean		
Characteristic	Event	Dream	T-test Results
Word count	62.73	54.15	t(24) = -1.68, n.s
Salience	1.131	.34	t(24) = -5.58, p < 0.001
Emotionality	.324	-.40	t(24) = -4.59, p < 0.001
Comprehensibility	1.128	.25	t(24) = -5.26, p < 0.001
Surprise	.398	.45	t(24) = 0.24, n.s.
No. Familiar	2.443	1.36	t(24) = -4.15, p < 0.001
No. Unfamiliar	.199	.75	t(24) = 5.04, p < 0.001

Table 5. Means (and SDs) for report characteristics in Experiment 1

		Dream	Event
Word count	Original	54.15 (21.26)	62.73 (32.85)
	Recall	39.27 (16.82)	54.63 (34.91)
Detail	Original	2.57 (.32)	2.80 (.21)
	Recall	2.31 (.60)	2.58 (.43)
Episodic Richness	Original	2.27 (.33)	2.22 (.20)
	Recall	2.13 (.63)	2.24 (.48)

A significant main effect of memory was also found, $F(1, 24) = 6.47$, $p < 0.05$, with event reports (58.68) being significantly longer than dreams (46.71). The interaction of these variables was not significant, $F(1, 24) = 1.50$, n.s.

Similarly for the detail scores, a main effect of time demonstrated the original reports to be significantly more detailed than the recalled reports, $F(1,24) = 13.28$, $p < 0.001$. Dreams were significantly less detailed than events, $F(1, 24) = 10.93$, $p < 0.005$, and interaction was far from significant, $F < 1$. Finally, the episodic richness scores were analyzed, although no significant effects were found (all F's < 1.43). The original dream reports were more episodically rich than the recalled reports, although for the events the recalled reports were similar.

A source monitoring task was included, with participants deciding whether the report that they were cued to recall was a dream or an event. Performance in this task indistinguishable for both dreams (85.6%) and events (84.0%), $t(24) = .36$, n.s.

If a presented target sentence (from an actual report) was judged to be "true", or a lure sentence, "false", that sentence had been correctly recognized. The percentages of correctly recognized dream and event sentences (out of the 40 items in each task) were compared and Table 6 details the percentage of hits (correct recognition) and false positives (FPs; incorrect recognition of lure sentences). Recognition performance was similar for both dreams and events. The means of 78.48 and 79.57 for dreams and events, respectively, did not differ significantly, $t(24) = -.96$, $p > .05$. Similarly, the source monitoring task for the target sentences produced high performance for both dreams (82.9%) and events (84.3%) that did not differ significantly from one another, $t(20) = -.43$, n.s.

Remembered and Forgotten Reports. The characteristics of all the reports that remembered in the recall task were compared with those that were not recalled for each individual. This aimed to specifically pinpoint which, if any, of the characteristics seemed to be most important in ensuring that a memory was recalled a month after being reported. For each individual, the dreams and events that were correctly remembered and those that were forgotten in the recall task were compared upon 9 dimensions: report length (word count), detail and episodic richness (both taken from the autobiographical memory interview; on a scale of 0-3), number of familiar and unfamiliar characters featuring in the original report, and salience, emotionality, comprehensibility, and surprise of the original reports. Table 7 illustrates the descriptive statistics for the remembered and forgotten reports for the characteristics measured.

Due to recall performance being relatively high, with a grand mean of 86.67%, there were few "forgotten" reports to be characterized and compared to the "remembered" reports, which were characteristically very similar to the overall trends described previously. This resulted in a small N as some participants remembered all dreams or events, and so they would not have a score for the forgotten reports, thus eliminating their values from the analyses, which produced few degrees of freedom. This, coupled with relatively high SDs, meant that repeated measures ANOVAs were, on the whole, not significant. Despite this the characteristics of the remembered reports were generally higher than the characteristics of the forgotten reports.

Table 6. Recognition performance (and SDs) for dreams and events in Experiment 1

	Hits	FPs	Overall performance
Dreams	91.11 (9.10)	21.49 (24.14)	82.87 (20.02)
Events	90.00 (10.00)	26.60 (24.43)	79.79 (21.16)
Means	90.56 (6.76)	24.04 (23.40)	81.33 (19.97)

Table 7. Mean characteristics (and SDs) of remembered and forgotten reports Experiment 1

Characteristic		Dream	Event	Total
Word count	Remembered	53.47 (21.21)	62.69 (31.76)	59.07 (22.03)
	Forgotten	44.58 (21.46)	76.58 (53.23)	59.04 (42.12)
Detail	Remembered	2.65 (0.29)	2.80 (.29)	2.76 (.21)
	Forgotten	2.27 (.60)	2.83 (.41)	2.71 (.48)
Episodic Richness	Remembered	2.42 (.31)	2.22 (.28)	2.32 (.20)
	Forgotten	2.20 (.59)	2.33 (.41)	2.13 (.52)
Number familiar	Remembered	1.44 (.86)	2.13 (.79)	1.75 (.66)

Table 7. (Continued)

Characteristic		Dream	Event	Total
Number familiar	Forgotten	1.42 (1.80)	2.00 (1.58)	1.40 (.93)
Number unfamiliar	Remembered	.64 (.69)	.37 (.66)	.49 (.46)
	Forgotten	.68 (.72)	.92 (2.01)	.98 (1.39)
Salience	Remembered	.25 (.83)	1.12 (.73)	.67 (.60)
	Forgotten	.38 (.88)	1.25 (.52)	.84 (.47)
Emotionality	Remembered	-.30 (.96)	.34 (.85)	-.01 (.61)
	Forgotten	-.18 (1.18)	.33 (.88)	-.03 (.93)
Comprehensibility	Remembered	.22 (.82)	1.09 (.65)	.64 (.58)
	Forgotten	-.13 (1.23)	1.00 (.89)	.28 (.52)
Surprise	Remembered	.50 (.84)	.35 (.93)	.43 (.72)
	Forgotten	-.23 (.85)	.08 (.49)	-.04 (.36)

Discussion

Memories for dreams were characterised by being less detailed than memories for waking events along a host of self-report measures, and were less detailed using the Autobiographical Memory Interview rating scale. Recall performance was high, with events being more recallable than dreams. Recognition and source monitoring performance was reasonable, indicating that memories for these experiences were accessible. Despite this, the retrospectively recalled memories may well have involved recalling thoughts or conversations about those experiences that had occurred since the actual dream or event, that is, recalling or recognizing a rehearsed experience rather than the original experience itself. The memories generated in Phase 1 of Experiment 1 may have been particularly salient events that had been thought or talked about since their occurrence. This may have increased their likelihood of being recalled at a later date. Further events could have been more rehearsed than dreams, as indicated by their higher salience scores, and considering that dreams are less likely to be discussed than salient events.

Although it is impossible to measure dream experiences without relying upon memory, it seemed necessary to employ a diary paradigm in order to recall experiences whilst they were occurring, at least in the space of a few hours as opposed to months and years. Experiment 2 aimed to investigate whether current dreams and events would show different patterns of recall and recognition to those obtained in Experiment 1. Memories for current experiences were expected to be less rehearsed that retrospective experiences, thus tapping into more valid processes in relation to everyday episodic and autobiographical memory. Coupling this idea with the continuity hypothesis (Schredl and Hoffman, 2003), comparable patterns of recall and recognition across the memory types were predicted.

EXPERIMENT 2

Investigating current dreams and events allowed everyday experiences to be characterized, whilst aiming to achieve greater validity of recalling and recognizing the original memory trace as opposed to a rehearsed version of a memory, which may have been the case for the retrospective experiences characterized in Experiment 1. Recent dreams and events ("current" memories) were instructed to have occurred during the previous night or day, for dreams and events, respectively. The numbers of dreams and events reported were matched in that participants reported the same number of events as dreams. In addition unlike the previous experiment, the recent dreams and events were also matched in terms of when they had occurred.

Design and Procedure. Experiment 2 was conducted in a largely similar way to Experiment 1, but differed in that participants were required to record a dream whenever they could remember one occurring. Thus, if a dream could be recalled from the previous night, they were to record it as soon as possible after waking. Whenever a dream template was completed, an event template was to be completed for an episodic event from the previous day. This meant that if two or more dreams were recorded from one night, a corresponding number of event templates were to be completed for an event that had occurred during the preceding day. This procedure was continued until as many dreams had been recorded as possible. Participants were instructed to keep the diary for at least 2 weeks. However, if participants could not recall any more dreams, the materials were returned. Again, if fewer than 5 dreams and events had been recalled, then the participant was excluded from further phases. Participants were encouraged to record information concerning the date of the diary report (both the date and the hour of occurrence) as well. The ratings for emotionality (whether positive or negative), comprehensibility, personal importance, and surprise were recorded in he same way as in Experiment 1. The same 25 participants completed all phases.

Results

Phase 1: Characteristics. A mean of 9.74 dreams and 9.15 events were reported in a matched design. Table 8 details the characteristics of dreams and events from Experiment 2. Events were significantly more salient, emotional (positively), comprehensible, surprising, and contained more familiar characters than the dreams, which were longer and contained significantly more unfamiliar characters than the events.

Phases 2 and 3: Recall and Recognition. No differences were found between the number of recalled events (70%) and the number of recalled dreams (67.5%; $t(23) = -.340$, n.s.). In order to ascertain how much information of the original reports had been recalled, length (word count), detail and episodic richness ratings were collected and compared over the original reports and at recall. As with the Experiment 1 data, a series of 2 x 2 repeated measures ANOVAs were conducted on these data measuring the main effects of time, memory type, and the time x type interactions. Table 9 details the descriptive statistics for these variables. For the report lengths, a significant main effect of time was found with the original reports being longer than those in the recall task, $F(1, 24) = 54.96$, $p < 0.001$. Experiences reported in the original diary phase (62.18) were significantly longer—about twice as long—as those reported in the recall task (30.47) for recalled reports. There was also a significant main effect of memory type, $F(1, 24) = 14.79$, $p < 0.001$, with dreams (53.07) being significantly longer than events (39.58). The interaction was also significant, $F(1, 24) = 23.68$, $p < 0.001$, illustrating that dreams decreased in length between the time of reporting the experience and recalling it, more than the events decreased.

The same analyses were conducted for the detail scores. The main effect of time, $F(1, 21) = 41.10$, $p < 0.001$, showed that the original reports were much more detailed than the recalled reports. There was no significant effect of memory type, $F(1, 21) = .02$, n.s., as means were very similar. The interaction also did not reach significance, $F(1, 21) =.33$, n.s. As detailed in Table 9, dreams were slightly more detailed than events, and the initial reports were more detailed than those of the recall task.

A significant main effect of time was found for the episodic richness scores, $F(1, 21) = 5.10$, $p < 0.05$. The original experiences (2.11) were more episodically rich than those in the recall task (1.86). The main effect of type was not significant, $F(1, 21) = .535$, n.s., but the interaction was, $F(1, 21) = 5.213$, $p < 0.05$. As for the length of the reports, dreams lost their episodic richness over time more than the events. The source of events were monitored significantly more accurately (83.2%) than dreams (72.8%), $t(24) = -2.40$, $p < 0.05$). Recognition performance was similarly high for both dreams and events, with 75.87% accuracy for dreams and 77.61% for events, $t(24) = -.76$, n.s..

Table 10 displays the hits (correctly recognised targets) and false positives (FPs; incorrectly recognised lures) for the two types of reports. Source monitoring accuracy for the targets in the recognition task did not differ significantly between dreams and events, $t(20) =-2.024$, n.s., although performance was nominally higher for the events than the dreams (means were 85.7% and 78.6%, respectively). Accuracy was comparable to that in the recall task.

Figure 3 illustrates the recall and recognition performances for both dreams and events, across both Experiments 1 and 2, so as to highlight the differences in trends for retrospective and current memories. An experiment*memory (dream/event) * retrieval (recall/recognition) ANOVA was conducted.

Table 8. Comparisons of the characteristics of dream and event reports in Experiment 2

Characteristic	Mean: Event	Mean: Dream	t-test Results
Word count	49.576	74.79	$t(24) = 5.59, p < 0.001$
Salience	.47	-.28	$t(23) = -4.45, p < 0.001$
Emotionality	.38	-.17	$t(23) = -4.53, p < 0.001$
Comprehensibility	1.34	.03	$t(23) = -7.84, p < 0.001$
Surprise	.62	-.27	$t(23) = 5.53, p < 0.001$
No. Familiar	1.95	1.67	$t(23) = -1.27$, n.s.
No. Unfamiliar	.11	.59	$t(23) = 5.57, p < .0001$

Table 9. Means (and SDs) for report characteristics in Experiment 2

		Dream	Event
Word count	Original	74.79 (31.93)	49.58 (23.77)
	Recall	31.35 (22.58)	29.59 (20.55)
Detail	Original	2.81 (.19)	2.74 (.26)
	Recall	2.18 (.60)	2.26 (.62)
Episodic Richness	Original	2.20 (.23)	2.01 (.23)
	Recall	1.82 (.62)	1.91 (.57)

Table 10. Recognition performance (and SDs) for dreams and events in Experiment 2

	Hits	FPs	Overall performance
Dreams	88.22 (18.62)	29.36 (26.08)	77.55 (21.44)
Events	80.67 (17.37)	33.83 (28.02)	71.70 (23.46)
Means	84.44 (15.23)	31.60 (25.90)	74.62 (21.43)

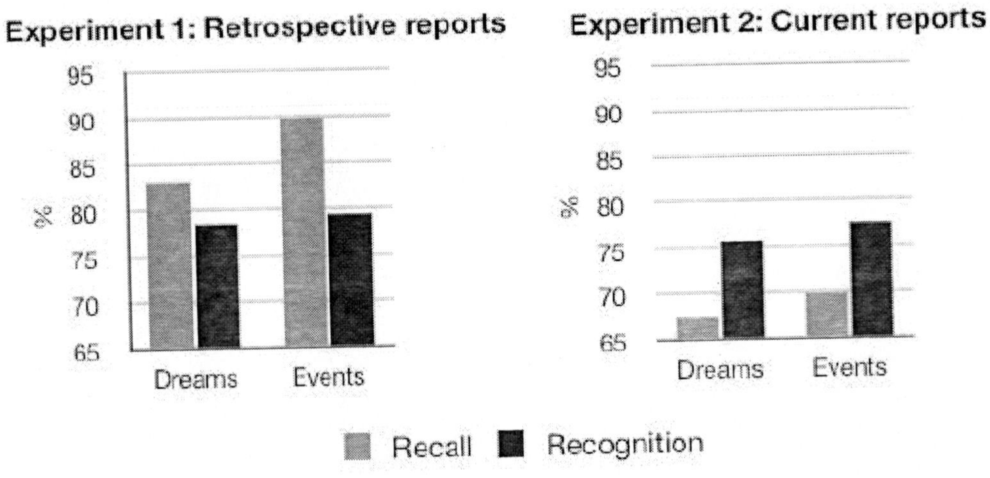

Figure 3. Comparable recall and recognition performance for retrospective and current reports.

A significant main effect of experiment was found, $F(1, 21) = 13.99$, $p<0.001$, demonstrating the higher retrieval performance for retrospective experiences. Specifically retrospective events were better recalled than retrospective dreams and current dreams and events were similarly recallable (experiment*retrieval: $F(1, 21) = 8.20$, $p<0.01$).

Remembered and Forgotten Reports. The same analyses were conducted as described in Experiment 1. The characteristics of all the reports that were recalled in the recall task were compared with those that were not recalled for each individual. Table 11 illustrates the descriptive statistics for the characteristics of the remembered and forgotten reports (dreams and events).

Table 11. Mean characteristics (and SDs) of remembered and forgotten reports in Experiment 2

Characteristic		Dream	Event	Total
Word count	Remembered	75.79 (31.82)	53.81 (29.31)	59.04 (42.12)
	Forgotten	79.64 (53.63)	52.45 (22.05)	65.73 (29.32)
Detail	Remembered	2.87 (.23)	2.86 (.26)	2.85 (.17)
	Forgotten	2.78 (.34)	2.67 (.41)	2.75 (.32)
Episodic Richness	Remembered	2.18 (.27)	2.08 (.27)	2.75 (.32)
	Forgotten	2.09 (.52)	2.03 (.34)	2.06 (.33)
Number familiar	Remembered	1.67 (1.18)	1.70 (.84)	1.58 (.54)
	Forgotten	1.60 (1.14)	1.75 (.66)	1.75 (.76)
Number unfamiliar	Remembered	.78 (.80)	.17 (.33)	.45 (.42)
	Forgotten	.52 (.62)	.18 (.53)	.30 (.43)
Salience	Remembered	-.15 (.98)	.78 (.86)	.38 (.70)
	Forgotten	-.21 (1.19)	.15 (1.12)	.16 (.86)
Emotionality	Remembered	-.39 (.52)	.41 (.83)	.05 (.47)
	Forgotten	-.27 (.69)	.24 (.84)	-.07 (.37)
Comprehensibility	Remembered	-.27 (.96)	1.23 (.86)	.42 (.75)
	Forgotten	-.34 (.95)	1.26 (.57)	.35 (.51)
Surprise	Remembered	.80 (.57)	-.35 (1.04)	.18 (.64)
	Forgotten	.74 (.80)	.18 (1.35)	.66 (.65)

There were few forgotten reports to be characterized and compared to the "remembered" reports. This again resulted in low degrees of freedom coupled with relatively high SDs so few analyses were significant. Main effects of memory were found for report lengths, $F(1, 10) = 8.46$, $p < 0.02$, number of unfamiliar characters described in the experience, $F(1, 9) = 6.82$, $p < 0.05$, for comprehensibility, $F(1, 8) = 51.78$, $p < 0.001$, and for surprise, $F(1, 8) = 7.66$, $p < 0.05$. These mirror the overall trends for the reports as described above. Furthermore, a significant memory x remembered interaction was found for the surprise ratings of the reports. Forgotten reports were less surprising overall. Remembered dreams were surprising, whilst remembered events were not (as indicated by their negative score). Remembered reports were also more salient than forgotten reports, $F(1, 8) = 5.42$, $p < 0.05$.

Discussion

Findings from Experiment 2 indicate that current dreams and events were similarly recallable and similarly recognizable, thus upholding predictions about the comparability of autobiographical remembering for these distinct types of experiences. This was found despite dreams being less characteristically detailed than the events. Of the targets that had been correctly identified in the recognition task of Experiment 2, a t-test revealed that events were rehearsed significantly more than the dreams, according to participants' subjective reports, $t(20) = -2.89$, $p < 0.01$. This supports the idea that events are ruminated upon or discussed more than dreams, which may account for their recall advantage (for retrospective experiences), and also that rehearsal itself is key in remembering (or not remembering) autobiographical experiences, and therefore, dreams.

Experiment 2 was designed to overcome concerns regarding the validity of memories reported at Phase 1 in Experiment 1. However, the same issue may well have been problematic in Experiment 2, although to a lesser degree. Participants were not informed that their memory would be tested for the dreams and events that they reported. However, reporting those experiences in a diary and considering their characteristics when rating the memories was highly atypical of normal experiences. Although the dreams and events had to be recorded in order that the validity of subsequently recalled memories could be checked, this process could well have consolidated those memories much more than would have occurred in everyday life. In addition, dream memories are lost rapidly upon waking, so matching the level of detail in dream memories with event memories at the time of initial reporting is extremely difficult. Matching the amount of detail in dream and event memories would likely involve comparing detailed dreams with vague waking memories, thus comparing experiences that are unrepresentative of everyday life.

Conclusion

Both Experiments 1 and 2 reaffirmed the findings that there are characteristic differences between memories of dreams and waking autobiographical experiences (Johnson et al., 1984; Kemp and Burt, 2006; Kemp et al., 2003), although the findings were extended to include current as well as retrospective memories. Differences were also found between the recallability of those experiences, with retrospective events being significantly better recalled than retrospective dreams. Dreams and events were similarly recognizable. Current dreams and events were comparably recallable and recognizable, indicating that both types of memories were similarly accessible.

Performance in the recall tasks for memories in Experiment 1 was high for both dreams and events (grand mean = 87%). These retrospective experiences were therefore able to be recalled with episodic richness, even though the recalled reports (as opposed to the originally reported experiences) were shorter and less detailed. Recognition performance was also high, although not as high as in the recall task (grand mean = 79%). While this may be surprising given that recognition performance usually far exceeds that of recall tasks, two explanations are offered for these findings. First, the retrospective nature of the task required participants to essentially freely recall memories during Phase 1; at the point of dream and event generation. As these experiences could have occurred at any time throughout the lifespan, it would be surprising for them to have been forgotten in the latency period between Phases 1 and 2. Second, the two measures (recall and recognition) are not directly comparable. The level of detail of the memory being retrieved differed in the two tasks as the recall task required the participant to generate general information about their experience, whilst the recognition task referred to highly specific aspects of a memory, which may have been sensory perceptual in nature. Despite this, the initial findings appear to indicate that dream memories are not lost. If they are reported, then they can be recalled. In addition, if they are especially emotional, comprehensible, salient, or surprising they might be able to be recalled indefinitely.

Performance in the recall task in Experiment 2 was reasonable (grand mean = 69%) and predictably was lower than the recall performance of retrospective experiences. Events were slightly better recalled than dreams on average, although not significantly so. Thus, current dreams and events are less recallable than retrospective dreams and events, with retrospective events being the most recallable. This implies that rehearsal of older experiences (especially events) greatly improved their subsequent recallability, although it was doubtful as to whether the actual experience was being recalled, or an elaborated version of it. Recognition performance of current memories was similar to that of Experiment 1 (grand mean = 76%). It therefore seems that highly detailed (episodic) autobiographical experiences can be recognized providing that adequate cues are present at the time of retrieval.

Dream reports in Experiment 2 were found to be longer than event reports both at the time of being initially reported and at recall, as they required more explanation. A daily event of going to the gym, for example, is clear and comprehensible. Dreaming of being in an unfamiliar gym with people that one would not normally attend with may warrant a lengthier report and, subsequently, a seemingly more detailed report. This does not reflect the intensity or detail of the original experience itself. The method of reporting dreams and events in this way should perhaps be defined more strictly. Nonetheless events were longer than dreams in Experiment 1, likely indicating their extent of rehearsal.

When comparing the characteristics of the experiences that had been remembered as opposed to forgotten, many of the analyses did not find significant effects. This may be due to a number of reasons. First, dream and event reports may not have any characteristic in particular that determines whether an experience is remembered or forgotten. Other factors determine this, such as conscious encoding upon waking, or subsequent rehearsal. Next, the sample size may have been too small, considering the low numbers of reports than had been forgotten, with much variability in the values, for any significant effects to emerge. As events were better recalled than dreams, and they were significantly more salient, positively emotional and comprehensible, it seems that these characteristics may be particularly important in determining the successful retrieval of an autobiographical memory. One noteworthy finding illustrated in Table 7 concerns the detail of the dreams. The remembered dreams were less detailed than the forgotten events. This may suggest that dreams are encoded differently to waking events, as little information about the recalled dreams are available. In Experiment 2, many of the comparisons of the remembered and forgotten reports were also non significant, however remembered (recalled) experiences were more salient than forgotten ones, and remembered dreams were more surprising than forgotten dreams (and indeed remembered events). This highlights the influence of salience upon subsequent retrieval of a memory (Cohen and MacNeilage, 1974).

Considering these differences in the characteristics of dreams and events, it was not surprising that source monitoring performance was similar for dreams and events, as it is assumed that the conscious strategies used in making a source or reality monitoring judgment would be the same for all kinds of experiences (Johnson et al., 1984) For example, this would include assessing the characteristic of that memory: if weak the experience could be a dream, whereas if stronger, it could be an actual experience. Overall, individuals seemed capable of ascertaining whether an experience refers is a dream or an event, as indicated by above chance source monitoring performances. This further implies that dream memories differ characteristically from waking event memories, and may include detail that is typically dream-like or improbable in waking life. Source monitoring performances were higher in Experiment 2 compared to those reported in Johnson et al.'s (1984) experiments, in which participants were required to identify whether presented dreams were their own or belonging to a partner. Findings from the present experiment refer to situations that are more typical of everyday reality monitoring decisions.

Both experiments raised methodological questions in terms of conceptualizing dream recall, and provided insights into its nature. Participants were able to recall dreams when required to do so, in great detail in the case of the current dreams. Thus, dream recall may not be as poor as some authors have suggested (Hobson et al., 2000; Reed, 1974). Still, participants who remained in the entire experiment may have been inclined to recall their dreams, as those who dropped out may have struggled more. Thus, measures of dream recall could often be muddied by sampling bias. Nevertheless, the trends regarding dreams' comparability to waking memories are clear and the two diary studies provide a novel and systematic design for the study of real world autobiographical remembering.

Overall, these data demonstrate that memories for dreams are autobiographical experiences that are recallable and recognizable, providing the dream memory trace is not initially lost. While dreams are characteristically less detailed than waking experiences, they are comparable to them. The relative difficulties in recalling retrospective dreams as compared to retrospective events may reflect how dreams are less rehearsed and less salient than memories for waking events. As to whether this is the result of problems at the level of encoding, likely due to physiology of the sleeping brain, or the result of attending to waking memories more than dreams, remains to be disentangled. Data from recognition tasks in both experiments described here has demonstrated that, if encoded and recorded, dream memories are as accessible as memories for waking events. However, their lack of characteristic detail, coupled with the effort taken to report the dream upon waking, indicates that reconstructive processes of the autobiographical memory system may typify dream recall. As the difference in recallability of dreams and events disappeared when measuring current experiences, it is implied that given the appropriate means to do so (a dream diary and intent), dreams can be recalled and are comparable to waking autobiographical in terms of retrieval trends in the medium term, at least.

APPENDIX A: DIARY TEMPLATE FOR DREAMS AND EVENTS

Date of occurrence: Date__________Month______________Year_________

Hour (time) of occurrence:____________________Time of writing:____________

Title:____

Report of event/dream:

Please continue overleaf if necessary.

Please list characters involved, and their relationship to you:

Character__________________________Relationship______________________
Character__________________________Relationship______________________
Character__________________________Relationship______________________
Character__________________________Relationship______________________

Detail of the setting: ____

Perspective: first person (field) ________________observer perspective__________

What was the main activity____

What was the most distinctive feature of this memory?______________________
____

Rating for personal importance/salience (-2 = extremely unimportant; 2 = extremely important)

-2 -1 0 1 2

Emotional intensity (-2 = extreme negative; 0 = not emotional; 2 = extreme positive)

-2 -1 0 1 2

Comprehensibility (-2 = totally incomprehensible, 2 = totally comprehensible)
-2 -1 0 1 2

How surprising was this event? (-2 = not at all surprising, 2 = very surprising)
-2 -1 0 1 2

APPENDIX B: UNRELATED LURE SENTENCES FOR RECOGNITION TASKS

For retrospective dreams and events (Experiment 1)

Dreams

- I was waiting for a train to arrive in an old quiet station.
- I went off to University and I met three boys from my course.
- I was at home with my family who were having a party and I had worn my best outfit for the occasion.
- I was with my friend and we were late for a meeting, so we ran and ran, although it felt like we weren't moving at all.
- There was a lot of fighting. Things were flying about everywhere. I couldn't see.

Events

1. I couldn't believe I'd left my wallet in there – I was so annoyed.
2. When we found her I was really upset, I couldn't stop crying.
3. My friend had been told not to go, but we went anyway.
4. We went to see a band that I really like, and we had a great time.
5. I had passed the test – I couldn't believe it!

For current dreams and events (Experiment 2)

Dreams

- Later we were at a party with the people I live with.
- My friend told us she was pregnant and we didn't know what to say, so we nervously congratulated her.
- At a Spanish themed bar, having some drinks with friends.
- I was rushing to get ready in time and suddenly I was changed and ready to go.
- I saw what was on the exam paper before I had sat the exam!

Events

* I had just nipped out to the shop to buy some milk and I bumped into an old friend.
* I watched TV with some friends and ate pizza.
* I went for a walk as I was feeling so stressed about it.
* We went out for something to eat, ended up staying out until 1am.
* I went to the lecture, fell asleep through most of it and then left with my friends.

REFERENCES

Barclay, C. R., and Wellman, H. M. (1986) Accuracies and inaccuracies in autobiographical memories. *Journal of Memory and Language*, *25*, 93-103.

Botman, H. I., and Crovitz, H. F. (1989-1990). Dream reports and autobiographical memory. *Perceptual and Motor Skills*, 9(3), 213-224.

Cicogna, P., and Bosinelli, M. (2001). Consciousness during dreams. *Consciousness and Cognition*, *10,* 26-41.

Cipolli, C., Bolzani, R., Cornoldi, C., De Beni, R., and Fagioli, I. (1993). Bizarreness effect in dream recall. *Sleep*, *16*(2), 163-170.

Cohen, D. B., and MacNeilage, P. F. (1974). A test of the salience hypothesis of dream recall. *Journal of Consulting and Clinical Psychology*, *42*(5), 699-703.

Cohen, D. B., and Wolfe, G. (1973). Dream recall and repression: evidence for an alternative hypothesis. *Journal of Consulting and Clinical Psychology*, *41*(3), 349-355.

Conway, M. A. (1990) *Autobiographical memory: An introduction*. Milton Keynes. Open University Press.

Conway, M. A. (2001) Sensory-perceptual episodic memory and its context: Autobiographical memory. *Philosophical Transactions of the Royal Society B: Biological Sciences. 356*, 1413, 1375-1384.

Conway, M. A. (2005) Memory and the self. *Journal of Memory and Language*, *53*(4),594-628.

Conway, M. A., Gathercole, S. E., Collins, A. F., and Anderson, S. J. (1996). Recollections of true and false autobiographical memories. *Journal of Experimental Psychology: General*, *125*(1), 69-95.

Conway, M. A., and Pleydell-Pearce, C. W. (2000) The construction of autobiographical memories in the self-memory system, *Psychological Review*, *107*, 261-288.

Conway, M. A., Singer, J. A., and Tagini, A. (2004) The self and autobiographical memory: Correspondence and Coherence, *Social Cognition*, *22*(5), 491-529.

De Witt, T. (1988). Impairment of reality constructing processes in dream experience. *Journal of Mental Imagery, 12,* 65-78.

Domhoff, G. W. (2001). A new neurocognitive theory of dreams. *Dreaming*, *11*(1), 13-33.

Domhoff, G. W. (2002) *The Scientific Study of Dreams: Neural Networks, Cognitive Development and Content Analysis*. APA Press.

Foulkes, D. (1962). Dream reports from different stages of sleep. *Journal of Abnormal and Social Psychology*, *65*(14), 14-25.

Foulkes, D. (1979). Home and laboratory dreams: Four empirical studies and a conceptual reevaluation. *Sleep*, *2*(2), 233-251.

Foulkes, D. (1982). A cognitive-psychological model of REM dream production. *Sleep*, *5*(2), 169-187.

Freud, S. (1900) *The Interpretation of Dreams*. London: Hogarth Press.

Godden, D. R, and Baddeley, A. D. (1975) Context-dependent memory in two natural environments: on land and underwater. *British Journal of Psychology*, 66, 325-31.

Grenier, J., Cappeliez, P., St-onge, M., Vachon, J, Vinette, S., Roussy, F., Mercier, P., Lortie-Lussier, M., and de Koninck, J. (2005). Temporal references in dreams and autobiographical memory. *Memory and Cognition*, *33*(2), 280-288.

Hartmann, E. (2000). We do not dream of the 3 R's: Implications for the nature of dreaming mentation. *Dreaming, 10*(2), 103-110.

Hicks, R. A., Bautista, J. and Hicks, G. J. (1999) Boundaries and level of experience with six types of dreams, *Perception and Motor Skills, 89*(3), 760-762.

Hobson, J. A., and McCarley, R. W. (1977). The brain as a dream state generator: An activation-synthesis hypothesis of the dream state process. *American Journal of Psychiatry, 134*, 1335-1348.

Hobson, J. A., Pace-Schott, E. F. and Stickgold, R. (2000). Dreaming and the brain: Toward a cognitive neuroscience of conscious states. *Behavioral and Brain Sciences, 23*, 793-1121.

Hodges, S., Williams, E., Berry, E., Izadi, S., Srinivasan, J., Butler, A., Smyth, G., Kapur, N., and Wood, K. (2006). SenseCam: A retrospective memory aid. In P. D. a. A. Friday (Ed.), *Ubicomp* (pp. 177-193). Berlin: Springer-Verlag.

Horton, C. L. and Conway, M. A. (in preparation). Psychometric validation of the Memory Experiences and Dreams Questionnaire.

Horton, C. L., Conway, M. A., and Moulin, C. J. A. (in preparation). A fluency task comparing the accessibility of dreams and autobiographical memories.

Johnson, M. K. (1988). Reality monitoring: An experimental phenomenological approach. *Journal of Experimental Psychology: General, 117,* 390-394.

Johnson, M. K., Hashtroudi, S., and Lindsay, S. (1993) Source monitoring. *Psychological Bulletin, 114*, 3-28.

Johnson, M. K., Kahan, T. L., and Raye, C. L. (1984). Dreams and reality monitoring. *Journal of Experimental Psychology: General, 113*(3), 329-344.

Johnson, M. K., Suengas, A. G., Foley, M. A., and Raye, C. L. (1988) Phenomenal characteristics of memories for perceived and imagined events. *Journal of Experimental Psychology: General, 117*(4), 371-376.

Kahan, T. L., LaBerge, S., Levitan, L., and Zimbardo, P. (1997) Similarities and differences between dreaming and waking cognition: An exploratory study. *Consciousness and Cognition, 6*, 132-147.

Kemp, S., and Burt, C. D. B. (2006) Memories of uncertain origin: Dreamt or real? *Memory, 14*(1), 87-93.

Kemp, S., Burt, C. D. B., and Sheen, M. (2003). Remembering dreamt and actual experiences. *Applied Cognitive Psychology, 17*, 577-591.

Kopelman, M. D., Wilson, B. A., and Baddeley, A. D. (1989) The autobiographical memory interview: A new assessment of autobiographical and personal semantic memory in amnesic patients. *Journal of Clinical Experimental Neuropsychology. 11*(5), 724-744.

Koukkou, M., and Lehmann, D. (1983). Dreaming: The functional state-shift hypothesis. *British Journal of Psychiatry, 142*, 221-231.

Koulack, D., and Goodenough, D. R. (1974). Dream recall and dream recall failure: An arousal-retrieval model. *Psychological Bulletin, 83*(5), 975-984.

Linton, M. (1982). Transformations of memory in everyday life. In U. Neisser (Ed.), *Memory observed: Remembering in natural contexts*. San Francisco: Freeman.

Maquet, P. (2000). Functional neuroimaging of normal human sleep by positron emission tomography. *Journal of Sleep Research, 9*, 207-231.

McNamara, P. (2000) Counterfactual thought in dreams, *Dreaming, 10*(4), 237-246.

Meier, C. A., Ruef, H., Ziegler, A., and Hall, C. S. (1968). Forgetting of dreams in the laboratory. *Perceptual and Motor Skills, 26*, 551-557.

Montangero, J., Ivanyi, C. T., and de Saint-Hilaire, Z. (2003). Completeness and accuracy of morning reports after a recall cue: Comparison of dream and film reports. *Consciousness and Cognition*, *12*, 49-62.

Montangero, J., Pasche, P., and Willequet, P. (1996). Remembering and communicating the dream experience: What does a complementary morning report add to the night report? *Dreaming*, *6*(2), 131-144.

Nielsen, T. A. (2000). A review of mentation in REM and NREM sleep: "Covert" REM sleep as possible reconciliation of two opposing models. *Behavioral and Brain Sciences*, *23*, 851-866.

Odegard, T. N., and Lampinen, J. M. (2004). Memory conjunction errors for autobiographical events: More than just familiarity. *Memory*, *12*(3), 288-300.

Reed, H. (1974) The art of remembering dreams. *Quadrant*, *9*, 48-60.

Rubin, D.C., Schrauf, R.W., and Greenberg, D.L. (2003) Belief and recollection of autobiographical memories. *Memory and Cognition*, *31*(6), 887-901.

Schredl, M., and Doll, E. (1998). Emotions in Diary Dreams. *Consciousness and Cognition*, *7*, 634-646.

Schredl, M., and Hofmann, F (2003). Continuity between waking activities and dream activities. *Consciousness and Cognition*, *12*(2), 298-308.

Schredl, M., and Montasser, A. (1996-7). Dream recall: State or trait variable? Part I: Model, Theories, Methodology and Trait Factors. *Imagination, Cognition and Personality*, *16*(2), 181-210.

Tulving, E. (1983) *Elements of episodic memory*. Oxford: Clarendon Press.

Wolman, R. N., and Kozmova, M. (2007). Last night I had the strangest dream: Varieties of rational thought processes in dream reports. *Consciousness and Cognition*, *16*(4), 838-849.

In: Applied Memory
Editor: Matthew R. Kelley

ISBN 978-1-60692-143-2

Chapter 17

OUR LIFE'S LONG TERM WORK WITH OUR SMALL SHORT-TERM MEMORY: BUILDING BASIC MEMORIES INTO MORE COMPLEX KNOWLEDGE

Robert B. Glassman
Department of Psychology
Lake Forest College, Lake Forest, IL, USA

ABSTRACT

Short-term memory, or working memory, remains fairly constant at 7±2 ("the magical number") chunks across tasks widely different in their time duration demands or their content modalities. Moreover, it remains constant across species—indeed, humans and lab rats have about the same working memory capacity! Why is that so? A close look at some specific "applied memory" episodes in the lives of a couple of young children helps us to understand how an individual's organized growth of knowledge is served well by the working memory capacity that our biological evolution has yielded. Evolutionary natural selection of living systems operates on developmental processes. Convergent evolution and diverse homeostatic regulations must support working memory capacity in its adaptive range, *no matter what* the timescale occupied by the particular memory task or the brain systems that support tasks of that type. In regulatory systems a small range of "play" or permissible error is necessary for stability; hence 7±2 is not an exact constant, but a "fuzzy" one. A modest working memory capacity also is implied by the fact that orderly growth or revision of any complex natural or engineered system requires serial processing in a single "path of attention." Widening our path of attention too much would cause a combinatorial "explosion" of possible orderings to be checked against criteria (e.g. 4 items have 24 possible orders, while 9 items have fully 362,880 permutations). This would weigh down a sequential process. Finessing the problem by processing a lot of information at the same time ("in parallel") can occur only within a system already highly prepared with stereotypical routines. Living systems solve this problem by means of *progressive levels* of development—in a sense, "larger" cognitive units come to be built from units that were built previously. This involves two phases of binding. In the more basic phase, attributes immediately converge from long-term memory into overlearned chunks, of which three or four can occupy working memory at any instant. Pairs of these chunk clusters quickly sequence in working memory to yield a working double cluster of 7±2 chunks. These then form "gists" that participate in a flow of meaning development, as some of the specific item and order information loses its distinctiveness. Such emergence of meaning sometimes leads to formation of a new chunk, which then becomes available for more advanced cognitive processes. There is an analogy here with the developmental phenomena of assimilation and accommodation.

INTRODUCTION

Growing your Memory

As you walk through life you grow. You explore and create in ways that suit you. How do you manage? Sometimes things are going well—but sometimes not, in one of two opposite ways: (1) *Too much* is happening at once, and you're not prepared. "*Get me out!*" (2) *Not much* is happening; restfulness wanes to deep boredom. "*Get me out!*" Between these unhappy extremes, your effortful, probing, problem solving is head-on meeting the challenges you encounter, and successes are often yours. The "chunks" of knowledge you have gathered and shaped, so far, turn out to be appropriate this time, so your abilities are riding high. You are now in the "flow" (Csikszentmilhayi, 1990), freedom exercised consciously and actively, eager partner with the world. Your *applied memory* is being applied well.

In this chapter, we are concerned with the important range between too little and too much as it concerns our cognitive abilities and limitations. In *our life's long-term work, our small short-term memory*—or *working memory*—is analogous to a small "workroom" where new long-term memories are built and where older long-term memories are revised. Further, it is where the most significant mental growth of the individual takes place. Much of what has been grown and tested repeatedly becomes fairly set, drifting into a sort of unconscious long-term "storage," and then another round of growth takes place. These matters stay with us in much the same way throughout life, but they are most obvious when we watch a child. As an entrance point, let us watch a particular little girl during her first year. These brief anecdotes will feed into our understanding of several fundamental questions about memory and begin to help us appreciate our conscious "growing edge" in our very remarkable working memory:

- How does your memory represent the real world?
- What are some of the *kinds* of memory?
- Why, as adults, have we almost completely forgotten our first three years?
- What aspects of memory work unconsciously even when we are adults?
- How does new learning build upon what you know and what you now experience?
- How important is it to *actively* explore, with intentions, in play and work?
- Why is your short-term memory, or working memory, so small in its capacity?

Keep these fundamental cognitive science questions in mind as we take a look now at a corner of the real world.

LIFE IS SHAPED IN FAMILY EVENTS

December 2007 generated good memories for mom and dad and for visiting grandma and grandpa (me). Cassie is all of nine months and three weeks old, more than double her "age" at birth, now crawling and beginning to get into amusing trouble. She's begun to play the "you pick it up I throw it down again game" says her Dr. Mom, having seen a pattern even without having to invoke any of the mathematical significance testing of her profession as a health statistician. Soon, sitting in her high chair, Cassie plays the game with grandma, and I'm a proud grandpa to notice that after throwing an object down Cassie peers around at the floor, apparently trying to track it. Yes, says mom, beating her father (me) by mere milliseconds, as she unfurls a developmental psychology term: "She's had *object permanence* for the past month." After a few more minutes, Cassie will visibly treat *me* as an object to track carefully. Things in the world are achieving independent existence in her mind. There is "objectivity" and persistence, memory's defining attribute.

A CHILD CARVES HER OWN MIND BLOCKS

Indeed, we adults have to take *a lot* of care with kids, for many years. We do much teaching. Yet, it is not we teachers who "work" the hardest. Active seeking is a crucial component of *applied memory*. Cassie's floor tossing looks a lot like experimental research. Little Galileo at work, leaning out from her high chair Tower of Pisa[14] (Pledge, 1959, p. 61), experiments again and again, with each object that dad playfully puts before her, every time trying to follow its fate and its sound on the floor. The spoon is fun. The box is fun. The cloth placemat is fun too, though it doesn't make much of a sound. When you put a new object before Cassie, she examines it for a while before sending it to its precipitous fate. Cassie's experimental method is simple but effective—a grab and toss, stiffly abducting her arm, a fairly ballistic response, yet intelligently flexible in her aiming the reach at the object and in the fact that, when she occasionally misses the grasping part (noticing the miss after her arm completes the abductive tossing movement), she goes for it a second time, now succeeding.

If I allow myself to think more technocratically than I now really care to about this tiny loved one, I notice Cassie's movements lack a certain fine, fluid, continuous control that we adults display when we reach, grasp, and then put (or toss). The baby seems to have a more discrete set of responses, separately turned on and off, yet they are clearly sequenced intelligently. That's my granddaughter there! If play is a child's work, as they say, Cassie seems to be showing us that it's a good thing to go on to more complex understandings well before you polish up your simpler sensory and motor abilities.

When grandma, sitting on the left, teases a little by catching the object and putting it back before it can hit the floor, Cassie is hardly fazed; she next tosses it down to the right.

> Ah. These objects have interesting properties! As a human being I can outwit the big caretaker animate objects in the way I handle the inanimate objects they put before me.

---

[14] The well-known story about Galileo dropping objects of different weights from the Leaning Tower of Pisa, to study how quickly they fell, may be apocryphal. What is more certain is that he slowed down the acceleration by rolling balls down various inclined planes.

We are a twenty-first century American family—living about 2000 airplane miles apart. Cassie likely does not remember my rocking her to sleep in my arms during my first visit when she was two weeks old. I am not yet *that* cohesively permanent in her long-term memory. But now, when I walk away from the kitchen, she cranes her head to the right, to pick me up again, about fifteen feet away in the living room. More peering intently, this time at me, a moving object that makes different sorts of sounds than the ones she tosses onto the floor. Excellent target acquisition! Her consciousness of the present has a good degree of persistence. Her working memory is doing just as it should with at least one "object" at a time (me).

Episodic Memories, Childhood Amnesia, and Growth of the Alert Unconscious

There is lots and lots of careful study going on here, mainly on Cassie's part. But you know what? Although the knowledge she is now acquiring will become part of many larger patterns of knowledge, none of this will be available for Cassie's reminiscing over tea and scones when she's an adult. As distinct events, they will be gone. As a cognitive psychologist would put it, none of this is likely to last in Cassie's *episodic* memory (Tulving, 2002), which probably is a very good thing. After all, imagine how distracting it would later be to remember these moments well enough to describe them. *All* these episodes are now so excitingly attention grabbing. Lest Cassie miss any of it, the loving adults around her insist, with high-pitched urgency, that each of these events is just amazing. We are pretending that she sees things the way we see them, *naming* each object and event as if merely reminding her. We insist that each such "reminder" is worth attention at this very moment! We squeal unashamedly. We are all so engaged in this dance with a baby that we hardly realize how important these lessons are. What fun it is to program a child's memory.

As we get older, we accumulate episodic memories. We *remember the past*, and that helps us to *see the future*, both clearly toward the fairly certain near future (*"oops, it seems icy here; if I don't walk more carefully I'll slip and fall again"*) and less clearly, but making good guesses about possible, more distant futures (*"mom's gotten good sleep on vacation this week; maybe this is a good time to ask for a car"*). In thinking such thoughts we consciously picture the timeline of our life. That timeline has historical markers of "main events" such as birthdays, such as school graduations, and such as "remember that time we …," (Neisser and Hyman, 2000).

We adults are not too bad at recalling our life's overall sequence or at judging when likely future events will occur. But such long-term autobiographical timelining would likely get in the way of a baby's main cognitive tuning up. She's busy with smaller, more local, close-up pieces of time, space, and stuff. First, set up the basic categories of objects, events, and controlling-the-world-around-me intentions. Then, later, these mind tools will be put powerfully to work into bigger plans. Many of them will become readily available memory "chunks."[15]

[15] "Chunk" has been adopted widely as a technical term in research on working memory, referring to any grouping of objects or attributes that has become so familiar that it has a unitary quality in your thinking.

These all-important early stages of mental building must be why we all eventually wind up with fairly dense *childhood amnesia* for events before about the age of three years (Bauer, 2007). That eventually comes of our baby and toddler memories when we grow up, even though any typically articulate two-and-a-half-year old can easily and clearly tell you about, say, her visit to the hardware store last month with dad!

Procedural Memories Drift out of Consciousness

There is also a great deal of additional memory whose details we adults usually leave out of consciousness—the memories of how to see and do things skillfully. Again, it would be distracting to keep concentrating on the minutiae of our perceptual and motor skills, once we have them down. Cassie does not yet see things the way we do, so on this visit grandma is working hard, with safety in mind.

Consider stairs. Upon achieving enough control over your spinal locomotor reflexes to use them for exploratory crawling, one quickly finds that stairs are fun. Strange but true: Much of our human ability to skillfully sequence locomotor movements is innate, born into us, just as with other creatures. Moreover, these skills largely are built right into our lowest-level neural circuitry, in the gray-and-white matter connections of the spinal cord itself (Bear, Connors, and Paradiso, 2007). Of course, we humans are not as good at birth as a swimming fish, or as a foal that stands and walks soon after emerging from its mother. More of the complex things we humans do skillfully wind up "upstairs," in higher brain regions.

For Cassie, it won't be for many years that her ol' rock-climbing mom declares—and hopes Cassie remembers explicitly—"it's a lot easier to go up than to come down!" Perhaps her ol' tree-climbing grandpa will have already mentioned that. Or her ol' surfer dad will have explained a somewhat similar property of big Pacific Ocean waves. For now, concerned about Cassie's north end—which will become the precious repository of such knowledge—grandma keeps a close hand on her diapered south end. Cassie negotiates upward on the stairs, blithely unaware that, unlike when crawling on the floor, one cannot just stop and sit up. There won't be any floor there to support your butt! Let's see if this is among the things doting grandma can help keep her from learning the hard way.

Eventually, Cassie will learn well how to integrate and modulate all these little routine behavioral units that currently yield such bright experiences. She will remember these and other vital skills so well that she won't even know she knows them. Older kids and adults hardly ever think explicitly about all our competent routines—what psychologists often call our *procedural memories* (e.g., Sternberg, 2003). Cassie will become more at home, in space and time, and with the objects and events that fill space and time. She may well some day relate, to her more earthbound friends, an episodic memory of how remembering grandpa's advice about coming back down a tree made her a little more observant on the way up, once upon a climbing time, and saved her from the embarrassment of having to use her cell phone to call the fire department from a high branch. Judging by the vigor and persistence of her present "DADADADADA" battle cry as she crawls to the kitchen, she will accumulate such stories and enjoy telling them. Each such explicit story will also contain an implicit lesson in living.

Declarative Memories for Remembering Generalities—Allocating Consciousness Well

It may be just as well not to remember all the details of the many lessons in stair climbing, crawling, grasping and throwing, and many more to come, of our most basic skills. Cassie will never tell the following story: "And listen to this: Not only the eighth time, but I remember how I almost fell down the stairs a *ninth* time as I was going up after that chirping bird toy, except that grandma fortunately had her hand under my bottom!" It would be boring and distracting later on to reminisce about such things. Better to occupy consciousness instead with more mature problems in life whose possible solutions are harder to predict. So, hooray for the *childhood amnesia* that winds up submerging our first three years.

Language is a handy device that helps us deal with such larger problems in life. Judging by Cassie's impish grin when she disobeys mom's smiling suggestion "no" not to toss her food on the floor, Cassie is well on her way into English phonemes, and beyond, to words and conversation. Her cousin Alex, six and a half years old this same December (and—modern American family—living 3000 miles away on the other coast), already has quite a mouth on him, handy for being agreeable, or disagreeable, or—wise guy—cleverly both at once. Grandma on the telephone one recent Sunday evening: "Did you and dad just have a good weekend?" Alex: "Have we ever not had a good weekend?" This generalized reminiscence is a nice example of what cognitive psychologists call a *declarative memory* (e.g., Sternberg, 2003).

In addition to learning to read, in first grade now, and to chatting about the Harry Potter stories dad has just read to him, Alex is finding language a handy device to parse space and time to hold discrete units in memory; his recitation aloud helps to mobilize these units in learning a manipulative sequential skill. "Hold the loop, wrap it around, push another loop through, etc." and bingo (well, actually, not quite bingo yet), his shoelace is nicely tied.

I will probably hold on to this particular *episodic memory*, which marks my oldest grandkid's entry into a new phase, longer than Alex himself will, once he has it down as a brisk, fluid automatic sequence of movements that partially overlap each other in time, a *procedural memory*. Alex is now well past the part of life when virtually all explicit details disappear into *childhood amnesia*, but there is no point in remembering all these instances of shoelace practice. Within another several years, they will probably blend together into more general *declarative* memories—less individual episodes, more general descriptions, such as "those times grandma and grandpa visited," "those times dad and I went camping together," or "those times we rode our bicycles together" or "have we ever not had a good weekend?"

An Important Duality of Memory

We have just considered some vivid examples of kinds of memory cognitive psychologists have identified, and have done so in a way that helps us see how conscious and unconscious processes can participate in individual growth. We are now in a good position to focus closely on the significance of human cognitive abilities and limits as they concern the relationship between *long-term memory* and *working memory*.

In a very real sense, your memory is who you are. Memory is the knowledge that enables you to grow along the journey through life. Cognitive psychologists have elucidated the structure of memory by naming and trying to explain its different parts and forms. Among the most fundamental categories are two: (1) *long-term memory*—which is to say all of the extremely many things that you know well—and (2) *short-term or working memory*—which concerns the relationship your long-term memory bears with the "now" moment of your life (Baddeley, 1986; Ericsson and Delaney, 1998; Richardson et al., 1996).

A Basic Fact about Working Memory

Over a half-century ago, in 1956, cognitive psychologist George A. Miller published what has become one of the most famous papers in all of psychological science, entitled "The magical number seven, plus or minus two: Some limits on our capacity for processing information" (see Ebbinghaus 1885/1964, for a precursor to this discussion). In this remarkable review, Miller whimsically spoke of being "persecuted" by the integer 7, which kept turning up in his own and others' studies of human cognitive capacity. For example, people can *reliably* rate any quantity whatsoever on a scale of about 1 to 7—loudness, brightness, the intensity of a particular taste, the length of a line, the degree of attractiveness of a scene, etc. Suppose you completed the same estimation task a second time without remembering your first rating—the new rating would probably come out the same. Indeed, the rating almost surely would come out the same if you used a scale of 1 to 5. If you tried to use a scale of 1 to 9, you would still be pretty reliable although there might be a little slippage from the first to the second attempt. But go beyond the range of 7±2, say to a scale of 1 to 12, and you surely would show unintended shiftiness in your judgments from one estimation to your next attempt to estimate the same quantity. The scale of seven seems to be about all you can keep in mind at once.

Miller also famously pointed out that the same "magical number seven" cropped up in laboratory studies of how many items you could hold at once in your immediate memory when someone gives you a list. Let's say someone reads seven random words to you, or presents you with seven randomly ordered digits. You can very likely reproduce them back right away, no problem. But try to do that with, say, 14 new unrelated items. Problem!

Many thousands of scientific papers have been published in attempts to better understand this basic fact about memory. But this fact is not reserved for the science laboratory, because it is such a fundamental aspect of *applied memory* in real life. A nice thing about this scientific fact: We need not warn each other, "Don't try this at home, kids." *Do* try it with a friend or a relative.

Working Memory's Dimensional Elasticity Preserves Numerical Constancy

In his famous paper, George Miller emphasized how strange it was that "the magical number seven" cropped up so often in so many different ways, in studying immediate memory and capacity to make conscious quantitative categorical judgments. Since then, the quantity range 7±2 has proven even more strange and "magical" than Miller recognized. We come now to two peculiar findings about the small capacity of working memory.

- First, this capacity is the same in lab rats (and several other vertebrates that have been studied) as it is in human beings.
- Second, this capacity seems largely independent of the time it takes to complete a working memory task.

Indeed, we first recognized that paradoxical finding about time durations in considering some of the work that had been done with working memory capacity in animals, so let us consider that first. We will then consider how that led to a closer look at our own and others' findings about working memory capacity in humans. Putting all that together will lead us to a deeper appreciation of how working memory participates in individual growth and also why working memory capacity *evolved* as it has. In turn, that reasoning will suggest the new hypothesis that working memory capacity is a *regulated* quantity. That is: *There must be a kind of higher-level homeostasis in many diverse brain systems, which maintains working memory capacity within its proper quantity range of about 7±2.*

Rats R us: The Comparative Study of Working Memory Capacity

During the same era in the history of science as George Miller published his famous article about human cognition, others were working hard developing the study of cognitive neuroscience in animals (Fessard, Gerard, and Konorski, 1961; Milner, 1970). Animals are extremely interesting for their own sake, but also for the ways in which observing their differences and similarities to humans give us new perspectives. Indeed, it is valuable when we find that a species of animal is similar to us in some way. We then have the opportunity to try out more varied observations with the animals (while exercising proper ethical concerns, of course). For example, the brain of our mammalian cousin, the ubiquitous laboratory rat, is very similar in its detailed structural features to the human brain (Braitenberg and Schüz, 1998). Among these ways is the fact that the most recently evolved and largest part of the human brain, our cerebral cortex, looks very much the same under a microscope as that of the rat—right down to its large, dense population of treelike "pyramidal" neurons and to its overall sheet-like shape, having a thinness of only about 2 millimeters (Glassman, 2002).

If rats could speak, we might then look very closely for possible cognitive similarities with humans in verbal memory tasks. Equally well, however, we might then hesitate to carry out studies involving experimental brain manipulations with creatures that were "so human" as to have language. As it happens, lab rats are good subjects for the lab because they are both same and different in comparison with humans. They are similar enough to study thoroughly for potential insights, while they have sufficiently less self-conscious sentience than a human being to imply permissibility of carrying out thoughtful research with them.

During the 1970s, research showed that laboratory rats, in a spatial memory task called the "radial-arm maze," displayed about the same working memory capacity, as do humans in a verbal task—however, this important connection between animal research and human research was not made for many years afterwards. In such spatial memory tasks, rats are trained simply by putting them in the center of an asterisk shaped platform every day for a few weeks, until their natural ratty foraging explorations lead them to learn that there is a sweet food morsel at the end of each of the arms (see Figure 1). Once they learn that, on any given day when they are put into the radial maze, they tend to visit the end of each arm only once, retrieving each piece of food and eating it.

Now, you or I, if placed in such a situation would probably retrieve each of the rewards efficiently, simply by going systematically in a clockwise or counterclockwise direction to each of the ends. Rats, for some reason, prefer to seek out the rewards choosing the arms in an order that looks random. Perhaps it is a very old, instinctive, "species memory" that tells them to be unpredictable in their movements while in an open space—a good principle for any little animal to follow, lest a hungry predator be watching and remembering. Whether or not the animals themselves understand why, biological evolution by natural selection has led them (and humans) to have various self-protective behavioral dispositions. At any rate, whether or not we have correctly guessed the reason, rats generally do choose to go down the different arms in a random order. Yet, they usually perform perfectly in a radial maze that has up to eight arms (Olton, 1979).

These rats appear to use *their working memory capacity* to accomplish that feat, rather than using any "cheap tricks" such as sniffing where they have already been (Dale and Innes, 1986; Olton, Collison, and Werz, 1977). In the cleverest proof, experimenters built a radial maze whose center area could be kept still, while the arms around it were rotated. The rat was put in, allowed to make his choice of the first four of the arms, and was then kept in the center (by a set of doors that closed) while the arms were rotated 180 degrees. When released, the rat finished out the task, with precision going to the remaining four unvisited positions in the space of the room, but in so doing, it went down some of the very same arms as it had gone down earlier—the ones that had moved into those previously unvisited spaces. This nice experiment illustrates the wonderful scientific problem solving that researchers sometimes succeed in, using clever experimental designs. Although rats usually carry out the eight-arm maze task without errors, they do make errors of returning to the same arm when there are 12 arms or 17 arms (Brown, 1992; Olton and Samuelson, 1976; Olton, Collison, and Werz, 1977). This suggests that we have again encountered "the magical number" 7±2, now in a nonhuman species. Can we possibly be the same as lab rats in this way?

A Fair Interspecies Competition

To make a closer comparison between the animal and the human studies, after completing a preliminary test with humans using a drawing of a radial maze (O'Connor and Glassman, 1993), we asked people to carry out a spatial memory task modeled after the radial maze, illustrated in Figure 2. On nice summer days on our college campus, we asked people to begin in the center of a 15-meter diameter (about 50 feet) asterisk-shaped set of lines painted on the grass and to try walk to the end of each "arm" once and only once, retrieving the place-marker that was under the inverted flower pot at the end of each arm.

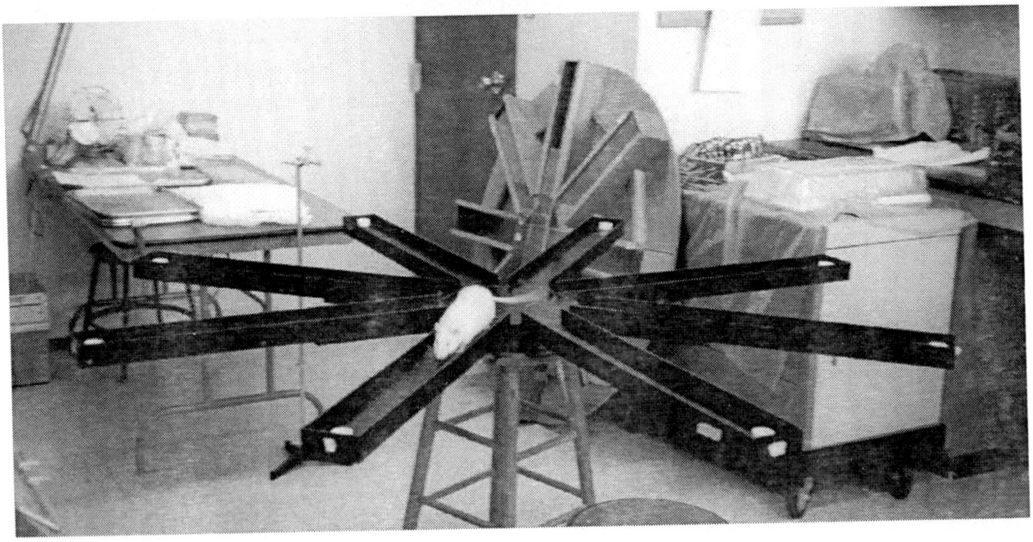

Figure 1. A laboratory rat retrieving food in one of the arms of a radial-arm maze.

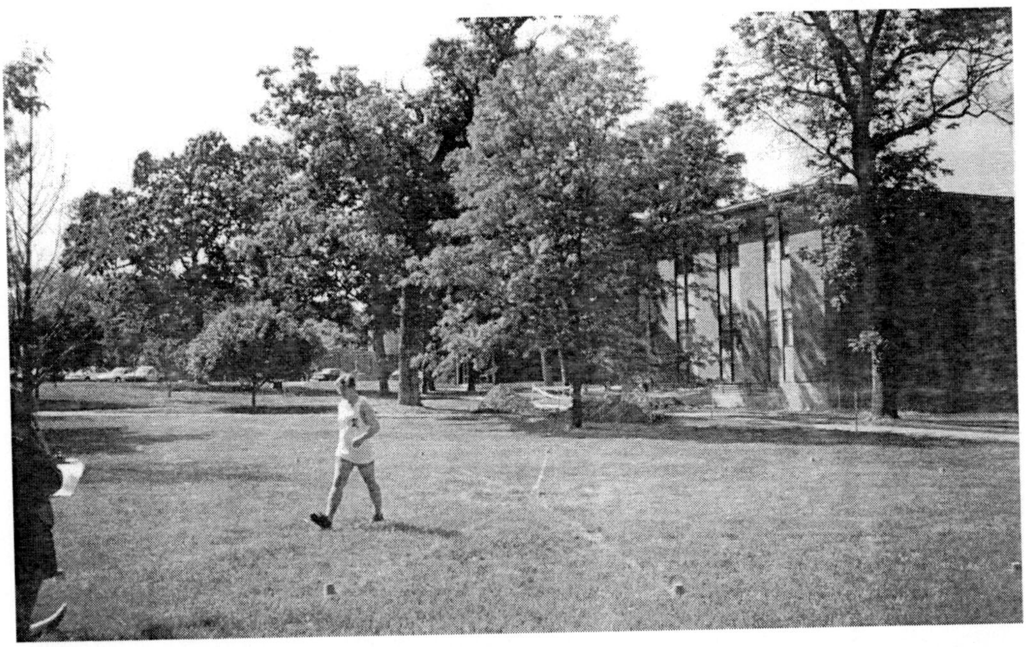

Figure 2. Illustration of a person in our outdoor radial maze.

We first explained to each participant the importance of making such comparisons across species, both for the sake of better understanding and for the new possibilities that it opens up for eventually finding treatments for human brain disorders that impair memory. We asked our kind volunteers, politely and with good humor, to "make it a fair contest" with the rats, by trying to choose arms in an unsystematic order, relying on memory not to repeat the same arm more than once.

We found that almost all the undergraduates could perform perfectly in the eight-arm maze (some professors did not do quite as well), but they made errors when asked to perform in a maze having thirteen arms or one having seventeen arms. Indeed, the number of errors humans made in those mazes was about the same as the number of errors lab rats make in the comparable tasks—about two errors in a 12- or 13-arm maze and about three errors in a 17-arm maze.

After puzzling over these data, we realized that probability mathematics would help in handling the likelihood that some of the arm choices were guesses, especially toward the end of a run-through, when only one or two unvisited arms remained. Indeed, it turned out that the scores in all the mazes implied that spatial working memory capacity was about eight or nine positions – very close to "the magical number seven" that had cropped up in so many human working memory experiments (Glassman, Garvey, Elkins, Kasal, and Couillard, 1994)! These findings with humans were soon replicated in other laboratories (Bohbot, Jech, Ruzicka, Bures, and Nadel, 1994; Ranck, Harris, Bleicher, Rotenberg, Stead, and Kubie, 1997). A comprehensive set of experiments in a large outdoor setting in the countryside of Russia revealed comparable capacity in a number of other animal species (Lipp et al., 2001).

In subsequent additional research at Lake Forest College, we compared human subjects to species of birds that are good at hiding food in caches and then finding it when needed. We learned that people who hid 12 place markers unsystematically under their selection of 42 inverted flower pots arrayed at random in a large open area could, afterwards, find about seven of those place markers (Glassman, Knabe-Czerwionka, Branch, and Brown, 2001; Glassman, 2003a)

Strange "Time Paradoxes" of Working Memory

That last experiment was a follow up on an additional set of radial maze experiments we had carried out in making a further comparison between the working memory of people and rats. They concerned a peculiar time elasticity, which has turned out to be an additional part of the "magic" of that "sevenish" range between 5 and 9 (that is, 7±2).

During the 1980s, researchers carrying out radial maze memory experiments with rats had stumbled across a surprising persistence over time of what they had been thinking of as "short-term" memory. Then, pursuing the issue, these experimenters learned that well-trained rats, after going down four of the arms of an eight-arm radial maze, could complete the task fairly accurately with the remaining four arms, on a day when they were actually removed from the maze for several hours (Beatty and Shavalia, 1980; Maki, Beatty, Hoffman, Bierley, and Clouse, 1984)! This seems incredible. Could human beings also do as well as rats if a delay were interposed at mid-task?

Rather than trying to keep undergraduate volunteers' attention long enough to see whether they could sustain a delay of several hours, we made a more practical decision to test people with a five-minute delay and then, when they succeeded in that, with a fifteen-minute delay. In an attempt to prevent people from turning this spatial memory task into a verbal memory task by naming the different positions, we filled the delays with an attention-occupying distracting task that required the use of spatial memory. We found that our undergraduate participants were indeed able to succeed in the eight-arm radial maze task, even with a fifteen-minute delay interposed midway (Glassman, Leniek, and Haegerich, 1998).

That finding is striking; however, on further thought, it simply confirms something we might have already realized about the mystery of "the magical number seven" when we began comparing radial maze memory to human verbal memory. That is, although a verbal working memory task can be done as quickly as you can hear and then say seven digits or letters or words—in well under a half a minute—the radial maze task takes several minutes, even when there is no deliberately imposed delay, because that's how long it takes for a rat or a person to walk down all the arms, also with a bit of pausing and deciding thrown in while surveying things from the center area. Further, the memory literature contains additional "time paradoxes." As background for grasping their significance, you have to know about the so-called *recency effect* in studies of working memory (e.g., Isarida and Isarida, 2006). If a person is given a list of words to remember that is long enough to exceed the usual "magical number seven" limits of working memory capacity—say fifteen words—they can remember only about seven of those words, and their recall is best for those words that were presented to them most recently, at the very end of the list. Of course, that's not surprising. Not surprising either is the fact that if the subject is made to delay recalling the list for 20-30 seconds while engaged in some distracting task, they forget those most-recently heard words of the list. We are all quite familiar with this tendency to forget things recently experienced.

But a surprising time paradox comes in under an experimental condition in which the list to be remembered is *presented slowly*, with a distraction-filled delay between each of the words and the next. That might seem to make everything more difficult, and it does, but only slightly. More interestingly, when an additional delay is then imposed before the subject is allowed to recall the words, the last few words are now remembered—the recency effect returns (e.g., Bjork and Whitten, 1974)! That finding has since been amply replicated and extended in studies with human beings carrying out verbal memory tasks, and there has been a vigorous search for the underlying explanation. Some of that work is described next.

Distinctiveness, the Serial Position Effect, and the "Ratio Rule"

Some attempted explanations of the slowly-presented list extended-recency effect have tried to replace our usual assumption about the importance of *absolute time durations*, when thinking about the degree to which forgetting takes place, with the issue of *distinctiveness* and with a related emphasis on *relative time durations* (Nairne, 2002). The relative time durations compare the amount of the delay required before recall with the amount of time that was present between each item of the list and the rest.

Such explanations concern the more general issue of the *serial position effect*, another of the most widely replicated findings in cognitive psychology laboratory studies of word list memory (e.g., Tan and Ward, 2000). This effect incorporates the *recency* phenomenon that we have just considered, together with its partner, *primacy*. That is, we tend to remember both the beginning and the end of a list better than the middle of the list. Among the plausible potential explanations of this effect is the idea that the beginning and end of the list are always *distinctive*. Yes, sometimes other parts of the list may be distinctive—for example, if the word "supercalifragilisticexpialadocious" occurs in the middle, you are likely to remember that (e.g., von Restorff, 1933). But the beginning and the end appear to be distinctive no matter what (Murdock, 1960).[16]

To study this issue much more carefully, Nairne, Neath, Serra, and Byun (1997) decided to look much more systematically than had been done before at the strange list-learning finding we discussed above—namely, that the serial position effect persisted, with a primacy effect at its head and a recency effect at its tail, even when lists of items are presented to the subject at a slow pace, with distractions in between each pair of items and a distraction at the end before being allowed to do the recall task. These researchers used a wonderfully simple testing situation in which undergraduates were asked to remember, in correct order, just a list of six randomly ordered letters. That's a pretty easy task, and the undergraduate subjects generally did well remembering letters in almost all positions at better than 50% accuracy. But they also made errors, and these errors nicely illustrated the serial position effect. As in the aforementioned studies demonstrating a peculiar flexibility of time, the serial position effect continued to show itself even when Nairne et al. (1997) stretched out the duration of presenting the letters by interposing random numbers in between each pair of letters in the list, and at the end of the list.

The comprehensive systematic variations that these psychologists carried out enabled them to look carefully and mathematically at a hypothesis, called the *ratio rule*, about the relative distinctiveness of individual items in each list. Other researchers had proposed this hypothesis earlier as an explanation of the recency part of the serial position curve (see Tan and Ward, 2000). Without going into all the detail, the basic idea is that our degree of distinct memory of each individual item depends on how far apart they seem from our current perspective in time. Thus, after hearing or reading a list, we are "closest" to the most recently heard items. Like looking at a parade of people marching but now beginning to disappear into the distance, it is easiest to see the few marchers who passed you most recently. Even if the marchers are spaced out from each other, you can distinguish the last few of them while earlier ones are starting to blend together in the "perspective" of your memory.

NATURE AND NURTURE: CHILDREN ALSO HAVE ABOUT THE SAME WORKING MEMORY CAPACITY

Although the line of investigation that concerns distinctiveness and the *ratio rule* is important, by itself it neglects the most striking and obvious fact about working memory capacity, that it almost always remains constant in the same range. Remember: The working memory capacity of humans seems to be only as great as that of lab rats! How can that possibly be? Yes, as scientifically educated human beings we have humbly learned how similar we are to "other animals" in physical makeup and in psychology. But it is also true that biological evolution has made us much greater than other animals—in our social intelligence, in our ability to use language, and in other ways. Indeed, one of the deep questions evolution researchers dwell on concerns the main natural selection factors that

[16] I should note that distinctness of time intervals to which a subject is asked to pay conscious explicit attention is also an interesting topic of psychophysical research (Grondin, 2002). Such studies, as well as ones that consider the fundamental bases of biological timing (Glassman, 2000; Palmer, 2002), might profitably be compared to these issues of primacy and recency, where timing is an important implicit factor.

created humans, from extremely ape-like ancestors only five million years ago, to our present human form less than 100 thousand years ago (Lumsden and Wilson, 1983). Consider that dinosaurs walked the earth for fully 125 million years or more (Colbert, 1965). Then, "a day later," in evolutionary time, we came along. Hello. Human beings really are something else.

We humans make and use tools. We pass knowledge around the world and down through historical time, by word of mouth, books, and for the past century, by electronic media technologies. We have culture. Yes, we have *nature*, just as other animals do, but we engage in so much more productive, long-term *nurture* than any other creature. At our best we use our human abilities to build civilizations in which we live larger and better lives. So how in the world can it be that creatures as intelligent as we are have a working memory capacity only equal to lab rats'? This question becomes poignant when we study cognitive development in children. Our working memory capacity is not all there is to our human intelligence, but there is a degree of correlation. Much research has shown that children become able to think more competently as their capacity to hold several items in mind increases (e.g. Cowan, 1997; Schneider and Pressley, 1997; Weinert and Schneider, 1995).

Because we are about to set this interesting and important fact to one side, it bears emphasis in all fairness: In these studies of development in children, as well as in studies of aging and of individual differences among young adults, many researchers have found that while there is little correlation between working memory capacity and measures of ability to think, or "fluid intelligence" when the simplest measures of working memory are used—lists of digits or short words—there is a more significant correlation (usually on the order of $r = 0.2$ to 0.5) when these simpler working memory measures are replaced with "complex working memory span" measures, in which each item to be remembered is preceded by a short distracting sentence ("sentence span") or simple arithmetic calculation ("operation span"). Many different variations of procedure have yielded results such as this, and they tend to be interpreted by the researchers as supporting a view of working memory that is both distinct from long-term memory and which has more than one component subsystem or process, a "primary" memory in which a few items are immediately available to the subject, and a "secondary" memory, from which another few items of material have to be retrieved (Engle et al., 2008).

Yet all these findings add up to a case of "a small difference making a small difference." Even a correlation as high as $r = 0.5$ accounts for only 25% of the variance; interesting, but not really a dominating effect. One wonders what sorts of intelligence or creativity may not be captured by the psychological tests that lead to these correlations. Moreover, it is *not* as if babies begin with a working memory capacity of *one* item and then it grows to *hundreds* by the time we are adults: The *biggest* our capacity ever gets is to "the magical number" 7 ± 2! There is a problem here. Cognitive scientists may have paid too much attention to small differences and not enough attention to this basic consistent fact, which they all know so well. We may have been "missing the forest for the trees." The "trees" are our thousands of interesting findings about memory capacity. Go browsing in your college library. Look at any of the psychology journals that include coverage of cognition. Do you see what I mean? Become engrossed in those "trees." Look up articles by the authors just cited, and delve into some of the factors that influence the numerousness of working memory capacity; besides a child's age, what other variables correlate with this quantity?

But next, again, take a few steps back. From this new vantage you can see the "forest"; all those working memory capacity variations come to about the same thing. Under all circumstances, working memory capacity is "*at most several* and *at least a few*." So what? So this: Understanding this fact requires looking at working memory capacity from a broader perspective than has been typical in cognitive psychology. *This fact must reveal a basic constraint that reality imposes on the evolution of intelligence.* As I explain below, that constraint has to do with *maintaining order in anything that grows*. It will help to get us to that point if we first further consider why the "forest" has remained insufficiently appreciated.

MISLEADING HEURISTICS CAN PLAGUE SCIENTISTS AS MUCH AS ANYONE ELSE

Why have cognitive scientists become so obsessed with small differences in working memory capacity that they have paid too little attention to its almost-constancy? I think it may be due to two ordinary thinking short cuts that are usually very handy both in science and in life. As with all heuristics, they can be mistakenly applied (Thaler and Sunstein, 2008).

The "Wealth" Heuristic. "More is better." This is often true. More is typically better in your scale of wages for an hourly job and for the length of a much-awaited vacation in Hawaii. Try to think of more examples. More is better when you are cramming for an exam in school; memorize as much as you can, hoping it sticks for at least a few days. But more is *not always* better. Think, for example, of how much you ought to stuff in your backpack before walking all the way to class. Or, how fast you can safely drive on a highway; if you're a driving athlete you may be able to do 80 miles an hour fairly safely, but what about 250 miles an hour? Maybe not!

"More is better" is *not* true in the *ongoing handling of information*. We ought to have realized this long ago because an inspiration for the development of cognitive science was the rise of computers. Beginning in the mid-twentieth century, psychologists noticed that computers provided ample proof that thought-like processes can be fully mechanistic while being complex and hidden (Anderson, 2000; Arbib, 1964). In their hypothetical generalizations from computers to organisms, cognitive psychologists have often acknowledged that computers are fundamentally *serial processing* devices (even contemporary ones with multi-core processors). Computers, even though extremely fast, manipulate and organize only a few pieces of information at one time, in their central processing units. This little-at-a-time quality was in evidence in an early groundbreaking proposal that, by working with an appropriate set of rules applied sequentially, a computer could become a "general problem solver" (Newell, Shaw, and Simon, 1960).

Cognitive scientists often contrast such serial processing with the *parallel processing* in the brains of organisms, where millions of neural communications are always occurring all at the same time. But a more appropriate human-computer comparison may be in the fact that in our human *conscious capacity* we are pretty much limited to a *single thread of attention*. Yes, most of us can walk, talk to a friend, and chew gum at the same time, but you also well know how readily your conversation can become disrupted and confused by a distraction more demanding than walking or chewing gum. This suggests (although computers are *not* organisms) that there is a fundamental limit in the logic of how any system, no matter what its size or type, can possibly process information, as structures of knowledge are grown.

The "Reduction to Unique Parts" Heuristic versus "Self-Similarity." We often analyze larger objects or systems in terms of *unique properties* of their *component parts*. You think this way when you fix your lawn mower or your mechanical pencil. Or, when the basement floor gets wet because the sump pump went out again. Is it merely because the float came loose, because the motor burned out, or something else? Scientists think in pretty much the same ways about "wholes and their parts." (Gregory, 1981, pp. 84-95; Wimsatt, 2007).

But there are other strange circumstances in which big things and the littler things of which they are composed are *very similar in their form*. This issue was made famous when so-called "chaos theory" and "fractals" became popular in mathematics and in more widely circulated news media about two decades ago (e.g. Gleick, 1987; Peitgen, Jürgens, and Saupe, 1992). Such ideas suggested how widely diverse starting conditions, which are quantitatively different in many details but are under certain qualitative constraints, may lead to precisely the same forms in the end (Peitgen et al., 1992); in other words, the parts of such a thing are "self-similar" to its whole. A widely used example concerned coastlines. When you see a coastline as it is photographed from outer space, it has meandering curves and inlets, etc. Then, when you zoom in closer, you again see coastal curves and inlets, this time smaller ones, yet shaped much the same as the larger ones of which they are part. Then, the same kind of self-similarity is seen on an even smaller scale when you continue to zoom in.

Strange though it is, this "self-similarity" phenomenon turns out to be pretty ubiquitous, if you focus on appropriate attributes (e.g., Eglash, 1999). For instance, self-similarity is present generally in the very fact that bigger whole things can so often be analyzed into their parts. And the parts have parts. And the parts of the parts have parts! Yes, there are differences between the wholes and the parts that compose them but yes, there is also sameness in the ubiquity of wholes and parts.

> So, naturalists, observe, a flea
> Hath smaller fleas that on him prey;
> And these have smaller still to bite 'em;
> And so proceed *ad infinitum*.
> ...
> (Jonathan Swift, 1667-1745, *On Poetry. A Rhapsody*)

Again, try to think of other examples: The branches of a tree divide and divide further in much the same way. This is also true of the branching capillaries of your blood vessels and true of the "trees" of dendrites that comprise the capacious receiving ends of most of the neurons in your brain. And this is also true in the metaphorical sense of your progressively "branching" interests in the things you are most deeply interested in.

"Scale Independence," not Always, but *Sometimes*

In recent years, scientists have identified more and more such cases of what is now often called *scale independence*. The world has a great deal of depth and diversity, so keep remembering that *scale independence* is not true of everything. For example, one of the fleas about which Jonathan Swift wrote his verse, can jump many times more of his body length than you can of your body length. A grasshopper can jump more body lengths than an elephant can. Such *scale dependence* is frequently true both in biology (e.g. Alexander, 2000; McMahon and Bonner, 1983) and in engineering such things as bridges and ships (Petroski, 1985). Very often the *relative proportions* of small things versus big things have to be very different. Consider the thinness of a grasshopper versus the thickness of an elephant, the sleekness of a sailboat versus the breadth of an ocean liner. But let us return to *self-similarity* and to scale *in*dependence. These things are extremely interesting when we come across them in biology and psychology (Brown, Neath, and Chater, 2007; Li, 2000; Schmidt-Nielsen, 1984).

CONVERGENT EVOLUTION

The vigorous search for *mechanisms* of memory, in looking at things up close (the "trees"), has diverted too much scientific attention from consideration of a way in which *functions* of memory (the "forest") are even more foundational. A key concept here is *convergent evolution* (Eibl-Eibesfeldt, 1975; Lewin, 1999). In nature, whenever a number of very different things turn out to have a remarkable similarity, there are only two possible reasons. (1) It may just be a coincidence. There are so many things going on at once in the world that accidents of all sorts, including striking similarities, are bound to occur. (2) It may be because ecological conditions have pretty much "forced" things, very slowly by natural selection, to evolve similar forms—in other words, "convergent evolution."

Examples of convergent evolution are all around us in nature, and all of them are examples of a peculiar *sameness* in the very same place as there is a dramatic *difference*. Some of the standard textbook examples of sameness in the face of difference via convergent evolution:

- The *fins* of fishes and the *flippers* of dolphins. They are different, in that fins are made of fin stuff, membranes supported by spiny struts, while flippers are made of the same flesh and bone as your own hands and feet. The vertebrate line that eventually led to mammals branched off from fish ancestors about 390 million years ago, and mammals arose about 70 million years ago (Colbert, 1965), but when some among mammals returned to the seas, their limbs eventually adapted to the requirements of locomotion in that medium, where a fin-shape is handy. So *voilà*. Flesh and bone took the shape of fins.
- The *wings* of birds and of bats are similar in shape. Birds' and bats' vertebrate ancestors branched away from each other eons before taking to the air in a later evolutionary coming together. Similarly, invertebrates existed for about 160 million years before vertebrates emerged, while insects arose about 280 million years ago (Simpson, 1949). Yet the wings of a butterfly evolved, in both shape and movements, to become more like the wings of a bird or of a bat than these vertebrates' locomotor limbs are like the limbs of their vertebrate cousins such as the elephant.
- The complex *eyes* of vertebrates evolved independently of the equally marvelous eyes of the advanced invertebrate cephalopod, octopus. There are some revealing prominent differences between octopus eyes and our eyes, such as the way the lens works and the arrangement of the retina at the back of the eye, yet the overall shape

and functioning of the eyes in both cases turned out remarkably similar. Natural selection of eyes occurred with respect to the properties of light. After evolutionary eons, *voilà*, an advanced eye became what an advanced eye had to be – because light is what it is (Gregory, 1997).

- There are also many examples of *convergent evolution in behavior*, just as impressive as the foregoing examples of bodily form. For example, in all social species, whether ants and bees or monkeys and humans, individuals have routines for *greeting* other individuals. We also have roughly analogous routines for nurturing young, for escaping predators, and many others (Eibl-Eibesfeldt, 1975; 1989).

Remember that all these examples of convergent evolution are instances of a prominent *constancy in the face of differences*. Different in some ways from the quantitative constants of nature in physical sciences, such *qualitative* constancies do have *quantitative* aspects. They are constrained by quantitative properties of the contexts in which they evolved, such as the very different resistances offered to a moving object by the water of the sea (fins, flippers), by comparison with the air to which flying creatures have adapted (wings).

Convergent Evolution and Working Memory Capacity

How might the principle of convergent evolution apply to the constancies among phenomena of working memory? The biological bases of memory, in neuronal structure, physiology, and biochemistry, imply that the detailed mechanisms by which the brain holds and transmits information inside of itself have very diverse time durations (Shepherd, 2004). For example, it takes thousandths of a second for ion channel activities to yield the electrical impulse of a neuron firing by which it communicates with other neurons and it takes fully tenths or hundredths of a second for a single brain wave to occur (Breedlove, Rosenzweig, and Watson, 2007; Nunez, 1995; Rosenzweig, 1996).

Those neurophysiological processes occur on much faster time scales than the memory phenomena that they support—but *some* of the brain foundations of memories *have to* take place on *exactly the same time scale as we experience* these memories, from large fractions of a second, to seconds, to minutes and hours, etc. That is a crucial assumption for any scientist seeking the material bases of mind (instead of unscientifically assuming a philosophical dualism of ghostly mind versus tangible matter), and it also identifies the greatest gap between what we know of cognition and what we know of brain. Nevertheless, brain researchers do know a good deal. Neuroscientists who have sought correlates in the brains of animals and people have described a diverse set of biological phenomena that seem to sustain memories. These include blood flow to particular brain regions, neuronal electrical activity, communication between neurons by chemical transmission, as well as changes over time in the strength of such communication, protein synthesis and changes in the branching patterns of neurons. All these take different amounts of time (Breedlove et al., 2007; Rosenzweig, 1996).

If there is, indeed, *scale independence* of memory phenomena across different time durations, that must be because the same reality of what memory can possibly accomplish imposes itself, wherever appropriate—via natural selection, the way evolution always works—across all these different biological mechanisms. If working memory, for some reason, *must* be in the range 7±2, then natural selection will have taken it there eventually, no matter what the time demands of the different underlying biological processes. This will have occurred just as flippers and fins converged in shape. There is also an important secondary implication here, that working memory capacity must be a neuropsychological *regulated* quantity. I explain this important hypothesis next.

REGULATION OF QUANTITY IN WORKING MEMORY

All living systems survive only insofar as they adequately anticipate and handle the challenges that come at them from their environments. The brilliant social psychologist Donald T. Campbell (1974; Kim 2001) made this point interestingly, by saying that organisms are replete with "vicarious selectors." *Vicarious selectors* stand in for the dangerous *natural selectors* that could easily interfere with organisms' viability, or perhaps just kill them outright. For example, your eyes and your reactions to things you see (approach or avoid) help to keep you in good shape. Indeed, every single physical and psychological aspect of animals and humans may be thought of in this way. We individual organisms occupy the earth for as long as our vicarious selectors (a) successfully keep us out of life-losing trouble, and (b) encourage taking life-sustaining advantage of good opportunities. Of particular interest at this point is the presence within us of diverse *regulatory mechanisms*. Regulatory mechanisms keep all our processes in their proper ranges—not too much and not too little (Breedlove et al., 2007; Eibl-Eibesfeldt, 1975).

We have myriads of regulatory mechanisms! Are you thirsty? You drink water. Are you afraid of getting hit by a train? You quickly move your car off the tracks at the railroad crossing. Are you cold? You put on a coat, or go inside, or shiver. Each of these examples, mentioned only briefly here, has a great deal more richness. You may elaborate from your own experience, and then be amazed at how much more you learn about these mechanisms when you read some of the ample explanations in textbooks of physiology and psychology. There are regulatory mechanisms faithfully working inside you to adjust the neurotransmitter levels among all your billions of neurons, to adjust your heart rate and blood pressure, your ear's response to the loudness of sounds, your hormonal levels, your immune system responses, your digestion, and so many others. Each of them always involves a kind of self-checking by means of "feedback loops" (Arbib, 1964; Ashby, 1960; Pierce, 1980). By far, most regulations are unconscious.

Most regulation *has to be unconscious*. If you had to consciously adjust your blood pressure, blood sugar levels, and everything else, you would be impossibly distracted! Your conscious capacity is reserved. Consciousness is specialized for dealing with larger problems that involve your direct interactions, as a whole organism, with your environment. Yes, there are exceptions. As we know, unfortunately, a regulation such as blood pressure, which is normally internal, does sometimes have to be *raised* to consciousness cognitively so that it can be *lowered* viscerally! Your physician warns you, advises you to purchase a sphygmomanometer to keep check, and prescribes pills. This routine does then, in fact, frequently distract you from the affairs to which you would much prefer devoting yourself.

As I suggested above, the aspect of reality that leads to the most significant constraint on the evolution of working memory capacity concerns the growth and maintenance of organization in any functioning structure. You cannot build a complex thing all at once. It "grows" as you work on it. Neither do complex natural things pop into existence all at once; they *grow*. The same is generally true any time you make controlled changes in a thing, or when nature makes changes. Accidental wounds take place suddenly, but healing takes time. A dropped vase breaks quickly – an uncontrolled change. Putting the vase back together (or making a new one) takes time.

The constraint of modest growth rate must be so inexorable that it has led to the convergent evolution of *many different regulatory mechanisms as secondary phenomena of working memory capacity*. Each of these regulations must be appropriate to the timescales, as well as to the scales of the other dimensions, or attributes, of the particular memory mechanisms it concerns. In the following parts of this chapter we will see why that constraint of reality is *combinatorial*. Elementary combinatorial mathematics suggests that working memory capacity of humans and other animals has to be only as modestly big as it is.

Parallel Processing only Under Special Conditions

Consider the obvious: There are only so many independent items a changing structure of any sort can cope with, while preserving organization. Only when there has been ample preparation can many things happen well at the same time. Our brains and bodies can be *parallel processors* at some levels only because they evolved over millions of years, so are now amply prepared. Similarly, lots of things move at once in concert in your car, because it is a product of many years of planning and trial and error research and development; now all its parts work together in the same way all the time. But if *you*, a single person, try to do too much at once, things disorganize. Similarly, "too many cooks spoil the broth."

Evolution must have "discovered" the a-little-at-a-time growth property of reality many times over, in different contexts, as new organizations evolved. Eventually humans evolved. Later, among us, eventually by nature and nurture cognitive psychologists emerged, who discovered that this property of reality concerns "the magical number 7±2." It is likely a constant of nature.

Constants of Nature: Precise Ones, Fuzzy Ones

Physicists, chemists, and engineers may object that a true constant of nature has to be much more accurately defined. Constants such as $e = 2.718\ldots$ and $\pi = 3.14159\ldots$ are defined precisely in a way that goes on to an infinite number of decimal places. As precisely defined also are the speed of light in a vacuum, Avogadro's number relating the exact number of atoms in a gram of any element to its atomic weight, and the gravitational constant that determines how quickly any falling object accelerates. There are more. Another constant that strongly emerges from a variety of mathematical premises is the so-called "golden ratio," or $\varphi=1.618\ldots$ (Huntley, 1970; Livio, 2002); indeed, a mathematical argument has been made for its specific relevance to brain waves and working memory capacity (Weiss and Weiss, 2003).

But deep in the nature of regulatory subsystems is that they have fuzzy margins, and "the magical number 7±2" seems to be a natural constant of this genre (MacGregor, 1987)—notwithstanding the point mentioned earlier that within that "small fuzzy region" researchers have found interesting modest correlations with measures of intelligence (Engle et al., 2008). A little "play," involving a small "permissible error," is crucial for the reliability and stability of regulatory systems. The thermostat that regulates the temperature of your home in winter turns the furnace on at one temperature and then off at a slightly higher temperature. Because that mechanical and electronic system is less precise than the temperature regulation neurochemical circuits built into your brain and body, you may experience this as feeling a little too cold just before the heat goes on and then a little too warm just before it goes off. Although we often think in terms of a regulatory "set point," it is always really a "set range" (Arbib, 1964; Ashby, 1960; Breedlove et al., 2007; Pierce, 1980).

The "magical number 7±2" must be such a regulatory set-range! If I am correct, it ought to be possible to show not only that a person does not function well if his working memory capacity is *too small,* but also if, for some tasks, working memory capacity were *too large*! A few years ago, undergraduates Joanna Bovee, Elaine Bregman, and I tried to empirically test this hypothesis by finding a circumstance under which *distracting* our research subjects would *improve* their ability to memorize. We were not successful, but one negative result need not require a scientist to abandon an interesting hypothesis! Please help think of ways to test it. In the following, final sections of this chapter we consider in more depth some of the reasons for the hypothesis that working memory capacity is a "natural near-constant" of 7±2.

A "Theory of Relativity" for Working Memory

Our findings with people in radial mazes, taken together with the peculiar findings about recency and time duration reported by others, were striking enough to suggest the need for a "working memory theory of relativity" (Glassman, 1998, 1999a, 1999b,2000, 2003a). It may have been brash to borrow a term from Albert Einstein, but it was an appropriate analogy, because Einstein's "theory of relativity," developed early in the twentieth century, focuses on *a quantity that remains surprisingly constant* (the speed of light), *while other things change* (e.g., the speed of an observer). This happens, according to Einstein (1931) in his explanation for laypersons, because physical time actually stretches or contracts.

In the "working memory theory of relativity," physical time does not actually stretch, but "memory time" does. What might account for the stretchiness of memory time? The "relativistic" time paradoxes I described above and other working memory phenomena keep returning us to the basic working memory numerosity itself, "the magical number 7±2." *Why* is our human working memory capacity, "the magical number seven," no more than that of the rat? Why is our adult human working memory capacity hardly more than that of a child? Looking more closely at a certain property of small numbers provides a compelling suggestion. First, we do so intuitively, then more quantitatively.

SEVEN IS MODEST

"The magical number seven" is a modest number. Seven is a "Goldilocks" number - "not too big and not too small." Did you ever notice that sentences seem to have about seven or so words in them? At the very foundation of any sentence are the subject, the verb, and the object—three terms. If you toss in an adjective and/or adverb modifier, an article or two, a preposition, there you are at about seven. "The big boy hit the ball hard." Seven words. Shorter sentences seem oddly tight-lipped. We tend to read longer ones as familiar phrases and shorter sentence-like clauses, which themselves have about seven units. If we do that well, the reader does not have to read twice, or the listener doesn't have to say, "Come again?" For example, my previous sentence has three major parts, "If we do that well" (5 words), "the reader does not have to read twice" (8 words), and "the listener doesn't have to say 'xyz'" (6 words plus a short quoted phrase). In the ballpark of seven is about how many things we can handle at once, digest and catch the gist of, before going on to the next moment. Thus, there seems to be something about that "magical number" that taps into the very structure of the interface between a cognizing organism and reality. It seems a logical necessity of cognition.

But *is* it logically necessary? Such a hypothesis demands rigorous examination. We have not *proven* it, but we can sketch in the beginning of a mathematical theory. Why should working memory capacity not be just a little bigger, let's say 8 plus or minus something, instead of 7±2? There is a reason! Consider the following progressive list of points about how many items we can reasonably handle in each moment.

- One object is too single-mindedly sparse; what's to decide – take it or leave it?
- Two items can be in either of two orders, A-B or B-A.
- Three items are present in predication: A acts on B. A simple sentence.
- Four items have many possible orderings. There are 4x2x3x1=24 permutations.
- Five items have 5x4x3x2x1=120 permutations—a lot of possibilities to examine.
- And then things really "explode."

ORGANIZING THOUGHTS: WORKING MEMORY CAPACITY MAXES OUT

This explosion is illustrated in Table 1. It would take too much room to illustrate comprehensively even all the permutations of four items, let alone five or six or more, but the table makes the idea of how to do that evident, should you want to give it a try. The main point of this illustration is that although seven is a "modest" number, seven and numbers close to it have a lot of "leverage" in the way they readily lead to much larger quantities. That "leverage" is combinatorial.

If you keep going with this scheme, you see that if you were confronted with a mere nine items, and had no preliminary way of constraining their conceivable relative positions, you would have 362,880 possible orderings to consider! This sort of issue is generally known as a *combinatorial explosion*. Looking at it as we just have, it is a *permutational explosion* of possibilities (see any textbook of discrete mathematics or probability for further explanation).

Table 1. Illustration Of "Exploding" Permutations

AB	ABC	ABCD	ABCDE	ABCDEF
BA	BAC	BACD	BACDE	BACDEF
	CAB	CABD	CABDE	…
	ACB	ACBD	ACBDE	…
	BCA	BCAD	BCADE	…
	CBA	CBAD	…	…
		ABDC	…	…
		BADC	…	…
		CADB	…	…
2	6	24	120	720

The burden such an explosion of possibilities suggests would wipe out the function served by our having a special working memory facility to handle the present moment! Remember we are considering a present moment in which an issue of *organization* is opened—either creation of a new memory or revision of an old one. Therefore, "parallel processing," of so many question-worthy details, is not a possibility. As explained earlier, simultaneous operations can maintain organization only with systems that are already highly prepared and specialized. So it is a good thing that our consciousness does not allow itself to be overwhelmed by too much at one time. Our elementary mathematical calculations help us understand what penalty in confusion might result from too much working memory capacity.

This line of reasoning suggests why working memory time intervals must be "relativistic" with respect to the particular task one is doing, as illustrated by our earlier comparison of word list tasks and the radial maze spatial task. Dealing with a sequence of words, heard at a normal rate of speaking, working memory focuses on short intervals under half a minute at a time. When dealing with a longer, more drawn-out spatial memory task, which requires walking about and remembering sites, working memory "steps back" to achieve its capacity allocation of about seven items, over longer time intervals of many minutes or more.

Developmental Shaping and its Evolution: Units Built of Units that Came Together Earlier

Let us return again to thinking about the growth of real people. At the beginning of this chapter, we saw Cassie developing some basic cognitive competencies that should someday become completely submerged and integrated, unconsciously, into the larger structures that then occupy her consciously. The word lists and other items typically used in the cognitive psychology laboratory study of memory are handy but incongruous. They are challenging to memorize at least in part because they are unfamiliar, not the kinds of things we ordinarily encounter. In one sense, this typical weakness of the cognitive psychology lab in addressing the *applied memory* of real life is also strength. We human beings evolved to constantly cope with new things not before encountered, and to constantly be learning, as we walk through life.

However, it is more accurate to note that, yes, we are always learning but, as we do so, we are always relying primarily on the competencies, or "chunks" of knowledge we have already developed. Too much newness is bewildering. As we walk through life our engagement with new experiences relies greatly on our older memories. We humans do so much of this that we have a much longer developmental period than any other species. Many other animals learn, and young animals of many species tune their skills by *playing*, but *children* emerge only with humans. We spend so many years as children, dependent on adult caretakers for support and protection, as we gather and polish our competencies. If you are reading this as a college student, let's face it; the age you are now is still very much a part of this process. You would have already gotten most of your life's tasks and adventures behind you if you were a dog, living "in dog years." Even a person my age (don't ask) retains childlike qualities in seeking new learning and growth.

There is a gap between studies of human development and of memory. Many studies reveal how memory for lists changes as children mature, but there is a gap of scientific scholarship between such research and other research traditions in child development, which concern how cognitive processes undergo a sequence of major changes in organization.

The seminal theory of the Swiss psychologist Jean Piaget remains foundational, although it has undergone revision by others since the mid-twentieth century (e.g. Piaget, 1952). Piaget's principles include the idea that development occurs primarily in four stages, but here I want to emphasize Piaget's foundational concepts of *assimilation* and *accommodation* as the ways in which our *cognitive structures* grow and reorganize as we mature.

The basic idea is this: As you walk through life, many things you encounter are sort of like other things you've already learned to deal with. At such times, you *generalize*. You simply remember that this somewhat new situation requires no really new problem solving; it can merely be added to the collection of things you think of and you respond to in such and such a way. So, you merely absorb or *assimilate* this new thing into your old remembered categories. However, every once in a while you have difficulty. At that point, in this Piagetian way of thinking, you have to *accommodate* by building a new mental structure. Your building of that new conceptual structure has nothing other to work with than (a) the mental structures (memories) you are already walking around with and (b) your current experience in this new encounter. (Plus, let's face it; you need a bit of luck.)

During your early childhood years, of course, there has to be a lot of accommodation. Enough of it and you move on to the next stage of development. For example, between ages two and three a child moves on, Piaget explained, from concentrating on "sensorimotor" skills such as reaching, grasping, and manipulating objects, to the "preoperational" stage (up to about age 6 or 7) of developing cognitive skills such as classification of objects and, of course, fluent use of language. Speaking of which: During our last visit to the west coast, a couple of months after December, for Cassie's first birthday, she was just beginning, hesitantly, to say some words. They seemed to come out only when Cassie "wanted to let them happen" (it's hard to know just how a toddler experiences this), and that seemed to encourage all the doting adults to keep pointing at things and repeating. Empathizing with Cassie, perhaps excessively, I asked whether grandma was trying to turn her into a trained parrot. But grandma succeeded at one point in getting Cassie to say "daisy" appropriately.

Soon, in a subsequent moment—you guessed it—Cassie *assimilated*, calling another flower a daisy.

Piaget's understanding of human cognitive development owes a great deal to an earlier, brilliant American psychologist, James Mark Baldwin, who, like Piaget, was fascinated by the principle of evolution put forth by Charles Darwin (Cairns, 1992; Plotkin, 2004; Weber and Depew, 2003). In an interesting historical analysis, Emily Cahan (1984) says:

> Central to both Piaget's and Baldwin's theory of knowledge is the conviction that transformations of the relationship between thoughts and things occur in an orderly progressive way (p. 129).

Cahan's subsequent comments illustrate how important it becomes for us to try to combine the cognitive psychology of human development with the cognitive psychology of memory. For example, she notes:

> From a biological point of view, assimilation represents the integration of external elements in to structures that are either evolving or completed... Baldwin refers to the assimilatory process as *habit formation.* However, a second process, accommodation, is required to guarantee adaptive change, and hence, development... (p. 130).

Thus, both for Baldwin and Piaget modification of cognitive structure, in the organized growth of accommodation, is elicited by conflict, or "confrontation between the old and the new" (Cahan 1984, p. 130) that occurs when *habit* no longer suffices.

A Brief Note on Possible Brain Foundations of Working Memory

Working memory capacity is like a short and narrow hallway that we must pass through during every waking moment of our life with no more than the several things we can carry through that hallway at once. No one yet has a comprehensive idea how working memory, or consciousness, is based in the brain, but there are hypotheses. Bjorn Merker (2007) thoughtfully reviewed a great deal of neuroanatomical literature, as well as clinical cases of children, sadly, born without a cortex ("anencephalic"). Merker argues that their emotional gestures suggest consciousness is deep in the brainstem—almost literally a narrow "hallway" of neural connections (also see my commentary, Glassman, 2007).

Another possibility: The extreme thinness (recall, a couple of millimeters) of our large-area cortical sheet (about 2600 square centimeters) might comprise the brain's structural basis for limited working memory capacity. It is the sheet upon which long-term memories are written. Taking this idea further, the relationships among psychological items held during a moment's working memory might have their dynamic neural counterparts in relationships among neighboring activated patches of cortex. The ability of such hypothetical memory-item representations to contact each other may be understood in terms of the so-called "four color theorem" of topology, or in terms of a related graph-theoretical mathematical principle concerning direct connections among up to four nodal areas (Glassman, 2003b). These ideas will turn out to be right or wrong when we discover good ways to test them.

Half of 7±2 Is 3 or 4: Two "Phases" of Memory, or "Levels of Binding"

These ideas connect with another important point about working memory that Miller had already touched on in his seminal 1956 paper: There are some indications that, when certain strict conditions of experimental observation are in place, working memory capacity is about *half* of "the magical number 7," that is, only about three or four items. Without going into great detail here, one common indication is that when we commit a new sequence of items to memory we tend to break it rhythmically into smaller groupings of about three or four. Watch yourself do that next time you copy your long driver's license number over onto a form.

That tendency to chop long sequences up into threes or fours might remind you that Western music generally uses 3/4 or 4/4 time. Using a different sort of musical analogy, I have also hypothesized that individual items in working memory might have a representation in our brain waves as different frequencies that have harmonic relationships among each other (almost as if they were pitches of sound or electrical wave "chords" in the brain). The reasoning here has to do with special mathematical properties of waves in harmonic relationships, which makes them advantageous as communicative signals (Glassman, 1999b, 2000). This idea is related to a great deal of recent brain research suggesting that when attributes are associated with each other in mind (e.g. redness and boxiness of a red box), the relevant neurons momentarily express closer relationships with each other by electrically oscillating in step—synchronized perhaps at 80 waves per second in what is now called the "gamma band" of EEG (Singer, 1994; Treisman, 1996). Recently, a prominent cognitive psychologist has reviewed evidence for "the magical number 4" (Cowan, 2001). However, to see why there must be two phases, or levels, to the operation of working memory, we must now return to an additional, important hypothetical generalization, made above.

The Secret of Life : Building Elements from Earlier Elements

We have already discussed the idea that complex systems grow in organization as later developing units encompass earlier, simpler (often smaller) ones. As you develop through life, your consciousness must enclose at least two "phases," by which smaller fragments of experience are bound together into your grasp of larger wholes. This is analogous to assimilation and accommodation. In one way of illustrating, a baby, during the first half-year or so of life, is busy tuning into the phonemes, or elementary accents, of the language of those around it. By late in that same year, even before saying its first whole words, the baby begins to sound to an outsider as if it were speaking that language. Baby is babbling with an accent. Bye and bye, those phonemes become built into larger units, the words and grammar of the parents' language. Still later, those words turn into sentences and then, perhaps, even book chapters. As with all other human constructions, larger parts come to be made up of smaller parts, which themselves were earlier composed from still more basic parts. (Remember my descriptions of Cassie's exploratory, memory-building adventures.) David Dirlam (1972) calculated that a chunk size between 3 and 4 items is mathematically most efficient for a memory search process. Indeed, how we manage a lifetime of memory accumulation is considered by Robert W. Doty (1998) to be one of the great "five mysteries of the mind" for brain scientists.

The principle that growth builds upon units of units of units (and so on) comprises the most basic essence of lifespan development. Working memory is always trying to build more comprehensive or general concepts into your long-term memory. Since it has to do that "in a narrow hallway," it somehow turns all the concept-items it is working with at any given time into things of a size that fit into that hallway, and which can pass through it while interacting in a fairly well-behaved way with the other up to six or so things that are passing through at the same time. Its ability to do that is both mysterious and familiar. It is easily understood, at least in rough outline, by considering those cases when a "chunk" passing through is labeled with a single word. Yes, words differ in length, but not that much. Significantly, a rather short word or phrase may sometimes conjure up a conception of something immense. Consider: "Whale," or "the world" or "the US Constitution." As concepts, words are all, democratically, about the same "size." You can consciously handle about seven such concepts at once.

To put this in another way, it seems that working memory has to involve, inherently, two levels of "binding" at any given time. At the "lower level," the attributes of objects in the world (i.e., those that you are presently attending to) "pluck" the systems of the brain that are tuned to those respective attributes, and set them to "ringing" together, in coherent brain wave oscillations. At the very same time, the physical relationships among those attributes in the objects themselves influence the binding together in mind and brain of coherent conceptions of those objects. At the "higher level" of binding, you consciously explore different possible meanings and relationships among the array of up to about seven thought-objects currently in mind. As you mature, with luck and judgment, those relationships grow more and more organized, complex, and useful.

There is not much question that language plays an important role here. But language remains enigmatic, even though it has been studied deeply and widely by academic types and others, including those who argue well that the emergence of language comprises much of what makes us human and is the main factor that drove the biological evolution of the large human brain (e.g., Pinker, 1994). Words solidify meanings and they cast a spotlight on those meanings. Naming something is like adding a hardener to the glue that is holding together the concept that the name represents or like building a closed cell membrane around the concept.[17] Language is so important that Cassie's entourage of adults spends much of their time eagerly pressing words upon her—and she is getting them. Words are such good tools. The ability of language to make chunks cohere and coordinate is so handy that Alex uses it in learning to tie his shoelaces—verbal strings and cotton strings.

Iggy, Alex's and Cassie's 4 ½-year old cousin, is another important member of this twenty-first century American family, also living a long distance away, with his dad and mom, from the rest of us. The fact that he has been pretty good with words and sentences for a long time already (one of his earliest utterances was "Bob Dylan.") might fool you—as it might with any child—that he understands all of what is going on around him. But, strangely, language is so important that our achieving a high degree of early skill with it actually *leads* the acquisition of most of our adult skills. We have gathered many thousands of words up into our fluency by the end of what Piaget called our "preoperational" stage (at about 7 years old)

[17] It is interesting that something so concretely useful as language has its essence best captured abstractly in metaphors.

even before going on to a higher, "operational" ability to judge the sizes and numbers of things by seeing past their most perceptually striking attributes. Indeed, although kids move on, at about two years old, from their "sensorimotor" stage to their preoperational stage, they still have a long way to go in developing the fluidly skilled sensorimotor coordinations that will serve them as older children and adults.

Hence, at four and a half, Iggy may well keep for a long time his *episodic memory* of joining grandpa in the exercise room of the hotel we grandparents stayed in during our visit in May 2008. Iggy has seen his dad (who keeps in pretty good shape) exercise, but there was something that intrigued him so much about old grandpa in the exercise room that he eagerly responded yes, when his dad asked him if he wanted to join in again, on the second day. And this became another wonderful example of a child actively reaching and stretching and *picking heavy things up*, both literally and figuratively, with eager, rough, cute approximations to grandad's curls, presses, and rowing movements, as dad gently nudged his hands into more proper form with the three-pound dumbbells he was holding. Iggy's speech is already fluent, and that requires highly skilled oral movements but, along with his cousins, he has many other things to become skilled at over the years. He has many "chunks," yet, to build.

Attention and working memory are something like the leading tip of a growing plant, with the difference noted before, that the developmental course of our mental growing depends more on our life's experiences than does the growth of a plant. The crucial role of working memory is to keep on organizing and reorganizing, little by little "the larger you," that is your long-term memory and your self.

REFERENCES

Alexander, R. M. (2000). Hovering and jumping: Contrasting problems in scaling. In J. H. Brown and G. B. West (Eds.) *Scaling in Biology* (pp. 37-50). New York: Oxford University Press.

Anderson, J. A. (2000). *Cognitive psychology and its implications: Fifth Edition*. New York: Worth Publishers.

Arbib, M. A. (1964). *Brains, machines, and mathematics*. New York: McGraw-Hill.

Ashby, W. R. (1960). *Design for a brain: The origin of adaptive behavior*. Revised ed. London: Chapman and Hall, Ltd./Science Paperbacks.

Baddeley, A. (1986). *Working memory*. New York, NY: Clarendon Press/Oxford University Press.

Bauer, P. J. (2007). *Remembering the times of our lives: Memory in infancy and beyond*. Mahwah, NJ: Lawrence Erlbaum Associates.

Bear, M. F., Connors, B. W., and Paradiso, M. A. (2007). *Neuroscience: Exploring the brain*. Third Ed. Philadelphia: Lippincott Williams and Wilkins.

Beatty, W. W., and Shavalia, D. A. (1980). Rat spatial memory: Resistance to retroactive interference at long retention intervals. *Animal Learning and Behavior, 8*, 550-552.

Bohbot, V., Jech, R., Ruzicka, E., Bures, J., and Nadel, L. (1994). Comparison of rat and human spatial memory performance. *Society for Neuroscience Abstracts, 20*, 361.

Bjork, R. A., and Whitten, W. B. (1974). Recency-sensitive retrieval processes in long-term free recall. *Cognitive Psychology, 6,* 173-189.

Braitenberg, V., and Schüz, A. (1998). *Cortex: Statistics and geometry of neuronal connectivity*. Second Edition. Berlin: Springer.

Breedlove, S. M., Rosenzweig, M. R., and Watson, N. V. (2007). *Biological psychology: An introduction to behavioral, cognitive, and clinical neuroscience*. Fifth Ed. Sunderland, MA: Sinauer Associates.

Brown, G. D. A., Neath, I., and Chater, N. (2007). A temporal ratio model of memory. *Psychological Review, 114,* 539-576.

Brown, M. F. (1992). Does a cognitive map guide choices in the radial-arm choice-maze? *Journal of Experimental Psychology: Animal Behavior Processes, 18,* 56-66.

Cahan, E. D. (1984). The genetic psychologies of James Mark Baldwin and Jean Piaget. *Developmental Psychology, 20,* 128-135.

Cairns, R. B. (1992). The making of a developmental science: the contributions and intellectual heritage of James Mark Baldwin. *Developmental Psychology, 28,* 17-24.

Campbell, D. T. (1974). Unjustified variation and selective retention in scientific discovery. In F. J. Ayala and T. Dobzhansky (Eds.) *Studies in the philosophy of biology* (pp. 139-161). Berkeley, CA: University of California Press.

Colbert, E. H. (1965). *The age of reptiles*. New York: W. W. Norton and Co.

Cowan, N. (Ed.) (1997). *The development of memory in childhood*. Hove, East Sussex, U.K.: Psychology Press.

Cowan, N. (2001). The magical number 4 in short-term memory: A reconsideration of mental storage capacity. *Behavioral and Brain Sciences, 24,* 87-185.

Csikszentmilhayi, M. (1990). *Flow: The psychology of optimal experience*. New York: HarperCollins.

Dale, R. H. I, and Innes, N. K. (1986). Interactions between response stereotypy and memory strategies on the eight-arm radial maze. *Behavioral Brain Research, 19,* 17-25.

Dirlam, D. (1972). Most efficient chunk sizes. *Cognitive Psychology, 3,* 355-359.

Doty, R. W. (1998). The five mysteries of the mind, and their consequences. *Neuropsychologia, 36,* 1069-1076.

Ebbinghaus, H. (1964). *Memory: A contribution to experimental psychology* (H. A. Ruger and C. E. Bussenius, Trans.). New York, NY: Dover. (Original work published 1885).

Eglash, R. (1999). *African fractals: Modern computing and indigenous design*. Piscataway, NJ: Rutgers University Press.

Eibl-Eibesfeldt, I. (1975). *Ethology: The biology of behavior*. Second Ed. New York: Holt, Rinehart, and Winston.

Eibl-Eibesfeldt, I. (1989). *Human ethology*. Hawthorne, NY: Aldine de Gruyter.

Einstein, A. (1931). *Relativity: The special and general theory*. New York: Crown Publishers/Bonanza Paperback.

Engle, R., Unsworth, N., Hale, S., De Alwis, D., Tamez, E., McCabe, D. P., Loaiza-Kois, V., Rose, N., Meyerson, J., and Roediger, H. L. III (2008). New insights from working memory research. Symposium at the 20th Annual Convention of the Association for Psychological Science, Chicago.

Ericsson, K. A., and Delaney, P. F. (1998). Working memory and expert performance. In R. H. Logie and K. J. Gilhooly (Eds.) *Working memory and thinking*. Hove East Sussex, UK: Psychology Press.

Fessard, A., Gerard, R. W., and Konorski, J. (1961). *Brain mechanisms and learning.* Springfield, IL: Charles C. Thomas, Publisher.

Glassman, R. B. (1998). A "theory of relativity" for paradoxical time span flexibility of limited item-capacity working memory. Involvement of harmonics among ultradian clocks? *Society for Neuroscience Abstracts, 24*(1), 166.

Glassman, R. B. (1999a). A working memory "theory of relativity": Elasticity over temporal, spatial, and modality ranges conserves 7±2 item capacity in radial maze, verbal tasks and other cognition. *Brain Research Bulletin, 48,* 475-489.

Glassman, R. B. (1999b). Hypothesized neural dynamics of working memory: Several chunks might be marked simultaneously by harmonic frequencies within an octave band of brain waves. *Brain Research Bulletin, 50,* 77-93.

Glassman, R. B. (2000). A "Theory of Relativity" for cognitive elasticity of time and modality dimensions supporting constant working memory capacity: Involvement of harmonics among ultradian clocks? *Progress in Neuro-Psychopharmacology and Biological Psychiatry, 24,* 163-182.

Glassman, R. B. (2002). "Miles within millimeters" and other awe-inspiring facts about our "mortarboard" human cortex. *Zygon: Journal of Religion and Science, 37,* 255-277.

Glassman, R. B. (2003a). Hypothesized temporal and spatial code properties for a moment's working memory capacity: Brain wave "harmonies" and "four-color" topology of activated cortical areas. In *Time and mind II: Information processing perspectives* (pp. 161-183). Hede Helfrich, Ed., Cambridge, MA: Hogrefe and Huber.

Glassman, R. B. (2003b). Topology and graph theory applied to cortical anatomy may help explain working memory capacity for three or four simultaneous items. *Brain Research Bulletin, 60,* 25-42.

Glassman, R. B. (2007). I Promethean, bound deeply and fluidly among the brain's associative robotic networks. *Behavioral and Brain Sciences, 30,* 95-96.

Glassman, R. B., Garvey, K. J., Elkins, K. M., Kasal, K. L., and Couillard, N. (1994). Spatial working memory score of humans in a large radial maze, similar to published score of rats, implies capacity close to the magical number 7±2. *Brain Research Bulletin, 34,* 151-159.

Glassman, R. B., Knabe-Czerwionka, J. J., Branch, A. M., and Brown, P. B. (2001). Proud to be a bird brain: Human working memory for caching and finding items in an outdoor area as good as birds in a laboratory. *Society for Neuroscience Abstracts, 27*(74), 4.

Glassman, R. B., Leniek, K. M., and Haegerich, T. M. (1998). Human working memory capacity is 7±2 in a radial maze with distracting interruption: Possible implication for neural mechanisms of declarative and implicit long-term memory. *Brain Research Bulletin, 47,* 249-256.

Gleick, J. (1987). *Chaos: Making a new science*. New York: Viking Penguin.

Gregory, R. L. (1981). *Mind in science: A history of explanations in psychology and physics.* New York: Cambridge University Press.

Gregory, R. L. (1997). *Eye and brain: The psychology of seeing.* Fifth Ed. Princeton, NJ: Princeton University Press.

Grondin, S. (2002). Sensory modalities and temporal processing. In *Time and mind II: Information processing perspectives* (pp. 61-77). Hede Helfrich, Ed., Cambridge, MA: Hogrefe and Huber.

Huntley, H. E. (1970). *The divine proportion: A study in mathematical beauty.* New York: Dover Publications.

Isarida, T., and Isarida, T. K. (2006). Influences of environmental context on the recency effect in free recall. *Memory and Cognition, 34,* 787-794.

Kim, K-M. (2001). Nested hierarchies of vicarious selectors. In C. Heyes and D. L. Hull (Eds.) *Selection theory and social construction: the evolutionary epistemology of Donald T. Campbell* (pp. 101-118). Albany: State University of New York.

Lewin, R. (1999). *Patterns in evolution*. New York: Scientific American Library.

Lipp, H-P., Pleskacheva, M. G., Gossweiler, H., Ricceri, L., Smirnova, A. A., Garin, N. N., Perepiolkina, O. P., Voronkov, D. N., Kuptsov, P. A., and Dell'Omo, G. (2001). A large outdoor radial maze for comparative studies in birds and mammals, *Neuroscience and Biobehavioral Reviews, 25*(1), 83-99.

Li, J. K-J. (2000). Scaling and invariants in cardiovascular biology. In J. H. Brown and G. B. West (Eds.) *Scaling in biology* (pp. 113-128). New York: Oxford University Press.

Livio, M. (2002). *The golden ratio.* New York: Broadway Books.

Lumsden, C. L., and Wilson, E. O. (1983). *Promethean fire: Reflections on the origin of mind.* Cambridge, MA: Harvard University Press.

MacGregor, J. N. (1987). Short-term memory capacity: Limitation or optimization? *Psychological Review, 94*, 107-108.

Maki, W. S., Beatty, W. W., Hoffman, N., Bierley, R. A., and Clouse, B. A. (1984). Spatial memory over long retention intervals: Nonmemorial factors are not necessary for accurate performance on the radial-arm maze by rats. *Behavioral and Neural Biology, 41,* 1-6.

McMahon, T. A., and Bonner, J. T. (1983). *On size and life*. New York: W. H. Freeman/Scientific American Library.

Merker, B. (2007). Consciousness without a cerebral cortex: A challenge for neuroscience and medicine. *Behavioral and Brain Sciences, 30,* 63-134.

Miller, G. A. (1956). The magical number seven, plus or minus two: Some limits on our capacity for processing information. *Psychological Review, 63,* 81-97.

Milner, P. M. (1970). *Physiological psychology.* New York: Holt, Rinehart and Winston.

Murdock, B. B. (1960). The distinctiveness of stimuli. *Psychological Review, 67,* 16-31.

Nairne, J. S. (2002). Remembering over the short term: The case against the standard model. *Annual Review of Psychology, 53,* 53-81.

Nairne, J. S., Neath, I., Serra, M., and Byun, E. (1997). Positional distinctiveness and the ratio rule in free recall. *Journal of Memory and Language, 37,* 155-166.

Neisser, U., and Hyman, I. E., Jr. (Eds.) (2000). *Memory Observed: Remembering in Natural Contexts:* Second Edition. New York: Worth Publishers.

Newell, A., Shaw, J. C., and Simon, H. A. (1960). A variety of intelligent learning in a general problem solver. In M. C. Yovits and S. Cameron (Eds.) *Self-organizing systems* (pp. 153-189). New York: Pergamon Press.

Nunez, P. L. (1995). *Neocortical dynamics and human EEG rhythms*. New York: Oxford University Press.

O'Connor, R. C., and Glassman, R. B. (1993). Human performance with a seventeen-arm radial maze analog. *Brain Research Bulletin, 30,* 189-191.

Olton, D. S. (1979). Mazes, maps, and memory. *American Psychologist, 34,* 583-596.

Olton, D. S., Collison, C., and Werz, M. A. (1977). Spatial memory and radial arm maze performance of rats. *Learning and Motivation, 8,* 289-314.

Olton, D. S., and Samuelson, R. J. (1976) Remembrance of places passed: Spatial memory in rats. *Journal of Experimental Psychology: Animal Behavior Processes, 2,* 97-116.

Palmer, J. D. (2002). *The living clock: The orchestration of biological rhythms.* New York: Oxford University Press.

Peitgen, H-O., Jürgens, H., and Saupe, D. (1992). *Chaos and fractals: New frontiers of science.* New York: Springer-Verlag.

Petroski, H. (1985). *To engineer is human.* New York: St. Martin's Press.

Piaget, J. (1952). *The origins of intellect in children.* New York: W. W. Norton and Co. (1963, by arrangement with International Universities Press).

Pierce, J. R. (1980). *An introduction to information theory: Symbols, signals, and noise.* Second, revised ed. New York: Dover.

Pinker, S. (1994). *The language instinct.* New York: HarperCollins.

Plotkin, H. (2004). *Evolutionary thought in psychology: A brief history.* Malden, MA: Blackwell Publishing.

Ranck, J. B. Jr., Harris, E., Bleicher, M., Rotenberg, A., Stead, S. M., and Kubie, J. L. (1997). Strategies humans use on radial-arm maze tasks. *Society for Neuroscience Abstracts, 23,* 2108

Richardson, J. T. E., Engle, R. W., Hasher, L., Logie, R. H., Stoltzfus, E. R., and Zacks, R. T. (1996). *Working memory and human cognition.* New York: Oxford University Press.

Rosenzweig, M. R. (1996). Aspects of the search for neural mechanisms of memory. *Annual Review of Psychology, 47,* 1-32.

Schmidt-Nielsen, K. (1984). *Scaling: Why is animal size so important?* Cambridge, UK: Cambridge University Press.

Schneider, W. and Pressley, M. (1997). *Memory development between two and twenty: Second edition.* Mahwah, NJ: Lawrence Erlbaum Associates.

Shepherd, G. M. (2004). Introduction to synaptic circuits. In G. M. Shepherd (Ed.) *The synaptic organization of the brain: Fifth Edition.* New York: Oxford University Press.

Simpson, G. G. (1949). *The meaning of evolution.* New Haven: Yale University Press.

Singer, W. (1994). Coherence as an organizing principle of cortical functions. *International. Review of Neurobioogy, 37,*153-183.

Sternberg, R. J. (2003). *Cognitive Psychology: Third Edition.* Belmont, CA: Wadsworth.

Tan, L., and Ward, G. (2000). A recency-based account of the primacy effect in free recall. *Journal of Experimental Psychology: Learning, Memory, and Cognition, 26,* 1589-1625.

Thaler, R. H., and Sunstein, C. R. (2008). *Nudge: Improving decisions about health, wealth, and happiness.* New Haven: Yale University Press.

Treisman, A. (1996). The binding problem. *Current Opinion in Neurobiology, 6,* 171-178.

Tulving, E. (2002). Episodic memory: from mind to brain. *Annual Review of Psychology, 53,* 1-25.

von Restorff, H. (1933). Analyse von Vorgangen in Spurenfeld. I. Über die Wirkung von Bereichsbildungen im Spurenfeld [Analysis of processes in the memory trace. I. On the effect of group formations on the memory trace]. *Psychologische Forschung, 18,* 299-342.

Weber, B. H., and Depew, D. J. (2003). *Evolution and learning: The Baldwin effect reconsidered.* Cambridge, MA: MIT Press.

Weinert, F. E., and Schneider, W. (Eds.) (1995). *Memory performance and competencies: Issues in growth and development.* Mahwah, NJ: Lawrence Erlbaum Associates.

Weiss, H., and Weiss, V. (2003). The golden mean as clock cycle of brain waves. *Chaos, Solitons, and Fractals* 18(4): 643-652.

Wimsatt, W. F. (2007). *Re-engineering philosophy for limited beings: piecewise approximations to reality*. Cambridge, MA: Harvard University Press.

INDEX

B

C

D

E

F

I

J

K

L

M

N

Q

R

S

T

U

V